Cambridge Technicals

Level **3**

Health and Social Care

Maria Ferreiro Peteiro, Judith Adams,
Mary Riley, Sarah Rogers and Peter Wedlake

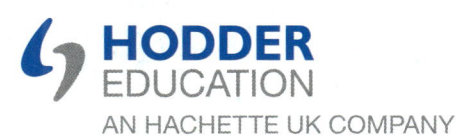

HODDER EDUCATION
AN HACHETTE UK COMPANY

Although every effort has been made to ensure that website addresses are correct at time of going to press, Hodder Education cannot be held responsible for the content of any website mentioned in this book. It is sometimes possible to find a relocated web page by typing in the address of the home page for a website in the URL window of your browser.

Hachette UK's policy is to use papers that are natural, renewable and recyclable products and made from wood grown in well-managed forests and other controlled sources. The logging and manufacturing processes are expected to conform to the environmental regulations of the country of origin.

Orders: Hachette UK Distribution, Hely Hutchinson Centre, Milton Road, Didcot, Oxfordshire, OX11 7HH. Telephone: +44 (0)1235 827827. Email education@hachette.co.uk Lines are open from 9 a.m. to 5 p.m., Monday to Friday. You can also order through our website: www.hoddereducation.co.uk

ISBN: 978 1 4718 7476 5

© Maria Ferreiro Peteiro, Judith Adams, Mary Riley, Sarah Rogers and Peter Wedlake 2016

First published in 2016 by
Hodder Education,
An Hachette UK Company
Carmelite House
50 Victoria Embankment
London EC4Y 0DZ
www.hoddereducation.co.uk

Impression number 13

Year   2024

Cover photo © plustwentyseven/Digital Vision/Getty Images

Illustrations produced by Barking Dog Art

Typeset by Aptara, Inc.

Produced by DZS Grafik, Printed in Slovenia

A catalogue record for this title is available from the British Library.

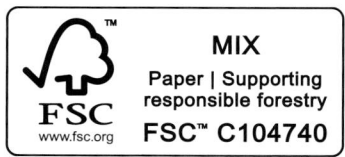

Contents

About this book

This book helps you to master the skills and knowledge you need for the OCR Cambridge Technicals Level 3 Health and Social Care qualification.

This resource is endorsed by OCR for use with the Cambridge Technicals Level 3 Health and Social Care specification. In order to gain OCR endorsement, this resource has undergone an independent quality check.

Any references to assessment and/or assessment preparation are the publisher's interpretation of the specification requirements and are not endorsed by OCR. OCR recommends that a range of teaching and learning resources are used in preparing learners for assessment. For more information about the endorsement process, please visit the OCR website, www.ocr.org.uk.

Using this book

Know what to expect when you are studying the unit.

Prepare for what you are going to cover in the unit.

Find out how you can expect to be assessed after studying the unit.

How will I be graded?

You will be graded using the following criteria.

Find out the criteria for achieving pass, merit and distinction grades in internally assessed units.

Understand all the requirements of the qualification, with clearly stated learning outcomes and assessment criteria fully mapped to the specification.

Try activities to start you off with a new learning outcome.

Carry out tasks that help you to think about a topic in detail and enhance your understanding.

Take the opportunity to share your ideas with your group.

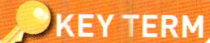
Understand important terms.

KNOW IT

1. Name three factors to take into account when using verbal communication.
2. Name three factors to take into account when using non-verbal communication.
3. How can you adapt your communication with others?
4. Name two communication theories.
5. Name four key aspects of reflective practice.

Answer quick questions to test your knowledge about the learning outcome you have just covered.

Unit 2: Assessment practice

Below are practice questions for you to try.

Try the types of question you may see in your externally assessed exam.

L01 Assessment activity

TOP TIPS

✔ Ensure you provide an explanation – detailed information about the different types of relationship and their context.
✔ Take the opportunity to present your evidence in a variety of formats, e.g. in a written or verbal format, as a poster or in a table.
✔ Ensure you provide detailed evidence about each care environment.

Start preparing for your internally assessed assignments by carrying out activities that are directly linked to pass, merit and distinction criteria. Top Tips give you additional advice.

Read about it

Suggests books and websites for further reading and research.

Acknowledgements

Every effort has been made to trace the copyright holders of material reproduced here. The authors and publishers would like to thank the following for permission to reproduce copyright illustrations and photographs:

Front cover © plustwentyseven/Digital Vision/Getty Images; **Page 8** © lassedesignen/Fotolia.com; **Page 15** © deanm1974/Fotolia; **Page 19** © John Birdsall/ Alamy Stock Photo; **Page 42** © Jules Selmes/Hodder Education; **Page 151** © Peter Titmuss/Alamy; **Page 178** © Picture Partners/Alamy Stock Photo; **Page 185** © Steve Meddle/REX/Shutterstock; **Page 157** © PhotosIndia.com LLC/Alamy; **Page 223** © Kirill Zdorov/Fotolia; **Page 225** © Photo Researchers Inc/ Alamy Stock Photo; **Page 247** © AlexRaths/iStockphoto; **Page 251** © Creatas via Thinkstock/Getty Images

This book contains public sector information licensed under the Open Government Licence v3.0.

Building positive relationships in health and social care

ABOUT THIS UNIT

Building positive relationships in the health, social care and child care sectors is essential for ensuring effective partnership working, both with individuals who require care and support, and with all those involved in their lives such as their advocates, families, friends, professionals and managers. Creating settings that are safe places for those who attend, live or work in them and where a sense of wellbeing is promoted is central to delivering high-quality, safe, effective and compassionate care and support.

In this unit, you will learn about the key features of different types of relationships in health, social care and child care settings. You will also learn more about the different factors that can impact on the building of these relationships and how a person-centred approach supports positive relationships.

Having the ability to reflect on your practices will help you to further develop your knowledge, understanding and skills in using communication and interactions effectively to build positive relationships.

LEARNING OUTCOMES

The topics, activities and suggested reading in this unit will help you to:

1 Understand relationships in health, social care or child care environments
2 Understand the factors that influence the building of relationships
3 Understand how a person-centred approach builds positive relationships in health, social care or child care environments
4 Be able to use communication skills effectively to build positive relationships in a health, social care or child care environment

How will I be assessed?

You will be assessed through a series of assignments and tasks set and marked by your tutor.

You will be graded using the following criteria.

Learning outcome	Pass assessment criteria	Merit assessment criteria	Distinction assessment criteria
You will:	To achieve a **pass** you must demonstrate that you have met all the pass assessment criteria	To achieve a **merit** you must demonstrate that you have met all the pass and merit assessment criteria	To achieve a **distinction** you must demonstrate that you have met all the pass, merit and distinction assessment criteria
1 Understand relationships in health, social care or child care environments	**P1** Explain different types of relationships that can be built in health, social care or child care environments	**M1** Analyse the role that context plays in different relationships in health, social care and child care environments	
2 Understand the factors that influence the building of relationships	**P2** Explain factors that can influence the building of positive relationships in health, social care or child care environments		
3 Understand how a person-centred approach builds positive relationships in health, social care or child care environments	**P3** Explain strategies to ensure a person-centred approach in health, social care or child care environments	**M2** Analyse how a person-centred approach supports the building of positive relationships in health, social care or child care environments	
4 Be able to use communication skills effectively to build positive relationships in a health, social care or child care environment	**P4** Demonstrate effective communication skills in a one-to-one interaction to build a positive relationship in a health, social care or child care environment	**M3** Review the effectiveness of the communication skills used during the interactions	**D2** Justify the use of reflective practice to ensure interactions build positive relationships in health, social care or child care environments
	P5 Demonstrate effective communication skills in a group interaction to build a positive relationship in a health, social care or child care environment		

UNIT 1 BUILDING POSITIVE RELATIONSHIPS IN HEALTH AND SOCIAL CARE

LO1 Understand relationships in health, social care or child care environments *P1 M1*

GETTING STARTED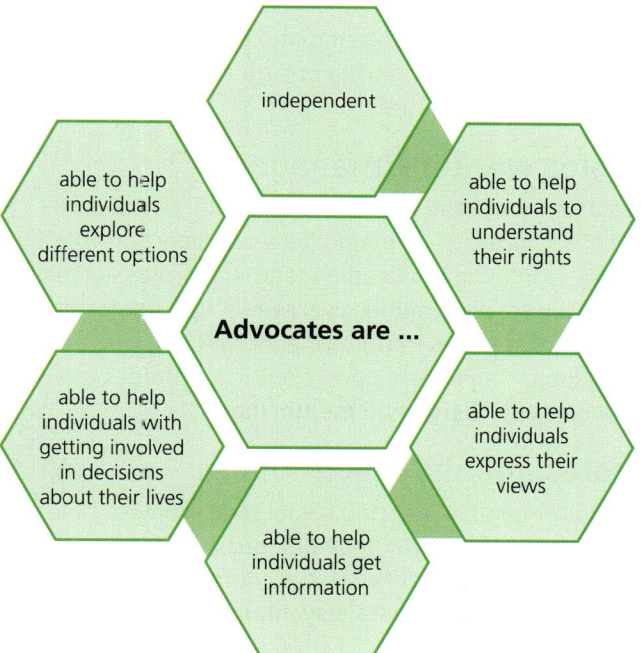

Relationship types (10 minutes)

Name as many types of relationships in health, social care or child care settings as you can. Share your ideas with the whole group.

🔑 KEY TERMS

Positive relationships – meaningful interactions that result in positive emotions such as happiness, enjoyment, peace and a sense of wellbeing. They are constructive and beneficial for all those involved.

Health environment – practitioners and organisations that provide diagnostic, preventative, remedial and therapeutic services in different settings.

Social care environment – professionals and organisations that provide care, support and protection to adults, young people and children at risk, or with needs arising from illness, disability, old age or other circumstances that place people at a disadvantage in society.

Child care environment – practitioners and organisations that work with children from birth–18 years in their own homes, in nursery or pre-school settings, schools, out-of-school clubs and activity clubs.

Working in partnership – a way of working that involves developing positive relationships between individuals, carers and professionals where individuals remain at the centre. Good quality care and support is developed through mutual respect and open and honest communication.

Advocates – those who represent the views, needs and interests of individuals who are unable to represent themselves.

1.1 Types of relationships

Individuals who require care and support

Building **positive relationships** with adults, children and young people requiring care and support is an essential part of effective practice. All work in **health, social care and child care environments** will involve **working in partnership** with individuals who are vulnerable, at risk of harm, or in need of support; for example, recovering from an operation in hospital, requiring assistance to live independently because of a mental health need or requiring support while living with a foster family.

These types of relationships require those who work with individuals to be effective CARERS with important qualities, such as being:

- **C**aring
- **A**pproachable
- **R**eliable
- **E**mpathetic
- **R**espectful
- **S**upportive.

Families/advocates of individuals who require care and support

Individuals have many different ways of defining what a family is and who they see as their family. For some, this may include their parents, brothers, sisters, aunts, uncles and grandparents. For others, their family may be their friends or neighbours who know them well over a long period of time and provide them with emotional and practical support.

Advocates also work closely with individuals and on some occasions with others who know the individual well. For example, this may be when there is a change in the health needs of an individual who has dementia or at a young person's support review meeting.

Figure 1.1 provides some more information about what advocates do.

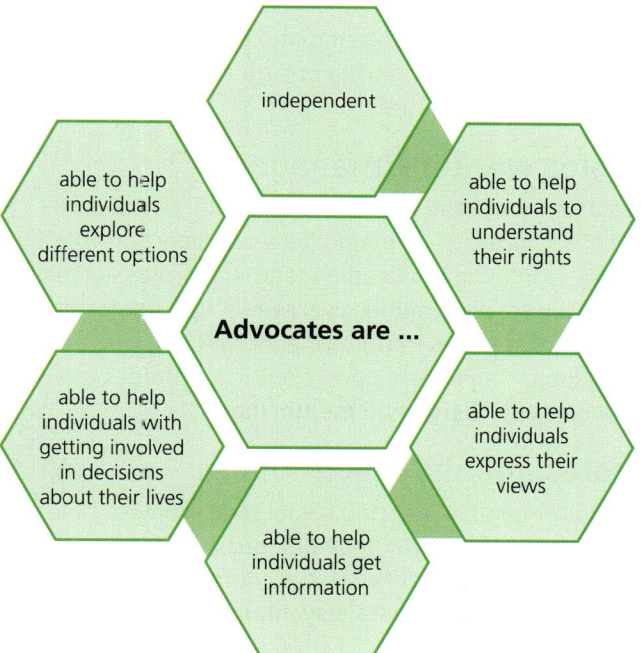

▲ **Figure 1.1** The role of advocates

Colleagues/peers

All health, social care and child care environments will consist of professionals who work in teams; this can include colleagues who work in the same job role or level in a work setting – these people are sometimes called peers. In these types of relationships, an element of friendship, peer-mentoring and support can often develop through the sharing of similar roles and working closely together.

Senior workers/managers

Senior workers and managers in health, social care and child care environments have an important role to play managing and leading teams of professionals. They have responsibilities overseeing the day-to-day running of services that provide individuals with care and support, and they support teams of professionals through **supervision** and **mentoring**.

Professionals/practitioners

A wide range of health and social care professionals and practitioners work in health, social care and child care environments, such as nurses, dieticians, therapists, **psychologists**, **psychiatrists** and social

workers. Practitioners can be identified with specialist fields or professions, for example medical, nursing and **allied health**.

Standards are in place to guide health and social care practitioners and professionals in carrying out their work duties and responsibilities to a high level, and include guidelines, values and principles that are relevant to health and social care professionals' working practices. For example, the Care Certificate was introduced on 1 April 2015 and is a set of standards for those who work in health and social care. It provides workers with guidance on the required skills, knowledge and behaviours that are required for compassionate, safe and high-quality care and support.

1.2 Relationship contexts

There are a number of contexts in which the different types of relationships in health, social care and child care environments take place.

Formal and informal contexts

Relationships can be both formal and informal. Formal relationships, such as those formed by senior workers and managers, are structured and usually arise out of an organisation's overall agreed aims. They are defined by rules, regulations and policies. Attitudes and behaviours that involve respect, empathy (understanding how others feel) and professionalism are also important characteristics of formal relationships.

Informal relationships, by contrast, are not defined by rules and regulations and are usually formed out of a friendship or a close personal connection, such as those between individuals and their families and friends. Knowing each other well, sharing common interests and intimacy are important characteristics of informal relationships.

One-to-one and group contexts

Relationships can develop in either one-to-one or group situations.

Read through the diary extract below. It is written by Alice, who works with children as a nursery worker. Note in particular the one-to-one and group relationships she has with others.

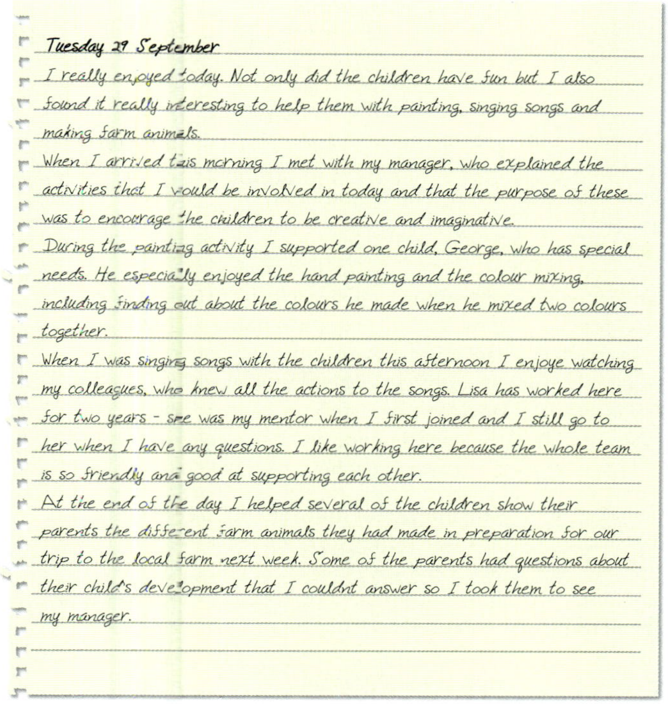

Tuesday 29 September

I really enjoyed today. Not only did the children have fun but I also found it really interesting to help them with painting, singing songs and making farm animals.

When I arrived this morning I met with my manager, who explained the activities that I would be involved in today and that the purpose of these was to encourage the children to be creative and imaginative.

During the painting activity I supported one child, George, who has special needs. He especially enjoyed the hand painting and the colour mixing, including finding out about the colours he made when he mixed two colours together.

When I was singing songs with the children this afternoon I enjoye watching my colleagues, who knew all the actions to the songs. Lisa has worked here for two years – she was my mentor when I first joined and I still go to her when I have any questions. I like working here because the whole team is so friendly and good at supporting each other.

At the end of the day I helped several of the children show their parents the different farm animals they had made in preparation for our trip to the local farm next week. Some of the parents had questions about their child's development that I couldn't answer so I took them to see my manager.

▲ **Figure 1.2** Alice's diary

Environment

In Section 1.1 you learned how relationships can take place in a variety of environments, such as in individuals' homes, in residential and community based settings.

Many individuals requiring health care do not need to move out of their homes as they can access the specialist care they need from home. For example, GPs can arrange for community nurses to visit an individual requiring end of life care at home and provide them with nursing care, advice on pain control, emotional and practical support. However, they could also choose to receive their care at a local **hospice**.

Individuals requiring social care can also access services and support from their homes or from a range of residential and community based settings. Individuals may require both health care and social care at the same time. For example, an individual who has a physical disability may require practical support with day-to-day activities such as personal care, cooking and shopping as well as support with managing their **asthma**, and may need to be referred to their GP for a medication review.

Child care can also be provided in a range of settings. A child whose parents are at work may be cared for on weekday evenings by a childminder, who ensures that the child is picked up from school, has a nutritious meal and takes part in activities like reading or creative play. A child may also access different clubs and classes in their local area such as Scouts, swimming and martial arts.

> **🔑 KEY TERMS**
>
> **Hospice** – a setting that provides support and end-of-life care to individuals and their families. Hospice care can be provided where individuals choose, for example at home, or in a hospice room in a hospital or nursing home.
>
> **Asthma** – a condition that can cause wheezing, coughing, chest tightness and breathlessness. It can develop in both young children and older people.

1.3 How context can impact relationships

Let us now think about how these different contexts can impact on the different types of relationships with, for example, individuals, their families, professionals and practitioners. Table 1.1 shows how different contexts can impact relationships both positively and negatively.

Table 1.1 Contexts and relationships

Context	Examples of positive impact on relationships	Examples of negative impact on relationships
Formal and informal situations – professional and personal relationships **Example:** an individual who has just been diagnosed with **Alzheimer's**	The individual may strengthen relationships with their family and friends as they work together to plan how best to manage the individual's changing needs. New positive relationships with professionals and advocates who can provide both practical and emotional support can also be built.	The individual may not be able to continue working and may have to depend on their family for managing day-to-day tasks such as cooking, shopping and paying bills. This can be a difficult change for the individual and their family, who may as a result experience frustration and loss.
One-to-one and group situations **Example:** an individual who has been diagnosed with **Parkinson's**	The individual may benefit from meeting regularly with a mentor as part of one-to-one peer support. Spending time with someone who has experience of a similar condition can provide the individual with hope, inspiration and ideas for how to maintain their independence. This will make the individual feel valued and listened to and continue to maintain their relationships with family and friends.	The individual may not feel ready to talk about their condition with others or may feel anxious about meeting people they do not know. This in turn may make the individual withdraw and not seek any support for living with their condition. Tensions between their family and friends may also arise.
The **physical environment** – independence in an individual's home and in a residential home **Example**: an older child who has a visual impairment	If their family home has been adapted for their **sight loss**, the child will feel safe and more confident. They may also be able to carry out tasks independently. Their family will also experience feelings of pride and belief in the abilities of their child.	If they have had to move from their home to a residential children's home, the child may feel insecure and anxious about the new environment. Their family may feel guilty and anxious that they have been unable to meet the child's needs and be unable to trust the professionals who are providing the child's care.
An individual's **social environment** – temporary dependency in an individual's home and hospital **Example:** an individual who has sustained a fractured hip and is in hospital	The individual may feel a sense of relief and security of being cared for rather than having to manage on their own at home. The individual may show appreciation and gratitude, making health care professionals feel valued for doing a good job.	The individual may feel uncomfortable and anxious if they have never stayed in hospital before. If they live independently, they may not be used to following routines and instructions from health professionals and may react negatively or aggressively. This may create tensions.

KEY TERMS

Alzheimer's – the most common cause of dementia and causes damage to the brain. Signs and symptoms include memory loss in the early stages; individuals may then develop difficulties with their communication, thinking, reasoning and perception skills.

Parkinson's – a neurological condition in which symptoms usually develop gradually. Signs and symptoms can include tremors or shaking, body rigidity or stiffness, feeling tired and weak, pain and depression.

Physical environment – surroundings or conditions, such as the space available, the positioning of furniture, amount of lighting and the level of noise.

Sight loss – individuals who are unable to see, i.e. 'blind', as well as individuals who are able to partially see, for example, shadows.

Social environment – the social conditions that influence building relationships, such as individuals and professionals' backgrounds, education, interactions with others.

KNOW IT

1 What are the common elements of relationships with colleagues/peers?
2 Name three differences between formal and informal relationships?
3 Identify three types of professionals who work in health care environments.
4 Name three settings where child care may be provided.
5 Identify two ways in which temporary dependency can impact on an individual's relationships.

LO1 Assessment activities

Below are suggested assessment activities that have been directly linked to the pass and merit criteria in LO1 to help with assignment preparation; they include Top Tips on how to achieve best results.

Activity 1 – pass criteria *P1*

Research your local area to find out about three care environments. One must be related to health care, one to social care and one to child care. For each environment, identify the different types of relationships and provide an explanation of their roles, required skills and qualities.

TOP TIPS
- ✔ Ensure you provide an explanation – detailed information about the different types of relationships.
- ✔ Take the opportunity to present your evidence in a variety of formats, e.g. in a written or verbal format, as a poster or in a table.
- ✔ Ensure you provide detailed evidence about each care environment.

Activity 2 – merit criteria *M1*

Examine how formal and informal situations, one-to-one and group situations and different environments can affect relationships both positively and negatively in health, social care and child care settings.

TOP TIPS
- ✔ Ensure you provide an analysis, i.e. a detailed examination of how context can affect relationships in health, social care and child care settings.
- ✔ Present your evidence in a variety of formats, e.g. in an assignment or as a presentation to the rest of the group.
- ✔ Ensure you provide detailed evidence of the positive and negative impacts on relationships in health, social care and child care environments.

LO2 Understand the factors that influence the building of relationships *P2*

GETTING STARTED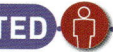

Positive relationships (10 minutes)

Discuss how different backgrounds, beliefs and needs can influence the building of positive relationships.

🔑 KEY TERMS

Tone – the strength of a vocal sound made by a person in a communication or situation, e.g. quiet or loud.

Pitch – the quality of a vocal sound made by a person in a communication or situation, e.g. low or high.

Body language – a form of non-verbal communication in which thoughts, feelings and intentions are expressed through the movement and position of the body.

Dialect – a form of language that is associated with a specific region or group of people.

2.1 Communication factors

Now you are now going to explore other important factors that influence the building of positive relationships in health, social care and child care environments. You will find this useful when studying other units, such as Unit 2 Equality, diversity and rights in health and social care, Unit 9 Supporting people with learning disabilities, Unit 14 The impact of long-term physiological conditions, Unit 22 Psychology for health and social care and Unit 23 Sociology for health and social care.

Verbal and non-verbal communication skills

Communication is a two-way process of sharing messages using both verbal and non-verbal methods. Effective use of verbal and non-verbal communication skills will ensure that messages are understood and received in the way that they were intended. Figure 1.3 includes information about different verbal and non-verbal methods of communicating.

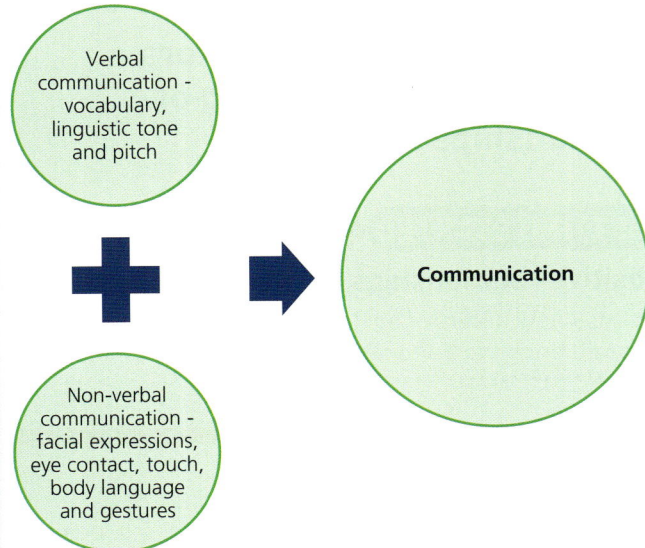

Verbal communication - vocabulary, linguistic tone and pitch

Non-verbal communication - facial expressions, eye contact, touch, body language and gestures

Communication

▲ **Figure 1.3** Different communication methods

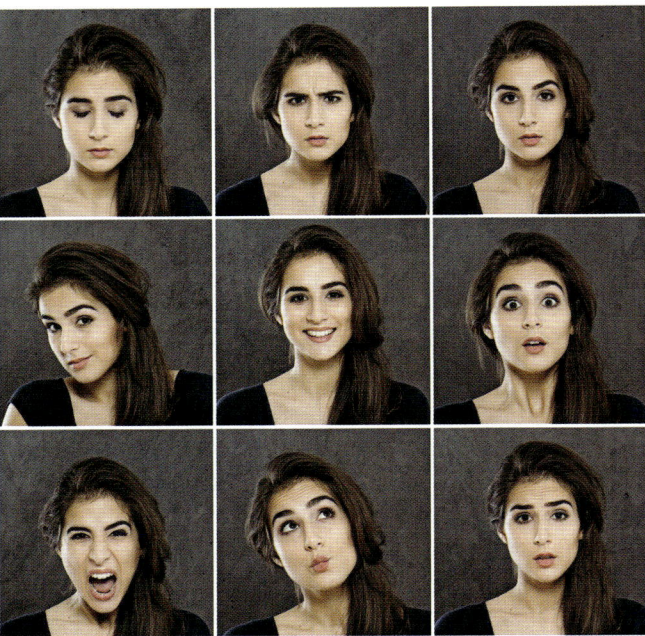

▲ **Figure 1.4** Our faces can convey many different meanings

How health, social care and child care professionals and practitioners communicate both verbally and non-verbally can influence the building of relationships with individuals, their families and advocates, colleagues, seniors, managers and other professionals. Here are some examples.

a A hospital consultant questions someone about the pain in his arm. They use a quiet **tone** and a medium **pitch**, language free from medical jargon and at a pace that can be understood. This will make the individual feel listened to and that any concerns raised have been taken seriously.

b A senior care assistant attends an individual's care review meeting about their changing needs. They use an empathetic tone and pitch when describing the individual's circumstances, use non-discriminatory and respectful language, and show through their **body language** that they are taking an interest in the discussions. They engage the individual and others present to create trust and make them more likely to raise other issues or questions.

c A special needs worker uses age-appropriate language, and avoids using slang and words from their own **dialect**. This will positively support a child's learning and development. A gentle touch on the shoulder and leaning towards the child can also reinforce positive behaviour.

PAIRS ACTIVITY

Watch me (30 minutes)

Write the following sentence on the whiteboard

93% of the information we give and receive is non-verbal.

Write different emotions on different cards: e.g happiness, anger, sadness, excitement, anxiety

One person in the pair picks a card without letting their partner see it. The person faces away from their partner and repeats the sentence on the board using the emotion on their card. The other person must guess what the emotion is but is not told if they are correct. The person repeats the sentence, this time facing their partner and using facial expressions and body language to convey the same emotion. The other person must again guess what the emotion is.

Swap roles and then discuss how information was conveyed verbally and non-verbally.

Written communication

Effective written communication is an important and necessary skill for health, social and child care professionals. It facilitates safe, effective and good quality care and support, and helps to avoid misunderstandings. For example:

● maintaining clearly written records that are free from slang and jargon
● updating records accurately with the correct information
● using non-discriminatory language; for example, using an individual's preferred name or title and avoiding offensive or stereotypical labels.

Figure 1.5 identifies other ways that written communication can influence the building of relationships.

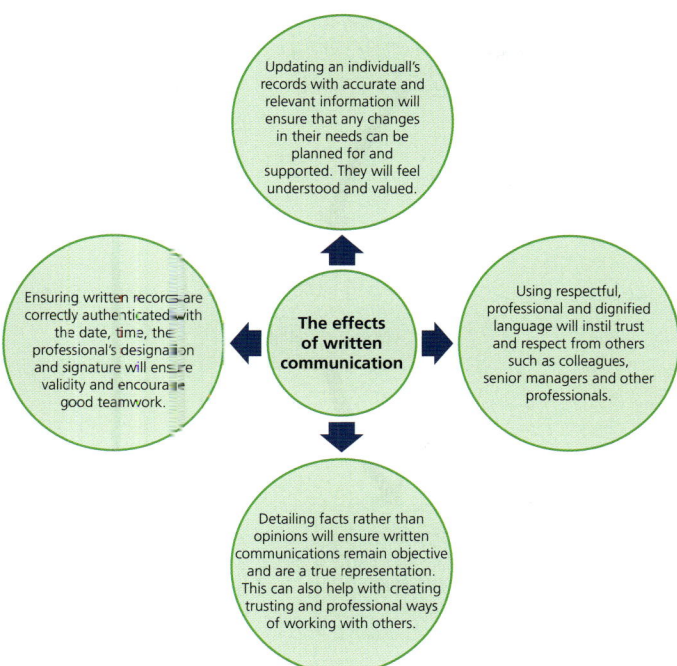

▲ **Figure 1.5** The effects of written communication

Special methods and adaptations

Knowing about and having the ability to use special methods of adapting communication is essential, as individuals who require care and support are all unique. In this way, meaningful and positive interactions can be developed with everyone.

Table 1.2 details some of the different ways that communication can be adapted to ensure effective two-way communication between individuals, their carers and others. Do you know about any others?

🔑 **KEY TERMS**

Deafblind – individuals who have a level of hearing and sight loss that, combined, severely impacts their daily life.

Hearing loss – refers to individuals who are unable to hear, as well as to individuals who are able to partially hear, for example just low tones.

Table 1.2 Examples of adapted communications

Adapted communication methods	What is it?	Who can use it?
Braille	Touching a series of raised dots and symbols that represent letters, numbers and punctuation marks.	Individuals who are blind and individuals who are **deafblind,** to read and write.
British Sign Language	A visual form that involves using hand signs, facial expressions and gestures.	Individuals who are deaf, to communicate with others.
Haptic communication	Using touch and tactile signs to a part of the body, such as on the individual's back or shoulder, to describe what is happening visually.	Individuals who are deafblind, to participate in their immediate environment.
Hearing aids	Small electronic devices fitted either in or on the ear to make sounds louder.	Some individuals who have **hearing loss,** to listen and communicate.
Makaton	A visual form that involves using speech with signs (gestures) and symbols (pictures). It is used alongside facial expressions, eye contact and body language to give as much information as possible.	Individuals who have learning and communication difficulties.
Signs and symbols	Signs are used with speech and symbols, often with pictures, to support spoken language.	Individuals who have learning and communication difficulties.
Speech-to-text reporters	A communication aid that converts spoken words into written words.	Individuals who are deaf and have hearing loss, to communicate with others.
Telephone relay service	A telephone service that enables individuals to place and receive telephone calls. Different types exist and include speech, text and symbols.	Individuals who have hearing loss, sight loss or difficulties with speaking.

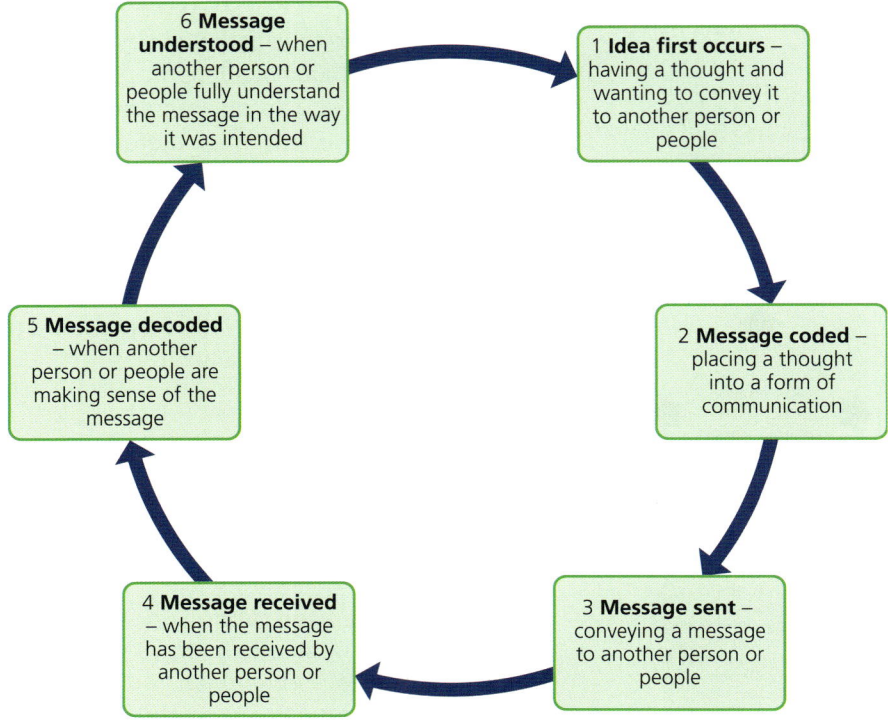

▲ **Figure 1.6** Argyle's communication cycle

Theories of communication, and application to health and social care contexts

Communication involves a number of different skills including listening, observing, understanding and making sense of different messages. Communication theories explain the process and can be useful for helping professionals and practitioners to understand how to apply effective communication skills to build relationships.

Argyle's communication cycle

British social psychologist Michael Argyle's research showed how non-verbal signals could be more important than verbal communication to convey individuals' feelings and attitudes. In 1972, Argyle developed a theory of how communication works in practice. It consisted of a communication cycle that contained six stages.

After the sixth stage, the communication cycle is repeated with more ideas and thoughts about the original message.

Argyle's communication theory is relevant to health, social care and child care professionals and practitioners as it is the basis of all meaningful interactions. It applies to both verbal and non-verbal communication and can be used to check that the communication method being used is understood, relevant and appropriate.

Tuckman's stages of group interaction

Bruce Tuckman was an educational psychologist. In 1965, he developed a four-stage model (he later added a fifth stage) after studying the behaviours of small groups of people in a range of environments. Tuckman's research showed how groups need to go through a series of processes or stages before they can reach their full potential and work effectively. These are as follows.

- Forming – group members are getting to know one another.
- Storming – group members begin to ascertain their views and ideas that may be similar to and/or in contrast to the views and ideas of others.
- Norming – the group establishes their aim and individual group members' roles and responsibilities.
- Performing – the group works effectively and collaboratively to a consistently high standard.
- Adjourning – the group achieve their aim and complete their work, recognise their achievements and move on.

His work has helped teams to understand how to work effectively together and in partnership.

SOLER

SOLER is a theory developed in 1975 by Professor Gerard Egan. It describes a number of key techniques that are essential for active listening, as follows.

- **S**quarely: how to position yourself in relation to the other person to show that you have a genuine interest
- **O**pen: how to maintain an open posture, e.g. uncrossed arms and legs to show that you are approachable.
- **L**ean: the effects that leaning slightly towards the other person can have, e.g. to show that you are interested.
- **E**ye contact: how and when to maintain eye contact to show that you are listening.
- **R**elax: the effects that being relaxed can have on the other person, e.g. to show that you have time for them.

This theory is used to ensure that non-verbal communication messages support the words that are spoken, otherwise resentment and misunderstandings may arise and prevent the building of positive relationships.

2.2 Cultural factors

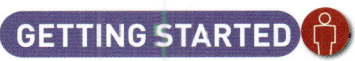 **GETTING STARTED**

Being an effective communicator (10 minutes)

Think about the skills that are essential for being an effective communicator. Share with a partner.

The people who access health, social care and child care settings are from different backgrounds, **races**, **religions** and cultures. It is important, therefore, that professionals and practitioners are aware of cultural factors when building relationships with individuals who require care and support and others involved in their lives. Not doing so may lead to misunderstandings.

Not every individual from the same culture will have the same preferences or beliefs; it is important to recognise, value and respect the great **diversity** within different cultures. For example:

- an individual brought up in a Jewish community may observe dietary requirements, such as kosher food, but choose not to observe traditions and weekly rituals like the Sabbath or Shabbat.
- an individual who belongs to the **LGBT** culture and is lesbian may not want to take part in **Pride** activities.
- an individual may prefer to communicate in a language other than English for important discussions relating to their care, such as when discussing treatment options.

You will read more about different cultures in Unit 2.

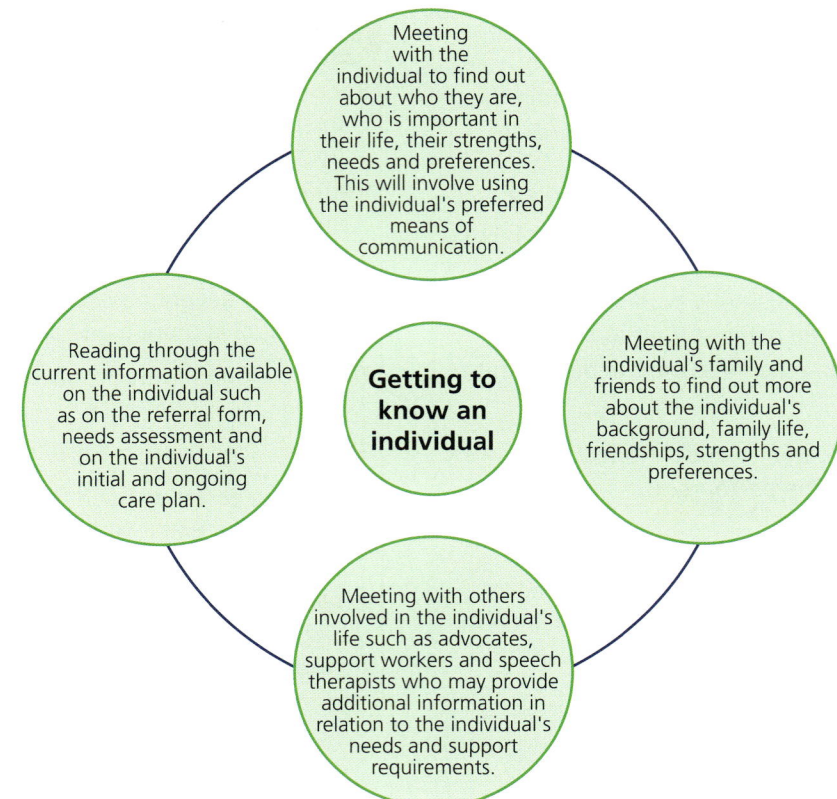

The following circles surround "Getting to know an individual":

- Meeting with the individual to find out about who they are, who is important in their life, their strengths, needs and preferences. This will involve using the individual's preferred means of communication.

- Reading through the current information available on the individual such as on the referral form, needs assessment and on the individual's initial and ongoing care plan.

- Meeting with the individual's family and friends to find out more about the individual's background, family life, friendships, strengths and preferences.

- Meeting with others involved in the individual's life such as advocates, support workers and speech therapists who may provide additional information in relation to the individual's needs and support requirements.

▲ **Figure 1.7** What does diversity mean to you?

2.3 Environmental factors

The physical environment

As well as communication and cultural factors, the physical environment plays a role in building relationships in health, social and child care settings. For example, in a health clinic, it is important that treatment rooms are private and located in quiet areas.

The social environment

The people who work in and access health, social care and child care settings have diverse backgrounds, experiences and education levels. This will affect how they interact and develop relationships with others.

For example, a health care worker who has completed their training in a hospital under the guidance of a qualified nurse will learn that providing individualised care to individuals involves being kind, caring, respectful and professional.

An individual who has been diagnosed with **depression** and who has had experience of caring for another family member with depression may have developed an awareness of the importance of seeking help immediately from others and they may also be more open to participating in talking therapies and self-help techniques.

2.4 Spiritual factors

Belief and value system

Having different sets of **beliefs** and **values** to others is not a problem if those differences are respected and tolerated. For example, an individual may value family life, including always putting family first and looking after family as an important aspect of their life, while another individual may not.

Avoiding assumptions and stereotypes

Celebrating differences, recognising the value they bring to our lives and avoiding making **assumptions** and using **stereotypes** that can impact significantly and negatively on building positive relationships is also important. For example, if people believe that everyone with mental health needs is dangerous to the public, it will be difficult for these individuals to be part of their communities and build relationships with others. Similarly, if individuals with mental health needs believe that professionals are not to be trusted, it will be difficult for them to build respectful and trusting relationships with professionals.

INDEPENDENT ACTIVITY

(10 minutes)

Read through the good practice tips developed by a mental health nurse, Liam, to avoid making assumptions and using stereotypes when providing care and support to individuals with mental health needs. Can you think of any other ways that assumptions and stereotypes can be avoided?

Good practice tips for mental health workers

- Always make it your goal to understand every individual better.
- Always treat every individual as a unique person.
- Always ask the individual – do not assume you know what they want, need or prefer.
- Always communicate directly with the individual. If you can't or don't know how to then ask, and get to know how they prefer to communicate
- Always respect the individual. Do not dismiss or ignore their views or beliefs because they are different to yours.

2.5 Physical factors

There are a range of different physical factors that may also affect the building of relationships between different people. Careful planning and specialist knowledge can help to overcome these. Table 1.3 provides examples of a range of physical factors as well as the effects that these may have.

Table 1.3 Physical factors and their effects

Physical factors	Examples	Effects on the building of relationships
Conditions	dementia, mental ill health, impact of pain	• The onset of dementia can change how an individual thinks and acts and others may misinterpret this and become upset. • Mental ill health can make an individual not want to interact with other people. • Pain can make an individual feel irritable and depressed, and withdraw from relationships.
Sensory impairment	hearing loss, sight loss, dual hearing and sight loss	• Hearing loss can make an individual feel frustrated and isolated. • Sight loss can make an individual feel isolated and anxious to communicate and engage. • Dual hearing and sight loss can make individuals feel isolated from others in their environment.
Physical disability	a person who uses a wheelchair, a person who has had a limb amputated, a person who is unable to move unaided	• A person using a wheelchair may find that others see the wheelchair before the person, and feel uncomfortable about building a relationship with others. • A person who has had a limb amputated may want to avoid building relationships because of their own view of their new body image. • A person who is unable to mobilise unaided may feel like a burden on others and this may change their interactions with others.
Language and perception needs	autism, English as a second language, learning disabilities	• A person who has autism may feel frustrated and have difficulty developing relationships with others. • Having English as a second language can affect how an individual expresses their thoughts and feelings, leading to misunderstandings. • A person with a learning disability may feel frustrated and embarrassed about being treated like a child.
Substance misuse	alcohol, drugs, prescribed medications	• Alcohol can make an individual aggressive and unpredictable, making it difficult to maintain relationships. • Drugs can make an individual lie, become defensive and abusive, making it difficult to maintain new and existing relationships. • Prescribed medications can affect how an individual thinks, feels and acts. The individual may as a result not want to interact with others.

KNOW IT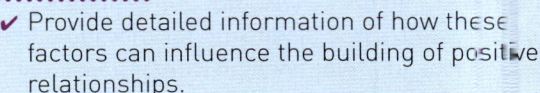

1 How can communication methods be adapted?
2 What's the difference between race and religion?
3 How can the environment influence relationships?

4 How can you avoid assumptions and stereotypes?
5 How can substance misuse affect relationships?

LO2 Assessment activity *P2*

Below is a suggested assessment activity that has been directly linked to the pass criteria in LO2 to help with assignment preparation; it includes Top Tips on how to achieve best results.

For one health, social care or child care environment, think about two different types of relationships and consider two factors for each that may influence these relationships.

TOP TIPS ✔

✔ Provide detailed information of how these factors can influence the building of positive relationships.
✔ You can present your evidence in a variety of formats, e.g. in a written or verbal format or as a recorded discussion.
✔ Include examples to show how these factors influence the building of positive relationships.

LO3 Understand how a person-centred approach builds positive relationships in health, social care or child care environments *P3 M2*

GETTING STARTED

Person-centred approach (10 minutes)

Think about what a person-centred approach means to you. Share with the whole group and agree on a definition.

The person-centred approach was developed from the work of the psychologist Dr Carl Rogers and recognises that individuals, rather than professionals or practitioners, are the experts. The individual's needs, views and wishes are the focus; they come first and become central to any care or support that is accessed.

3.1 Strategies to ensure a person-centred approach

All strategies to ensure a person-centred approach will involve putting into practice the following eight person-centred values that underpin all health, social and child care work:

1 individuality
2 choice
3 privacy
4 dignity
5 respect
6 rights
7 independence
8 partnership.

Understand an individual's needs and preferences

Developing an understanding of an individual's needs and preferences will involve building up a picture about their unique strengths and wishes. This will involve not only the individual but also all those other people that are important in their lives. Figure 1.8 details some of the different ways health, social care and child care professionals can do this.

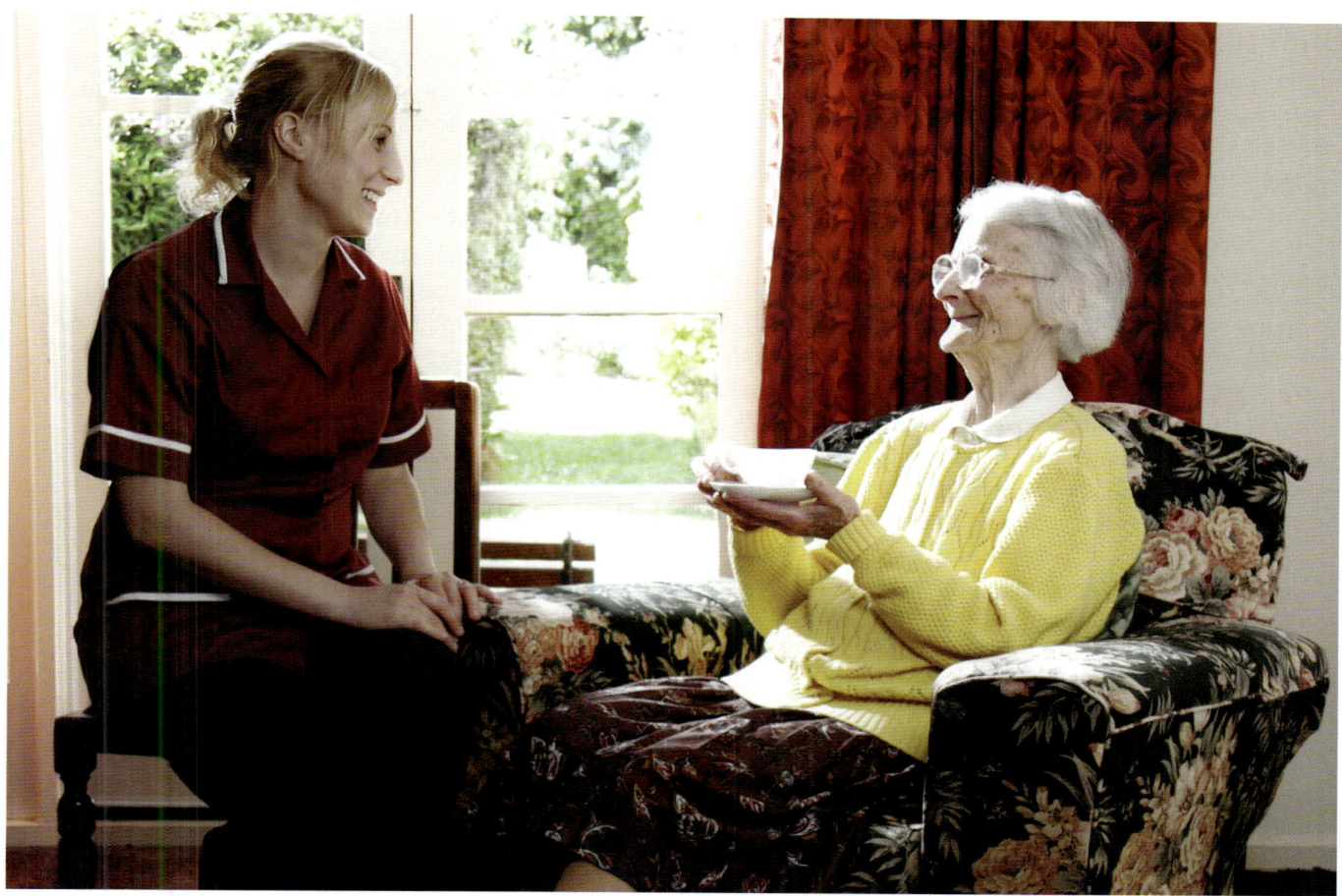

▲ **Figure 1.8** Getting to know an individual

Enabling and supporting an individual

It is very satisfying and enjoyable to enable an individual to be in control of their life and how they want to live it. This involves supporting them to learn and develop skills for themselves as well as maximising their independence.

Individuals can be enabled and supported to build positive relationships by:

- making themselves understood
- understanding others
- having their views heard
- making their own choices
- having their decisions respected.

Person-centred strategies to do this could include using advocates, **interpreters**, **translators** and **signers**. Technological aids such as a **Dynavox** or a **Lightwriter** could also be used to make communications with others easier.

Staff training

Staff training is another way of ensuring a person-centred approach as it includes information on the required skills, knowledge and ways of working. Through an induction programme, new staff joining an organisation can learn about person-centred ways of working while building up positive working relationships.

Statutory and mandatory training can also ensure that staff refresh their knowledge and keep up to date with current practices and thus build positive relationships. Person-centred ways of working are embedded in all the training that health, social care and child care workers receive. Additional or specialist training, such as stroke care, dementia care and **autism** awareness, can also provide opportunities for workers to learn more about person-centred approaches.

> ### 🔑 KEY TERMS
>
> **Autism** – a condition that is also known as autism spectrum disorder (ASD). It affects children, young people and adults with respect to their communication, social interaction and behaviour.
>
> **Agreed ways of working** – an organisation's policies and procedures.
>
> **Code of conduct** – a document that contains guidance on the behaviours and attitudes that reflect best practice and are expected from workers.

Demonstrate professional behaviour

It is also essential that staff demonstrate professional behaviour, for example in standards such as those in the Care Certificate (see page 34) and as stated in different organisations' **agreed ways of working** and **codes of conduct**. This involves maintaining confidentiality by only sharing information about individuals in a concise and informative manner with those who need it, as well as keeping verbal and written information in a safe place so others who are not authorised cannot access it. A commitment to being a reflective practitioner involves thinking about and learning from situations, incidents, issues and concerns.

The promotion of care values such as respect, empathy and compassion that underpin the skills and knowledge of all those who work in health, social care and child

care settings with children, young people and adults is also essential to professional conduct. Read through the Code of Conduct below of an after-school club and note what behaviours and attitudes are expected from staff, visiting activity providers and volunteers:

Code of conduct – Stars After-School Club

- Promote and uphold the privacy, dignity, rights, health and wellbeing of the children who attend.
- Promote and uphold equality, diversity and inclusion.
- Be polite and show respect for others.
- Communicate in an open and effective way.
- Respect confidentiality.
- Provide high-quality and safe care.
- Be committed to improving the quality of care through training and reflective practice.
- Maintain a relaxed and pleasant environment.
- Be aware of own and others' health and safety at all times.

3.2 How a person-centred approach supports positive relationships

Putting into practice these person-centred strategies will enable individuals who require care and support to have their needs met, and feel valued, respected and fulfilled. A person-centred approach also supports positive relationships through the following.

Empowering the individual

If an individual is empowered to be more aware of their own strengths and abilities, they will feel more confident and take more control of their life. Learning new skills will enable them to become more independent and work positively with professionals and others to achieve their goals.

Building trust

Trust is a key factor in building positive relationships. Using a person-centred approach involves open and effective communication and instilling confidence – two key ingredients for developing positive relationships. Listening attentively, honouring commitments and behaving in a professional manner will also instil trust and a sense of security. Remember: trust is earned!

Developing mutual respect

Developing mutual respect through respecting people's individuality and different cultural backgrounds can also help build strong, positive relationships. Showing respect for others' views and preferences, their opinions and roles within a team will support the development of positive relationships.

Recognising diversity

Respecting and valuing people's differences will lead to an **inclusive environment** in which people feel valued and want to actively take part. Treating people fairly and challenging discrimination when it occurs will further support the building of positive relationships.

Developing confidence

Person-centred approaches can develop individuals' confidence in making informed decisions about their care and support. Professionals who involve individuals' families and friends in their care and support will also develop confidence in how relatives' needs can be met.

Developing teamwork

Working in partnership is part of developing good teamwork. Working in a team also involves working alongside individuals, their families and advocates, colleagues and other professionals, all of whom have different skills, abilities, views and levels of knowledge. Doing so will give everyone a greater sense of belonging, lead to collective decisions and be a good way of learning from one another and developing positive relationships.

Leading to additional benefits

Other benefits can be the development of new relationships, the sharing and development of new skills, knowledge and approaches as well as a good environment for developing innovative ideas and ways of working.

KEY TERM

Inclusive environment – somewhere where everyone feels valued, their differences respected, and able to reach their full potential.

CLASSROOM DISCUSSION

Making positive relationships happen (25 minutes)

In two groups, discuss what's important in developing positive relationships. Focus on the five best ways of supporting positive relationships in health, social care and child care environments.

Then join together as a whole group to discuss supporting positive relationships.

? THINK ABOUT IT

Case study Lina

Lina is 75 years old and is finding it difficult to continue to live at home on her own due to gradual sight loss. Her son visits twice a week and she stays with her daughter most weekends. Lina is feeling isolated at home and would like to live somewhere with other people around her. A friend who works in a local care home has suggested that she moves there, but Lina does not feel that she would be happy living with strangers and would prefer to live with her son or daughter. Lina has already contacted the local advocacy group and has been matched with an independent advocate who will be visiting her next week to discuss her plans and to support her to take the next steps.

Imagine you are Lina's advocate. Think about the following.

1 What types of positive relationship does Lina have in her life?
2 How can you support Lina to discuss her plans for her future?
3 Make a list of what you may want to discuss with her or ask her about.
4 How might you adapt your communication with Lina? Why?

1 What's the meaning of a person-centred approach?
2 How can technological aids support an individual?
3 How can an individual be empowered?
4 What does diversity mean?
5 Why is teamwork important?

LO3 Assessment activities

Below are suggested assessment activities that have been directly linked to the pass and merit criteria in LO3 to help with assignment preparation; they include Top Tips on how to achieve best results.

Activity 1 – pass criteria *P3*

Produce a staff guide for new workers in a health, social care or child care setting about the different agreed ways of working for ensuring a person-centred approach.

> **TOP TIPS**
> ✔ Include detailed information with a clear rationale of how a range of strategies can ensure a person-centred approach.
> ✔ Ensure you provide detailed evidence about each strategy and include examples of how each strategy can ensure a person-centred approach.

Activity 2 – merit criteria *M2*

Identify a health, social care or child care environment and then describe a fictional individual who may live in or access services from it. Analyse how and to what extent a person-centred approach can support positive relationships for that individual in that environment.

> **TOP TIPS**
> ✔ Ensure you provide an analysis – a detailed examination of how a person-centred approach supports the building of positive relationships.
> ✔ Ensure you provide detailed evidence about each aspect of supporting positive relationships and include examples of how each can work in practice.

LO4 Be able to use communication skills effectively to build positive relationships in a health, social care or child care environment
P4 P5 M3 D2

4.1 Communication skills

GETTING STARTED

(15 minutes)

Read through the examples in Table 1.4 of the health, social care and child care professionals and practitioners who use a range of skills and methods to communicate effectively in both one-to-one and group interactions to build positive relationships.

Think about the following.

● What communication skills and methods do they share? Why?
● How are these used? Why?
● What effects do you think these skills have in building positive relationships in one-to-one interactions?
● What effects do you think these skills have in building positive relationships in group interactions?

Remember, every person and interaction is unique, so it is good to explore different ways of communicating. What works for one person or one interaction might not work for another.

> 🔑 **KEY TERMS**
>
> **Dietician** – a trained professional who provides advice and guidance on diet and nutrition.
>
> **Body mass index** – a calculation of a person's weight in kilograms divided by the square of their height in metres to determine if they are overweight or underweight.
>
> **Review** – a formal meeting where an individual's care or support plan is reviewed.

Table 1.4 Using communication skills

Type of interaction	Communication skills used
One-to-one interaction Steven, a **dietician**, meets Maureen who is 65 years old, has Parkinson's disease and has a low **body mass index** that shows she is underweight.	Verbal – Steven uses open questions to find out about Maureen's eating habits since she's been diagnosed with Parkinson's. Non-verbal – Steven listens attentively and shows his empathy for Maureen's difficulties with maintaining a constant weight. Written – Steven shows Maureen some guidelines for healthy eating. These have been written in plain and clear language and are jargon free. Application of communication theories – Steven ensures that he maintains an open and relaxed posture during his meeting with Maureen and that he observes her body language when questioning her.
One-to-one interaction Jessica, a senior support worker, meets with Yoruba, a support worker, for supervision.	Verbal – Jessica books an interpreter for the supervision as she is aware that English is Yoruba's second language and that in formal situations he prefers to communicate via an interpreter. Jessica uses plain language and terms while speaking, and gives Yoruba plenty of time to speak and respond to her questions. Non-verbal – Jessica uses eye contact and leans towards Yoruba whilst listening and speaking to him. Jessica also avoids looking at the interpreter when communicating with Yoruba. Written – Jessica shows Yoruba a copy of his supervision record form, written in clear language, and gives him an accurate record of today's discussions. Application of communication theories – Jessica sits at a slight angle in front of Yoruba so that she can look at and interact with him directly.
Group interaction Graham, a senior residential child care worker, participates in Anming's **review** with the residential manager and Anming's social worker.	Verbal – Graham adapts the language he uses and the questions he asks to ensure that all his verbal communications can be understood by everyone including Anming, who has a learning disability. Non-verbal – Graham maintains an open posture, uses eye contact and a seated position when listening and speaking to each person in turn. Written – Graham has supported Anming to include her ideas in her care plan in the form of pictures, photographs and plain words. Application of communication theories – Graham acts in a confident manner when trying to resolve the concerns of his manager and the social worker by taking into account their different views and ideas.

4.2 **Effectiveness of interactions**

In LO2 you learned about the different communication factors that can influence the building of relationships, including verbal and non-verbal communication skills, written skills and the application of theories of communication. How these are used in different situations will have a direct effect on relationships with individuals and others involved in their lives.

You will work with a wide range of people who all have unique needs and preferences. If these are not understood or taken into account then misunderstandings can arise and can make interactions difficult and unproductive. The quality of relationships will also be affected.

Self-awareness and reflection

Self-awareness involves being honest and understanding who you are, what influences you and why you interact with others in the way you do. It is a continuous process.

Reflection involves gaining insight by thinking about and learning from situations, incidents, issues and

concerns that may arise. It involves thinking about what happened as well as the reasons why. It helps you to identify both good practice and what needs to be changed to make it work better next time. This can in turn develop stronger working relationships between the team and others.

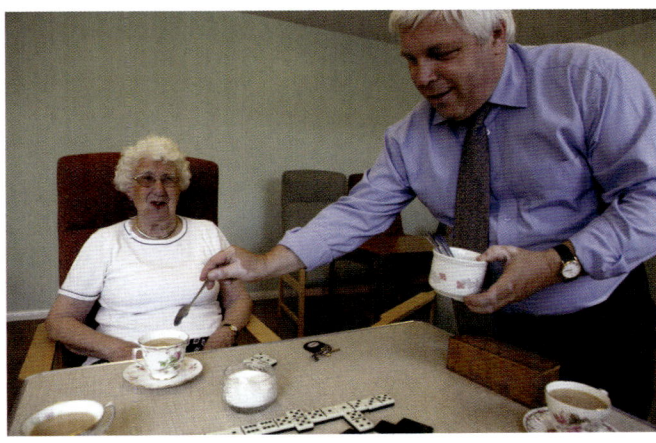

▲ **Figure 1.9** It is useful to reflect on why and how you did things

Use of strategies, support and aids to overcome barriers

Barriers to effective interactions in health, social care and child care environments may arise due to:

- a lack of insight into one's strengths and weaknesses
- a lack of knowledge and skills
- a lack of understanding of new or different approaches.

Feedback is very important as often others can tell you strengths and areas for development that you were unaware of. It involves others sharing their views, thoughts and feelings about how your knowledge, understanding and skills have affected them, the aspects they liked and they thought worked well, the aspects they didn't like and why they thought they didn't work as well. Receiving feedback positively will help you to develop as a **reflective practitioner**.

> ### 🔑 KEY TERMS
>
> **Reflective practitioner** – a professional who looks back over the work they do on a regular basis, and spends time thinking about and making improvements to their working practices.
>
> **Communication board** – a board with symbols and pictures that enables individuals to communicate by pointing to or looking at them.
>
> **Speech therapists** – trained professionals who assess an individual's communication difficulties and provide advice on how to address them.
>
> **Speech and language teams** – trained teams of professionals who provide support with enabling individuals to develop effective communication skills, and can also provide training and support to those working with individuals.

Training and development can involve attending training days and conferences and reading about updates and current research in the sector. Making the most of the knowledge and experience of those who work with you, such as your manager and colleagues, can be a useful way of ensuring that you maximise the benefits of training and development. For example, observing a colleague support an individual can help you to develop alternative communication strategies or to better understand how to use their adapted **communication board**.

Sometimes you may need to seek advice and information from other professionals with specialist knowledge such as **speech therapists,** and agencies such as **speech and language teams**, for example in relation to an individual's communication and language needs. This may be due to a change in an individual's needs, for example a stroke, dementia, loss of hearing or speech.

Being open to learning about new approaches to situations and considering different ways of practising is essential for developing more effective ways of working. Similarly, encouraging open discussions and talking through difficult and sensitive situations, considering options and the potential impact of these can create a service that promotes effective interactions and reflects current good working practices.

4.3 Aspects of reflective practice

How you reflect on specific incidents or activities will depend on how much experience you have had. It will also depend on your own preferences for learning – whether you prefer to learn and develop your practices when incidents and activities unfold (reflection-in-action) or whether you prefer spend some time after the incident or activity has happened thinking through on your own and discussing it with others (reflection-on-action). Donald Schon (1930–97) was a philosopher whose was influential in developing the concepts of 'reflection-in-action' and 'reflection-on-action'. The reflection-in-action concept is more commonly known as 'thinking on your feet'.

A model often used by health, social care and child care professionals for reflection is Gibbs' (1988) reflective cycle.

- **Stage 1 – What happened?** Think about the activity or situation you experienced. It is important you do this not too long after it happened as it is easy to forget important details.
- **Stage 2 – What did you think and feel?** Think about your thoughts and feelings at the time. How did you react? What did you say? Why?
- **Stage 3 – What worked well and what didn't?** Think through the positives and negatives of what happened including the actions that worked well and those that didn't.
- **Stage 4 – What happened and why?** Think through the reasons behind what happened, including the

factors behind individuals' and others' actions and words. Also think through whether you or anyone else contributed to what happened, whether it was intentional or not.

- **Stage 5 – What else could have been done?** Look at other ways that the activity or situation could have been done and dealt with differently. This will involve honest and careful reflection.
- **Stage 6 – What would you do next time?** Plan how you can make improvements if the activity or situation occurs again. This will involve considering other options that may work better but you will need to be prepared to be flexible in trying different methods and having a range of options in mind.

All six stages can be worked through at the time of an activity or situation occurring (reflection-in-action) or after it has happened (reflection-on-action).

Being a reflective practitioner can involve many elements, including wanting to learn, knowing how to learn, being able to make use of development tools such as training and being prepared to find out as much as you can about yourself, both personally and professionally.

GROUP ACTIVITY

(45 minutes)
Draw me

1 Using your textbook, the internet and other resources work in small groups to find out about other models of reflection.
2 Discuss and write down the key points associated with each model.
3 Draw a picture that represents each of the models.
4 Share these pictures with the rest of the groups and describe how these relate to models of communication.

KNOW IT

1 Name three factors to take into account when using verbal communication.
2 Name three factors to take into account when using non-verbal communication.
3 How can you adapt your communication with others?
4 Name two communication theories.
5 Name four key aspects of reflective practice.

LO4 Assessment activities

Below are suggested assessment activities that have been directly linked to the pass, merit and distinction criteria in LO4 to help with assignment preparation; they include Top Tips on how to achieve best results.

Choose one of the scenarios below.

A health care scenario

Part 1 – Marie has an appointment with the neurologist at the hospital to discuss the medication she is taking for epilepsy. Marie is unsure about continuing with her medication as she is experiencing many side effects including drowsiness, weight gain and difficulties concentrating.

Part 2 – Following Marie's hospital appointment Marie, her brother and advocate meet to discuss how best to support her.

A social care scenario

Part 1 – Liam has learning difficulties. He is not happy about spending most of his evenings at home. He wants to go out with his friends and try new activities.

Liam's support worker Mark is meeting him today to discuss this.

Part 2 – Liam and his support worker are meeting Liam's parents and social worker to discuss Liam's wishes and plans.

A child care scenario

Part 1 – Yana is 3 years of age. You notice that she finds it difficult to share the equipment used in activities when she is in a large group with other children and when asked to do so gets very angry.

Part 2 – You, your manager and Yana's parents are meeting to discuss the support that has been put in place for Yana.

Activity 1 – pass criteria *P4 P5*

Using your chosen care scenario **(Part 1)** role play effective communication skills in a **one-to-one interaction** to build a positive relationship.

Using your chosen care scenario **(Part 2)** role play effective communication skills in a **group interaction** to build a positive relationship.

Activity 2 – merit criteria *M3*

Reflect on both your role plays and for each one review how effective the communication skills that you used were by answering the following questions.

Care scenario – Part 1

1 What communication skills did I demonstrate in the one-to-one interaction?
2 Why did I use these communication skills?
3 How did I feel using these?
4 What went well?
5 What did not go well?
6 What did I learn?

Care scenario – Part 2

1 What communication skills did I demonstrate in the group interaction?
2 Why did I use these communication skills?
3 How did I feel using these?
4 What went well?
5 What did not go well?
6 What did I learn?

Activity 3 – distinction criteria *D2*

Complete a project that justifies the use of reflective practice to ensure interactions build positive relationships in health, social care and child care environments.

Read about it

Knapman, J. and Morrison, T. (1998) *Making the Most of Supervision in Health and Social Care*, Pavilion Publishers.

Leach, J. (2014) *Improving Mental Health through Social Support: Building Positive and Empowering Relationships*, Jessica Kingsley Publishers.

Morris, C., Ferreiro Peteiro, M. and Collier, F. (2015) *Level 3 Health and Social Care Diploma*, Hodder Education.

Moss, B. (2015) *Communication Skills in Health and Social Care*, 3rd edition, Sage Publications.

Schön, D. (1983) *The Reflective Practitioner: How Professionals Think in Action*, Temple Smith.

Unit 02

Equality, diversity and rights in health and social care

ABOUT THIS UNIT

Individuals using health, social care and child care services may be vulnerable and/or dependent on others, so it is very important that practitioners are aware of, and supportive of, people's rights and differences. The focus of this unit is to examine how health, social care and child care environments support individuals' rights, value their diversity and provide them with equal opportunities in order to meet their needs.

You will learn about the possible causes of discriminatory practices, the effects discrimination can have on individuals in care situations and the role of legislation and national initiatives in promoting anti-discriminatory practice. You will consider strategies and approaches that practitioners working in health, social care and child care environments can use to promote equality, respect diversity and protect the rights of individuals in their care.

LEARNING OUTCOMES

The topics, activities and suggested reading in this unit will help you to:

1 Understand the concepts of equality, diversity and rights and how these are applied in the context of health, social care and child care environments
2 Understand the impact of discriminatory practices on individuals in health, social care and child care environments
3 Understand how current legislation and national initiatives promote anti-discriminatory practice in health, social care and child care environments
4 Understand how equality, diversity and rights in health, social care and child care environments are promoted

How will I be assessed?

You will be assessed through an external assessment set and marked by OCR.

LO1 Understand the concepts of equality, diversity and rights and how these are applied in the context of health, social care and child care environments

🔑 KEY TERMS

Values of care – core principles that underpin care work. They aim to eliminate discrimination, reduce inequalities and help to ensure individuals' care needs are met.

GETTING STARTED

How am I valued and respected? (10 minutes)

In pairs, discuss ways that your college or school shows respect for and values individuals.

Share an example with the rest of the group that demonstrates how the following are promoted:

- equality
- diversity
- rights.

1.1 Concepts

Equality

Promoting equality means ensuring people are treated fairly and equally. All individuals must be given the same choices and opportunities regardless of their specific needs and differences. They must not be discriminated against due to their age, race, sexuality, disability or gender, for example.

Diversity

Diversity encompasses recognising and valuing that every individual is unique. Valuing diversity involves accepting and respecting individual differences, for example differences in religion, beliefs or race.

Rights

Rights are what everyone is legally entitled to and are enshrined in legislation, such as the Equality Act (see page 32). Examples of rights are given below.

- Choice. Choice gives individuals control over their lives and increases their self-esteem because it promotes independence. In a residential care home, choice can be whether or not to join in activities, choosing what to wear and which TV programme to watch. In health care an individual has the right to go to the GP of their choice. People with a sensory impairment should be able to choose whether they live in a supported environment or independently with support tailored to their needs.
- Confidentiality. Information should only be shared on a need-to-know basis, for example with other workers involved in an individual's care. You should not share information with anyone else, even a person's family or friends, without an individual's permission. The only exceptions to this are if a person:
  - is at risk of harming others
  - is at risk of harming themselves
  - is at risk of being hurt by others

or

  - when there is a risk of a *serious* offence being carried out.
- Protection from abuse and harm. Safeguarding procedures should be followed at all times to protect adults and children in care environments. Health and safety legislation should be adhered to. Fire and evacuation procedures should be in place. Risk assessments should be carried out for activities, trips and use of equipment, for example using a hoist to lift an individual into the bath.
- Equal and fair treatment. Individuals should be treated in accordance with the law and their needs. Everyone should be given the same opportunities to access education, health and social care. It is important to realise that providing the same treatment does not always guarantee equality, because different individuals are in different situations and have different needs. Treating everyone the same does not mean equality is being promoted.
- Consultation. Individuals in health, social care or child care environments should be asked for their opinions and views about the type of care and activities they would like, and their views and opinions taken account of wherever possible.
- Right to life. An individual's life is protected by law. This means that no one is allowed to harm you and equally you are not allowed to harm anyone else. Everyone's life should be valued and respected.

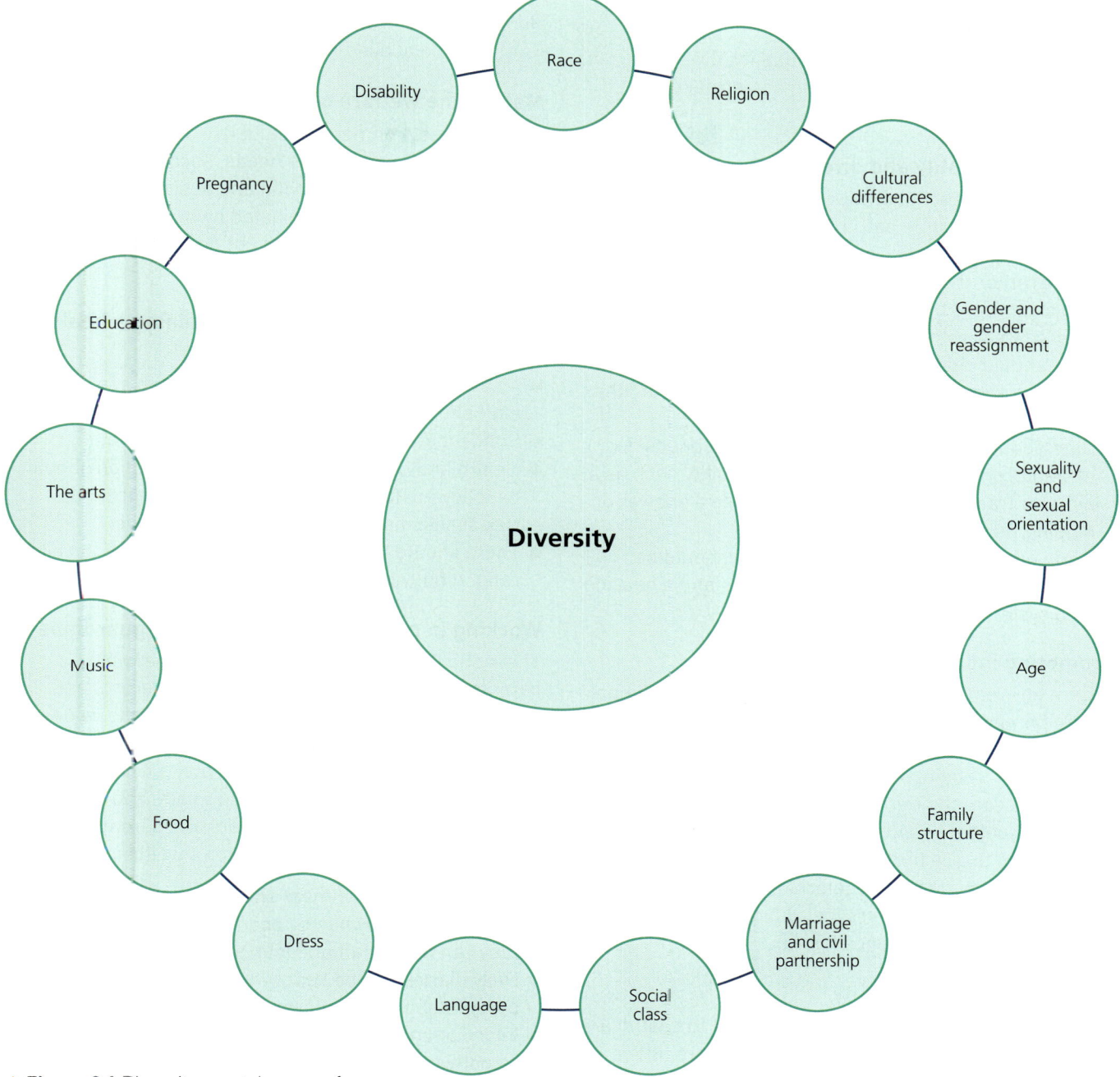

▲ **Figure 2.1** Diversity can take many forms

1.2 Application of the concepts

Applying the **values of care** ensures that all individuals using health, social care and child care environments receive appropriate levels of care, attention and treatment and that they have equal opportunities and are free from discrimination. Their diversity is valued and their rights supported.

The values of care provide clear guidelines to inform and improve practice so that staff know how to provide effective care. They also guide staff about legal requirements. Applying the values of care also helps to maintain or improve quality of life, for example helping a child to reach their full potential and providing access to those with mobility problems or communication barriers.

The values of care in health and social care services

Here are some examples of how equality, diversity and rights can be applied in health and social care environments.

Promoting equality and diversity

- Care workers should always use non-discriminatory language and not be patronising to the individuals they are caring for. For example, use a patient's name rather than referring to them as 'dear', or allowing a care home resident to choose what they want to wear rather than telling them.
- They should challenge discrimination, such as racist or sexist remarks made by a staff member or another individual.
- Care should meet an individual's specific needs; for example, providing assistance with mobility such as a Zimmer frame, helping someone to take a shower or helping them to get dressed.
- A trip out for residents of a care home should be somewhere that has wheelchair access and a hearing loop system.

Promoting individual rights and beliefs

- Care environments, such as hospitals and residential care homes, could provide access to a prayer room or transport to church, for example, to support individuals' religious beliefs.
- In health care the right to choice of a pregnant woman could be supported by asking her whether she wants to give birth at the hospital or at home.
- Providing a menu with vegetarian, gluten free, halal and kosher options caters for all types of dietary needs and provides choice for all.

Maintaining confidentiality

- It would not be appropriate for care staff to chat in a corridor about one of the residents in a care home, or to leave a resident's personal file lying around in the lounge.
- Documents containing personal information should be filed away in a locked cabinet or in password-protected electronic records.
- Information should only ever be shared on a 'need to know' basis with practitioners involved with the individual's care.

The values of care in child care services

Here are some examples of how equality, diversity and rights can be applied in child care environments.

Making the welfare of the child paramount

Child care environments should use a child-centred approach where the child's needs, such as being healthy, staying safe, enjoying and achieving, come first. A child must never be humiliated by being publically told off or made fun of and should not be verbally abused or smacked.

Keeping children safe and maintaining a healthy environment

- A safeguarding procedure should be in place and all staff should be DBS checked.
- Staff should wear lanyards for identification.
- Health and safety procedures and legislation should be followed, for example having regular fire drills, risk assessments and first aiders available.
- There should always be an appropriate staff to child ratio. A bullying policy should be in place.

Working in partnership with parents/guardians

There should be a two-way relationship between parents/guardians and the care setting. Parents and practitioners need to listen to one another and value one another's views to achieve the best outcomes for the child. Parents have the right to play a central role in making decisions about their child's care, and successful relationships between practitioners and parents will have a beneficial impact on children's wellbeing.

- A child care environment should welcome parents and guardians by having open days or evenings where they can meet staff and look around the setting.
- Daily diaries can be kept by nursery staff to keep parents/guardians informed of progress.
- Information sessions could be provided on topics such as potty training, dealing with tantrums or picky eaters.
- Awards certificates could be sent home.
- Parents/guardians could be invited in to discuss behaviour or other issues.

Encouraging children's learning and development

- Activities should be stimulating and interesting for the children and suited to their developmental progress.

Valuing diversity

- Displays, toys, resources such as books and DVDs, and food should reflect different cultures, beliefs and needs.
- Celebrate a range of festivals with all the children, for example Diwali, Christmas, Chinese New Year. Welcome signs should be in different languages.
- Meeting individual communication or mobility needs shows all children are valued.

Ensuring equality of opportunity

- Meeting children's individual needs, whether those are cultural, religious, to do with mobility, dietary or communication.
- Staff should be aware of, and follow, the equal opportunities policy.
- Activities should be accessible to all with adapted resources if required or one-to-one support if needed.
- All areas should be accessible to all; this may require adjustable tables to accommodate wheelchairs, and ramps to ensure physical access.
- All children should be treated fairly with no 'favourites'.

Anti-discriminatory practice

- Staff should be good role models by using non-discriminatory language – no racist or sexist comments.
- Discriminatory comments or behaviour should be challenged.

Maintaining confidentiality

- Information should be shared on a need-to-know basis only.
- Children's personal information should be kept secure in a locked filing cabinet or password protected if electronic.
- It is important that staff do not have conversations about the children where they can be overheard. Such conversations should take place privately.

Working with other professionals

Sometimes it is necessary to work with other practitioners or agencies that support children. The school nurse, a health visitor or a social worker are examples. Information should be shared openly but sensitively.

1.3 Support networks

A number of support networks ensure that equality, diversity and rights are promoted in care settings.

Advocacy services

Advocacy means getting support from another person in order to help an individual express their views and wishes, and ensures their voice is heard.

Table 2.1 gives some examples of organisations that provide advocacy services.

Table 2.1 Examples of organisations that provide advocacy services

Organisation	Activities
SEAP (Support, Empower Advocate Promote)	A charity that provides free, independent and confidential advocacy services. It helps resolve issues or concerns about health and wellbeing or health and social care services. SEAP's aim is to ensure that individuals are in control of decisions that are made about them and that their experiences, views, wishes and feelings are heard.
Mencap	A charity that works in partnership with people with a learning disability, and supports people to live life as they choose.
Empower Me	An organisation that develops advocacy and service user involvement projects. It supports mental health service users and people with learning difficulties to have a voice, which allows them to challenge stigma, and promotes social inclusion and community cohesion.
British Institute of Learning Disabilities	A body that campaigns for people with learning disabilities to be valued equally, participate fully in their communities and be treated with dignity and respect.

Support groups

Table 2.2 gives some examples of support groups.

Table 2.2 Examples of support groups

Organisation	Activities
Mind	A charity that provides advice and support to empower those experiencing a mental health problem. It campaigns to improve services, raise awareness and promote understanding.
Age UK	A charity that raises awareness of the difficult situations faced by many older people, and keeps relevant issues in the public eye and relevant in parliament. Campaigns vary from calling for the reform of the care system to trying to improve the bus route in a local community. Factsheets and advice guides for older adults are produced on a range of topics such as claiming benefits and planning care.
Headway	An association that promotes understanding about brain injuries and provides information, support and services to survivors, their families and carers.

Informal support

Individuals may receive informal support from people they know, such as friends, family and neighbours. Often these people provide essential services such as shopping or driving the individual to medical appointments. This type of support can, for example, support an older person to maintain their independence and help them continue living in their own home.

LO2 Understand the impact of discriminatory practices on individuals in health, social care and child care environments

KEY TERM

Discrimination – when people judge others based on their differences and use these differences to create disadvantage or oppression.

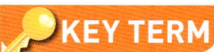

GETTING STARTED

Who are they? (5 minutes)

Write down the following three headings:

- A 78 year old man
- A teenage boy with multiple face piercings and tattoos
- A 16 year old single mum

Underneath each heading quickly write down any words that immediately come to mind to describe that person.

Share and discuss your descriptions. Are the descriptions based on fact or opinion? Are the descriptions fair? Have any judgements been made? What have you assumed about each person?

2.1 Discriminatory practices

Discriminatory practice involves treating someone unfairly or less favourably compared to others. Discriminatory practice can take many forms, such as excluding someone from activities, or verbal or physical abuse.

Basis of discrimination

Discriminatory practice develops from uninformed attitudes and beliefs that result in unfair treatment of certain individuals or groups of people. **Discrimination** can occur on the basis of an individual's race, culture, disability or social class.

Race

Race refers to a group that is considered to have distinct characteristics based on their skin colour, nationality or ethnic origin. The NHS, emergency services and local authorities ask people to classify their race as White, Asian, Black, Mixed Race, Chinese/any other ethnic group. Data and statistics gathered using the classification system can be used to monitor, for example, use of services by different ethnic groups or the effectiveness of equal opportunities policies. Discrimination on the basis of race is called racism.

Culture

Culture refers to a group of people in society who share the same customs, language, dress, beliefs and values. Cultural groups perceived by some people as being different, such as Traveller communities are often victims of discrimination.

Disability

A disability is defined as a physical or mental impairment that has a substantial and long-term negative effect on a person's ability to do normal daily activities. Discrimination on the basis of a disability is called disablism.

Social class

Social class is usually defined by economic or educational status, where people are grouped into hierarchical social categories. People sometimes have unfavourable views of others and make judgements because of their social class.

Age

People are sometimes discriminated against because of their age, and despite being an ageing society there are still negative perceptions about older people being frail or confused. Discrimination based on age is called ageism.

Gender

This refers to whether someone is male, female or transgender. Discrimination that occurs because of someone's gender is called sexism.

Sexual orientation

Discrimination due to someone's sexuality, if they are bisexual, gay or lesbian, is known as homophobia.

Religion

Religion is a system of beliefs and values. Religious beliefs can be very important to people and influence the way they live their life. Religious discrimination could involve a person's religious needs not being met, for example kosher food not being available for a Jewish patient at a hospital.

You will come into contact with a wide variety of different individuals from many walks of life. It is essential that you examine and reflect on your own attitudes and beliefs to ensure that you do not unfairly discriminate against the individuals in your care.

Direct and indirect discrimination

Direct discrimination involves intentionally putting someone at a disadvantage or treating them unfairly based on their differences. For example, a woman who is told that she did not get a job because she is female is a victim of direct sex discrimination.

Indirect discrimination is when a policy, practice or a rule applies to everybody but it has a detrimental effect on some people. The discrimination is accidental or unintentional. For example, if a job advertisement stated that male applicants must be clean shaven, this would discriminate against men whose religious beliefs prevent them shaving their beards.

Types of abuse

The term 'abuse' refers to a wide range of negative and harmful ways of behaving.

Types of abuse which may be found in health, social care and child care environments are shown in Figure 2.2.

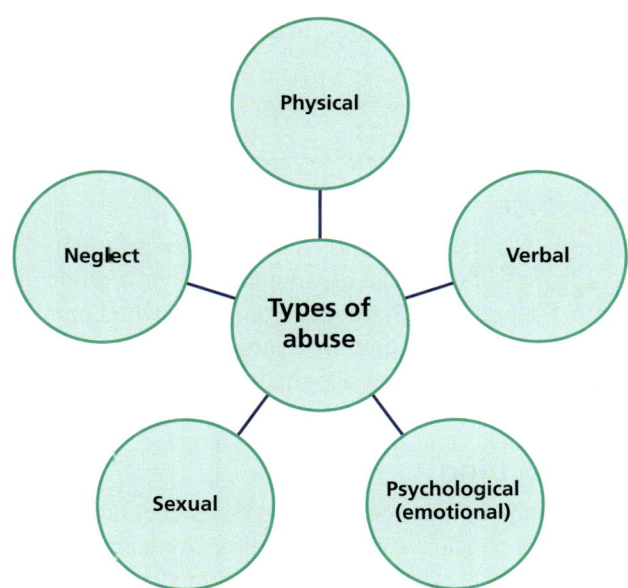

▲ **Figure 2.2** Types of abuse in health, social care and child care environments

- Physical abuse. This occurs when someone causes physical pain or threatens to hurt an individual. A carer could handle a child roughly when changing a nappy. This could cause physical injuries such as bruising or, if very roughly handled, broken bones.
- Verbal abuse. This could be name calling, insults or swearing to try to humiliate someone or reduce their dignity or security. An example could be a care assistant in a residential home using foul language and raising her voice because a resident is taking too long to finish her meal when the carer wants to go off duty.
- Psychological (emotional) abuse. Threats and constant criticism are examples of psychological abuse. The aim is to undermine and control the person being abused.

- Sexual abuse. This would include any type of unwanted sexual contact, such as touching breasts, genitals or buttocks when the victim is either dressed or undressed.
- Neglect. This is when a carer fails to care for someone properly. Their basic needs for warmth, food, clean clothing are not met.

INDEPENDENT ACTIVITY

Recent abuse scandals (30–40 minutes)

Research the cases of abuse at Hillcroft Nursing Home, Stafford Hospital and Orchid View Care Home, or other recent abuse scandals in health, social care or child care environments.

1 What type of abuse occurred?
2 Consider the reasons why these incidents of abuse happened.
3 What could the care setting have done to prevent them from happening?

Prejudice

Prejudice is when someone has a negative attitude towards, or unfair dislike of, an individual or a group of people. Prejudice is often based on ill-informed opinion or on inaccurate information. Examples include racial prejudice or punishment of people because of their sexual orientation.

Stereotyping

Stereotyping involves making judgements about individuals or groups of people based on prejudices. It means making unfair assumptions that people with certain characteristics are the same. For example, 'girls are better behaved than boys' or 'midwives are always women'.

Labelling

Labelling means to identify people negatively as part of a particular group. The assumption is that 'they are all the same'. For example, 'all old people are frail and need to be looked after'. Some older adults are indeed frail and need support; however many older adults continue to live independently into their 90s.

Bullying

Bullying describes a range of negative behaviours that can intimidate or harm individuals. It can involve humiliating, insulting or harassing someone by constantly criticising them, making inappropriate comments or repeating offensive jokes and nicknames. Bullying may be carried out by a person who is in a position of power, such as a manager, supervisor or carer. It may involve bullying another care worker, or bullying service users.

2.2 Individuals affected

Discriminatory practice can affect anyone within a health, social care or child care environment, not just those who use the services. Hospital practitioners may be subject to discriminatory practice from their supervisor, from the patients or patients' families. A child attending a nursery may be discriminated against by the nursery staff, other children or their families.

Examples of three main groups of individuals who can be affected by discriminatory practice in health, social care and child care environments are shown in Table 2.3.

Table 2.3 Who is affected by discriminatory practice?

Individuals who require care and support	Family, friends, relatives of individuals	Practitioners
• Patients • Clients • People with disabilities • Babies • Children • Young adults • Older adults	• Parents • Grandparents • Sons and daughters • Step-family members • Best friends • Neighbours	• Nurse • GP • Physiotherapist • Midwife • Surgeon • Health visitor • Social worker • Care assistant • Counsellor • Nursery assistant

2.3 Impact on individuals

Being discriminated against can negatively affect an individual's physical, intellectual, emotional and social wellbeing. This can lead to health problems and social exclusion.

Disempowerment

Individuals who have suffered discrimination can feel disempowered. They will feel a lack of control in their life, particularly if they are in residential care where they are dependent on a carer who is abusing them.

Low self-esteem and low self-confidence

Self-esteem and self-confidence can be destroyed by discrimination, leading to an individual feeling worthless.

Poor health and wellbeing

An individual's wellbeing may be affected; they may become withdrawn and isolate themselves to avoid the situation, feeling frightened about further discrimination and ill-treatment. Health problems can develop, such as high blood pressure or anxiety, and if the individual is already ill, their condition may deteriorate and their recovery be delayed. Physical abuse can have serious, and in some cases fatal, consequences.

The effects do not occur in isolation; they are interrelated. For example, if a nurse experiences bullying in the workplace it can lead to loss of concentration when completing tasks, due to worry and stress. Socially the nurse may become withdrawn and not want to go to work, or they could become agitated or aggressive with other staff or patients. This could reduce confidence causing further emotional effects such as the nurse becoming frustrated and developing low self-esteem.

? THINK ABOUT IT

Case study

Read the newspaper article 'Former Male Nurse Wins Sex Discrimination Case', which can be accessed via the following link.

http://tinyurl.com/gotsclj

1 Describe the discriminatory practice that Mr Moyhing experienced.
2 What assumptions were the basis for the discriminatory practice?
3 What has been the impact of this discriminatory practice on Mr Moyhing?

KNOW IT

1 Explain the difference between 'direct' and 'indirect' discrimination. Give an example of each.
2 Name and give an example of four types of abuse.
3 In your own words write a definition of the following terms:
   a social class
   b prejudice
   c culture
   d disempowerment
   e ageism.

LO3 Understand how current legislation and national initiatives promote anti-discriminatory practice in health, social care and child care environments

GETTING STARTED

A good initiative? (10 minutes)

From April 2016, all nurses and midwives have had to 'revalidate' to maintain their registration with the Nursing and Midwifery Council (NMC).

Work in pairs to research and discuss the introduction of revalidation. Consider the impact of this initiative for nurses and midwives, for care providers and for people who use health care environments. Share your thoughts with the rest of the group.

KEY TERM

Legislation – provides individuals with rights to which they are entitled through laws passed by parliament. Law is upheld through the courts.

3.1 Key aspects of current legislation

Legislation protects the rights of both individuals receiving care and providers of care and support; it also states their responsibilities to society. Laws provide a legal framework for care and provide individuals with the right to access and to receive care and support. The government uses legislation to create regulatory arrangements for monitoring care organisations and to set standards for service delivery.

The Care Act 2014

This Act relates to those being assessed or receiving social care, and their carers. Key aspects include the following.

- Duty on local authorities to promote an individual's 'wellbeing' when making a decision about an individual, e.g. their personal dignity, protection from abuse and neglect, physical, mental health and emotional wellbeing, social and economic wellbeing, suitability of living accommodation and control by the individual over day-to-day life (including over care and support).
- Continuity of care must be provided if someone moves from one area to another, so that there will be no gap in care or support.
- Duty on local authorities to carry out Child's Needs Assessments (CNA) for young people where there is likely to be a need for care and support after they reach the age of 18.
- An independent advocate is to be available to facilitate the involvement of an adult or carer who is the subject of an assessment, care or support planning or a review.
- Adult safeguarding. This includes: responsibility to ensure enquiries into cases of abuse and neglect, establishment of Safeguarding Adults Boards and responsibility to ensure information sharing and inter-professional working.

- Local authorities have to guarantee preventative services which could help reduce or delay the development of care and support needs, including carers' support needs.

The Health and Social Care Act 2012

This Act is underpinned by two main principles: enabling patients to have more control over the care they receive and that those responsible for patient care – the doctors, nurses and others who work in the NHS and social care – have the freedom and power to commission care that meets local needs. Key aspects include the following.

- No Decision About Me Without Me is intended to be the guiding principle by which patients are treated. Patients will be able to choose their GP, consultant, treatment and hospital or other local health service.
- Clinical Commissioning Groups are GP-led bodies that commission most health services, including primary care services such as GPs, dentists and pharmacies, and secondary care services such as those provided by hospitals.
- Health and wellbeing boards bring together health and social care commissioners, councillors and a lay representative to promote joint working and tackle inequalities in people's health and wellbeing.
- Public health: increased focus on prevention with local councils taking over responsibility for public health services and population health improvement, for example obesity, anti-smoking, screening, vaccinations.
- Healthwatch is an independent service created by the Act, which aims to protect the interests of all those who use health and social care services. It has a role in communicating the views of patients to commissioning bodies and regulators.

The Equality Act 2010

When the Equality Act came into force it simplified the existing laws covering discrimination, such as the Sex Discrimination Act, Race Relations Act and Disability Discrimination Act and put them all together in one piece of legislation. Key aspects include the following.

- Makes direct and indirect discrimination on the basis of a protected characteristic illegal. The nine protected characteristics are: age, disability, gender reassignment, marriage and civil partnership, pregnancy and maternity, race, religion, sex, sexual orientation.
- Prohibits discrimination in education, employment, access to goods and services and housing
- Covers victimisation and harassment on the basis of a protected characteristic.
- Reasonable adjustments have to be made by employers or providers of goods or services for those with disabilities. For example, installing a ramp to access a building, aids such as computer software to help a person to do their job or providing information in a suitable format.
- Women have the right to breastfeed in public places. It is against the law for a woman to get less favourable treatment because she is breastfeeding when receiving services. However, there is no right to breastfeed at work.
- The Act encourages positive action. One form of positive action is encouraging or training people to apply for jobs or take part in an activity in which people with that protected characteristic are under-represented.
- Discrimination due to association is now an offence. This means that there is now protection for carers of an individual who has a protected characteristic.
- Pay secrecy clauses are now illegal.

The Mental Capacity Act 2005

'Capacity' is the ability to make a decision. This Act provides a legal framework setting out key principles, procedures and safeguards to protect and empower those who are unable to make some of their own decisions. This could include people with learning difficulties, dementia, mental health problems, strokes or head injuries. It has five statutory principles.

1 A presumption of capacity. Every adult has the right to make their own decisions and must be assumed to have capacity to do so unless it is proved otherwise. So a care worker must not assume someone cannot make a decision for themselves just because they have a particular condition or disability.
2 Support to make own decisions. A person must be given all practicable help before anyone treats them as not being able to make their own decisions. This might include presenting information in a different format for those with learning disabilities, for example.

3 Unwise decisions. People have the right to make what others may regard as an unwise or eccentric decision. Everyone has their own preferences, values and beliefs which may not be the same as those of others; they cannot be treated as lacking capacity for thinking differently.

4 Best interests. Action taken or decisions made under the Act or on behalf of a person who lacks capacity must be done in their best interests. So care workers should provide reasons showing the decision they are making is in the individual's best interests. They should try to involve the person, or consider whether the decision could be put off until the person regains capacity.

5 Less restrictive option. Anything done for or on behalf of a person who lacks capacity should be least restrictive of their basic rights and freedoms. So while it would be reasonable for a care worker to insist on accompanying an individual with learning disabilities who lacks capacity on a visit to the shops or to see friends, it would not be reasonable to lock them in their room to prevent them from going out.

The Children Act 2004

Key aspects of the Children Act include the following.

- Protecting children at risk: this may involve taking a child away from their family using an emergency protection order or care order.
- The paramount principle is that the child's needs must come first. For example, taking a child away from their family may adversely affect the adults but may be in the child's best interests. Children have the right to stay within their wider family circle wherever possible.
- Child has a right to be consulted. Children who are mature/old enough have a voice and their wishes should be taken into consideration.
- Children have a right to an advocate.
- Staying safe, being healthy, enjoying and achieving, make a positive contribution and economic wellbeing are universal ambitions for every child and young person, whatever their background or circumstances.
- Encourages partnership working. Practitioners need to ensure information is shared to help avoid miscommunication, particularly in child protection situations.
- Created the Children's Commissioner and set up children's safeguarding boards to represent children's interests.

The Data Protection Act 1998

The act states that information and data should be:

- processed fairly and lawfully: information should be collected only with an individual's permission. The information should only be shared on a 'need to know' basis
- used only for the purposes for which it was intended: information should only be gathered for a specific and necessary purpose and only used for that purpose
- adequate and relevant but not excessive: care workers should only collect and use information that is needed. For example, a detailed case history would be required by a social worker in order to inform a care plan but not by a nurse treating someone who has injured their ankle playing football
- accurate and kept up to date: inaccurate data should be destroyed or corrected. Care workers have a responsibility to ensure information is correct and systems should be in place for checking accuracy, for instance checking with patients
- kept for no longer than is necessary: delete or destroy information when it is no longer needed. For example, securely deleting or shredding sensitive or personal data
- processed in line with the rights of the individual: 'processed' means how the information is used. People have a right to know if information is being held about them and how their information is being used. They have the right to have any errors corrected, and to prevent any data being used for advertising or marketing
- secured: non-authorised people should not be allowed access to the information. The information, for example patient records, should be kept in secure conditions. Clear guidelines should be in place for who can have access to the information and there should be a confidentiality policy
- not transferred to other countries: information should not be transferred outside the EU unless the service user has given consent. This is because other countries may not have the same data protection legislation as the EU and so the data may not be secure.

PAIRS ACTIVITY

What are the benefits of legislation? (30 minutes)

Work in pairs to discuss the benefits for health, social care and child care environments of one of the pieces of legislation listed above.

Share your ideas with the rest of the group explaining how the law relates to supporting individuals' rights and the provision of quality care.

3.2 Overview of national initiatives

The Care Certificate 2014

The Care Certificate consists of set of standards that health and social care workers must follow in their daily working life. It provides clear evidence to employers, patients and people who receive care and support that the health or social care support worker in front of them has been assessed against a specific set of standards and has demonstrated they have the skills, knowledge and behaviours to ensure that they provide compassionate and high-quality care and support.

Quality assurance

External bodies, such as those listed in Table 2.4, are involved in regulating and inspecting the quality of health, social care and child care environments.

Table 2.4 Examples of quality assurance bodies

Care Quality Commission (CQC)	The regulator of health and social care for England. It registers and licenses care services to ensure that essential standards of quality and safety are met, and monitors them to ensure they continue to meet these standards. Inspection reports are published and if settings are found not to meet the required standards the CQC can take action such as warning notices and fines.
Ofsted (Office for Standards in Education)	Inspects and regulates services that care for children and young people and publishes a report that will identify good practice and areas for improvement. If a child care setting, which could be a childminder, a nursery or a school, is graded 'inadequate' the setting is placed in special measures. The setting will be provided with support from the local authority, additional funding and resourcing to aid improvement.
Equality and Human Rights Commission (EHRC)	Provides information to individuals so that they know their rights. It also provides information to organisations such as care homes, schools and hospitals to ensure that they know about their responsibilities under equality law. The commission can provide legal advice in cases of discrimination and will support individuals to take cases to court. It has powers to force organisations to fulfil their equality responsibilities.
NICE (National Institute for Health and Care Excellence)	Improves outcomes for individuals using the NHS and other public health and social care services. NICE considers whether a treatment benefits patients and will help the NHS meet its targets for example by improving cancer survival rates, and whether the treatment is value for money or cost effective. It also provides evidence-based guidelines on how particular conditions should be treated, on how public health and social care services can best support people and provides information services for those managing and providing health and social care.

3.3 The impact of legislation and national initiatives

Person-centred approach to care and provision and individual needs met

Legislation and national initiatives are focused on promoting and protecting the rights and needs of the individual. The values of care embed person-centred practice and ways of working to meet individual needs. This allows individuals using health, social care and child care environments to say what is important to them, gives them more control and improves their quality of life. For more on person-centred care, see Unit 6 (page 123).

Empowerment

This is how a carer encourages an individual to make informed choices and decisions so that they can take control of their own life. Care settings that implement legislation, initiatives such as the Care Certificate and carers applying the values of care will empower individuals to make informed choices and make decisions for themselves.

Accessible services

According to the Equality Act (page 32), reasonable adaptations have to be made to health, social care and child care environments to accommodate disabilities whether these are mental, physical or sensory. For example, information can be provided in large print or in Braille for individuals with visual difficulties and PECs (picture exchange communication systems) used for children with learning disabilities. Ramps, automatic doors and lifts assist those with mobility difficulties or who have children in a pushchair. Adaptations such as these all contribute to making all settings accessible for all.

Provides a system of redress

Each piece of legislation outlines the rights that individuals are entitled to. If those rights are breached then the law can be enforced by taking legal action through the courts so that individuals have their rights restored or the person or organisation breaking the law is penalised, e.g. with a fine or imprisonment.

Clear guidelines for practitioners to follow

The Mental Capacity Act, for example, makes it clear who can take decisions, in which situations, and how they should go about it. The Data Protection Act provides detailed regulations about how to handle information about individuals in health, social care and child care environments.

The Care Certificate has 15 standards against which a health or social care support worker is assessed. These include 'Understand your Role', Duty of Care', 'Privacy and Dignity' and 'Health and Safety'. Completing the Care Certificate demonstrates that the care worker knows exactly how to carry out their work to the highest standard.

Raises standards of care

Ofsted, for example:
- promotes service improvement/raises standards
- ensures services focus on the interests of their users
- identifies good practice
- identifies areas for improvement
- ensures that services are efficient and effective
- establishes whether services promote value for money.

The CQC, for example:
- registers services
- monitors and inspects services
- regulates services – hospitals, GP practices, walk-in centres, out-of-hours services and care homes
- sets out the standards of care required
- checks that services meet the required standards of quality and safety
- publishes inspection reports
- awards ratings – outstanding/good/requires improvement/inadequate; by law service providers have to display their CQC rating.

Staff selection and interview procedures must comply with the Equality Act

The provisions of the Equality Act impact on the way that staff are selected and interviewed. For example, the advertisement must not state requirements that discriminate against certain groups, such as women. Questions asked at interview must be non-discriminatory, the same for all candidates and cannot be personal questions. Asking the same questions gives everyone a fair chance. It would not be appropriate, for example, to ask questions about an individual's disability; questions should relate to the job requirements and the skills they can offer.

The interview panel should be trained in equality and diversity to avoid any bias or discriminatory practice. The interview must take place somewhere accessible with facilities for all candidates including those with a disability. Candidates should be selected on merit and not, for example, on lack of mobility, appearance or age. Care settings should have policies and procedures in place to ensure best practice to provide equal opportunities for all candidates.

Organisational policies

There are many benefits to having organisational policies on, for example, bullying, confidentiality, equal opportunities and data handling. They ensure that health, social care or child care environments have attended to how they will provide the best quality of care in a way that promotes equality and supports individuals' rights. Some of the benefits are summarised below.

Benefits for the individual requiring care or support
- They help to prevent an individual being discriminated against.
- They ensure they are treated fairly.
- They ensure they are treated according to their needs.
- They promote opportunity through access to the service.
- They develop their self-esteem/confidence, their feelings of being empowered and valued.
- They help the service user feel safe and secure.

Benefits for the care worker
- They help them do their job more effectively.
- They guide them on good practice and help them to provide quality care at all times.
- They help to protect them (from accusations of bullying or discrimination) if they have followed the policy.
- They ensure that all staff are working to the same high standards and consistency of care.

Benefits for the organisation
- They help them to provide a quality service to children/parents/patients etc.
- They ensure that staff are working within the law.
- They help the organisation run smoothly/effectively as staff have common/clearly understood procedures to follow.
- They protect the organisation against complaints and help it to develop a good reputation.

KNOW IT

1 Name three different pieces of legislation that would apply in a health care environment.
2 What is meant by a 'system of redress'?
3 State four standards included in the Care Certificate.
4 What do the initials CQC stand for?
5 Describe the role of the CQC.

LO4 Understand how equality, diversity and rights in health, social care and child care environments are promoted

Best practice at a lunch club for older adults? (5 minutes)

Consider this scenario:

Staff provide the same meal for all of the older adults attending the lunch club. They think this is important so that everyone is treated the same. The staff make sure the food provided is soft or cut into small pieces. This is because older people struggle to chew because of wearing dentures and they suffer from arthritis making it difficult for them to cut up their food.

Is this best practice? Justify your answer.

4.1 Applying best practice in health, social care or child care environments

By following the underpinning principles of the values of care (see LO1, page 26) practitioners in health, social care and child care environments will be able to provide high-quality, personalised, safe and compassionate care that promotes the equality, diversity and rights of individuals in care environments. Key aspects of best practice include:

- being **non-judgemental**
- respecting the views, choices and decisions of individuals who require care and support
- anti-discriminatory practice
- valuing diversity
- using effective communication
- following agreed ways of working
- training and **professional development** opportunities for staff
- mentoring, **monitoring** and **performance management** of staff
- attending staff meetings to discuss issues/practice.

It is the care setting's and the individual care worker's responsibility to ensure understanding and awareness of how to promote best practice. This can be achieved by various methods. An individual care worker may carry out a skills audit or reflect on their own practice and produce a personal development plan. The setting could provide opportunities for staff to share best practice, sessions where they can discuss what went well and what could be improved in the future, and targets could be set. Inexperienced staff could have a mentor or a coach to help develop their practice. Provision of training and adequate resources to do a job to the required standard are essential.

Applying best practice involves providing the care that is required to meet the needs of individuals. This improves the individual's self-esteem, making them feel valued, and enables them to have trust and confidence in the practitioners providing their care. This in turn can improve the individual's wellbeing by helping them to maintain their independence, make progress or have a speedier recovery.

Emily's cup of tea (20 minutes)

Follow the link below and watch the clip. Then split into small groups to discuss the aspects of applying best practice that you have seen the practitioners use.

http://tinyurl.com/jfqaane

Each small group can then feed back to the whole class identifying key aspects and examples of best practice.

KEY TERMS

Non-judgemental – respecting a person's feelings, experiences and values, even though they may be different from yours. Not judging or criticising someone because of your own attitudes or beliefs.

Professional development – the process of improving and increasing the skills and capabilities of staff.

Monitoring – to measure and check the progress or quality of something over time. Methods of monitoring can involve observations, inspections, analysis of surveys given to service users or staff, for example.

Performance management – an ongoing process between a care worker and their supervisor involving meetings and observations over time to provide feedback on performance and identify targets for improvement where appropriate.

4.2 Explaining discriminatory practice in health, social care or child care environments

An understanding of how discrimination and unfair treatment can be detrimental to individuals and their wellbeing is essential for an informed care worker to provide high-quality care.

You should be able to identify the basis of the discrimination and the form it takes. You should be able to evaluate the possible impact of the discriminatory practice on the individual concerned and, if appropriate, effects on the individual's family or care workers.

While considering the lunch club scenario (Getting Started activity page 36), you may have recognised several examples of discriminatory behaviour and attitudes. For example, the staff believe that 'treating everyone the same' promotes equality and is fair – no one is treated differently. In fact, it is important to treat people according to their needs, and this may mean treating them differently. Some of the older adults may require a gluten-free or vegetarian meal, so would not be able to eat the same food as everyone else. Being provided with soft or cut-up food is patronising and may well make the older adults feel embarrassed, as though they are being treated like children. Not all older adults struggle to cut up food, so it is unacceptable to stereotype and label all of the older adults in this way.

Further examples of discriminatory practice are explained in Table 2.5.

It is the responsibility of all practitioners, in all care environments, to recognise discriminatory practice when it occurs and to respond with appropriate action.

4.3 Choosing appropriate action/ response to promote equality, diversity and rights in health, social care or child care environments

Raising concerns about discrimination and examining current practice are important ways of promoting equality, diversity and rights. Appropriate action may involve:

- reporting an incident to the relevant authorities
- reporting to management
- reflecting on your own attitudes
- changing your practice, or encouraging this in others.

It is important that the action is appropriate and that all internal steps have been taken before reporting to the authorities. Many issues can be resolved by simple changes within the health, social care or child care environment, but others require more drastic action such as reporting to authorities such as the Care Quality Commission (CQC) or Ofsted. The Stafford Hospital scandal led to the Department of Health producing a guidance booklet for health service staff about how to raise concerns to help prevent a similar situation ever happening again.

Department of Health: Raising Concerns at Work booklet: http://tinyurl.com/hza3wt8

The Social Care Institute for Excellence has produced a short film about raising concerns and how the process can improve the quality of care provided. The link is given below.

http://tinyurl.com/q8p6y8x

Table 2.5 Examples of discriminatory practice

Discriminatory practice	Examples
Prejudice (see also, LO2, page 30)	• Avoiding people who are perceived as different, for example a nurse who is reluctant to attend to patients from certain ethnic backgrounds. • A nursery nurse who thinks that children from a certain postcode are 'common' and treats them less favourably than others.
Inadequate care	• A childminder sitting a child in front of the television all day to keep them quiet. • Hospital patients' physical needs not being met, such as having to wait too long for food and drink, or not being taken to the toilet when needed.
Abuse and neglect	• This could be verbal abuse, such a day centre staff mocking and making jokes about young adults with learning disabilities. • Care assistants causing bruises due to handling residents roughly while giving them a bed bath. • A residential home for adults with dementia not providing any activities because 'there is no point, they won't remember anything'.
Breach of health and safety	• A care setting not having any trained first aiders. • Staff not trained in manual handling. • Equipment not regularly checked for damage. • Inadequate hygiene practices. • Activities not being risk assessed.

Revisit the lunch club scenario (Getting Started activity, on page 36).

What action should be taken to improve this situation? Appropriate treatment of the older adults attending the lunch club would involve applying the values of care to meet their individual needs.

For example, cutting up food may well be awkward for someone with arthritis in their hands. This issue could be addressed by offering choices on the menu that do not need so much cutting, such as pasta with a sauce. This gives the individual the opportunity to select food that they know they can manage themselves. This would promote independence and empower the person rather than patronise and humiliate them. It also means that everyone's right to choice is being provided for.

Also, the staff need training about equality and diversity as they think that 'treating everyone the same' is fair. Lack of training is often a reason for staff not providing an acceptable level of care, as they are not aware of what they should be doing. It is the role of the organisation's management to arrange and provide the training so that the staff are fully aware of how to promote equality and diversity. A supervisor could then monitor the lunch club sessions to check that the situation has improved.

In addition, those who attend the lunch club could be given a satisfaction survey and information about the complaints procedure to feed back to the lunch club organisers and give them an opportunity for the older adults to have their views heard. This maintains their right to consultation.

Some further examples of appropriate actions and responses to promote equality, diversity and rights in health, social care and child care environments are given below.

Methods of challenging discrimination

- Challenge at the time – explain to the person how they are discriminating, to raise their awareness of what they are doing, enabling them to reflect on their actions. The person could be supervised so that the quality of their work is monitored.
- Challenge afterwards through procedures – tell the person to read the organisation's policies, on equal opportunities and bullying for example. Senior staff could be consulted for advice on how to address the issue. In a serious case, disciplinary action could be taken against the person. This would make everyone aware of the importance of the issue and provides a basis for changing individuals' attitudes.
- Challenge afterwards through long-term campaigns – awareness sessions could be provided for staff on equality, diversity and rights or effective communication, for example. This training would be a professional development opportunity that helps to improve understanding of correct ways of working.

Whistleblowing

This involves raising concerns with a more senior member of staff such as a supervisor or manager. In an environment with an open culture where concerns can be raised without fear of repercussions, such as victimisation or bullying, managers will listen and act upon the issues raised in order to make improvements for staff and the individuals using their services. In extreme circumstances a person may need to 'whistleblow' to outside authorities such as Ofsted or the Care Quality Commission.

Providing information about complaints procedures and advocacy services

This enables a member of staff or someone who uses health, social care or child care environments to take action about poor treatment, for example. The organisation's complaints procedure should be provided so that the individual knows who to complain to and whether to make an internal complaint or involve an outside agency such as the CQC, a solicitor or the Equality and Human Rights Commission. Some individuals are unable to speak up for themselves, for example someone with dementia or learning difficulties. Having support from an advocate can enable them to obtain their rights and have their care needs met.

Dealing with conflict

Active listening, remaining calm, being objective and empathetic are ways of resolving conflict in care environments. It is important to see both sides of an argument and positively look for solutions.

Other responses could be applying values of care (see LO1), implementing policies, codes of practice and legislation (see LO3), and mentoring and monitoring (see LO4).

PAIRS ACTIVITY

PAIRS ACTIVITY

(90 minutes)

Working in pairs or small groups investigate what you could do to promote equality, diversity and rights if you were setting up a new nursery or a residential care home. If possible, visit a local nursery or care home and interview a care worker. Alternatively, you could research local care settings on the internet.

You could look at, for example, policies, procedures, training and staff recruitment. Consider the activities provided, environment (e.g. displays), food, facilities, etc. You could share your ideas with the rest of the group as a poster or PowerPoint presentation.

KNOW IT

1 List four different kinds of discriminatory practice.
2 Explain potential effects of inadequate care on an individual.
3 Produce a mind map showing different ways health, social care and child care environments could promote equality, diversity and rights.
4 What is meant by 'agreed ways of working'?
5 How could a care setting ensure that a member of staff correctly follows the 'Moving and Handling' procedure?

Read about it

Fisher, A. *et al.* (2012) *Applied AS Health & Social Care for OCR*, revised edition, Oxford University Press.

Gaine, C. (2010) *Equality and Diversity in Social Work Practice*, Learning Matters.

Lindon, J. (2012) *Equality and Inclusion in Early Childhood*, 2nd edition, Linking Theory and Practice, Hodder.

Moonie, N. *et al.* (2007) *Core Themes – Health and Social Care*, Heinemann.

Thompson, N. (2012) *Anti-Discriminatory Practice: Equality, Diversity and Social Justice* (Practical Social Work Series), Palgrave Macmillan.

Unit 2: Assessment practice

Below are practice questions for you to try.

Read the following job advertisement for a family support worker.

> **Checkleigh House Children's Centre**
>
> **Family Support Worker**
>
> **Job description:**
>
> To provide support and advice to families tailored to their individual needs, within the Children's Centre and through home visits.
>
> You will work as a part of the team delivering family support services in this ethnically diverse area.
>
> **To apply you should be:**
>
> - Level 3 qualified or equivalent
> - able to speak Urdu
> - clean shaven (male applicants)
> - over 18 years old

1 Which one of the following requirements in the job advertisement is an example of indirect racial discrimination. Choose **one** only: (1)
   a applicants must be Level 3 qualified or equivalent
   b applicants must be able to speak Urdu
   c male applicants must be clean shaven
   d applicants must be over 18 years old.
2 Explain the reasons for your answer to question 1. (4)
3 a Identify a piece of legislation that could be used to challenge indirect racial discrimination. (1)
   b Outline key aspects of the legislation you have named. (5)
4 In a recent Care Quality Commission inspection report, the staff at Checkleigh Residential Care Home were criticised for not valuing the diversity of their residents.
   Evaluate ways the management could ensure that the diversity of their residents is valued. (10)
5 Identify two early years values of care. Give an example for each of how a nursery nurse could apply them in their day-to-day work with the children. (4)

Total marks: 25

Unit 03

Health, safety and security in health and social care

ABOUT THIS UNIT

Promoting wellbeing and ensuring safe and secure environments in the health, social care and child care sectors is essential not only for individuals who require care and support but also for all those who are involved in their lives, such as their visitors, advocates, families, friends, professionals and managers. Creating settings that provide protection from danger, risk or injury and promote a sense of safety, free from danger, threat or fear is central to delivering high-quality, safe and effective care and support.

In this unit you will learn about the different types of hazards in health, social care and child care settings as well as their potential impact on others. You will also find out about the key legislation and organisational policies and procedures that promote health, safety and security as well as the roles and responsibilities of employers, employees and individuals who require care and support to comply with these. Knowing how to respond to different incidents and emergencies will help you to further develop your understanding of the procedures to follow in health, social care and child care settings.

LEARNING OUTCOMES

The topics, activities and suggested reading in this unit will help you to:

1 Understand potential hazards in health, social care and child care environments
2 Understand how legislation, policies and procedures promote health, safety and security in health, social care and child care environments
3 Understand the roles and responsibilities involved in health, safety and security in health, social care and child care environments
4 Know how to respond to incidents and emergencies in a health, social care or child care environment

How will I be assessed?

You will be assessed through an external assessment set and marked by OCR.

LO1 Understand potential hazards in health, social care and child care environments

GETTING STARTED

Hazards (10 minutes)

Look around you and see how many potential hazards are in the room. Share with a partner and discuss why you think these may be hazards.

1.1 Types of hazards

Health, social care and child care settings can be sources of potential **hazards** that, if ignored or not minimised, could cause ll-health and harm to the people who live, visit and work in them as well as damage to the environment These are environments where accidents can happen due to the frailty of individuals, which can make them more susceptible to falls and to acquiring infections.

> 🔑 **KEY TERMS**
>
> **Hazard** – a potential source of harm or adverse health effect.
>
> **Dementia** – a condition that is caused when the brain is damaged by diseases such as Alzheimer's or a stroke.

Table 3.1 outlines types of hazards that may occur in health, social care and child care environments.

Table 3.1 Types of hazards that may be found in care settings

Type of hazards in health, social care and child care environments	Examples
Environmental hazards, such as crowded areas and wet floors that can cause slip and trip hazards in settings' surroundings	• Worn vinyl flooring in the shower room in a hospital • A wet bathroom floor in a residential care home • Frayed carpet in the hallway entrance of a children's centre
Biological hazards, such as waste and body fluids that can cause the spread of infections and affect people's health	• A used bandage left on a bed in a clinic • Soiled laundry left on the floor in a bathroom of a nursing home • Vomit on the floor of a children's play area that has not been cleared up
Chemical hazards, such as cleaning agents and medication that can cause harm if not used and stored correctly	• An unlocked medicine trolley on a hospital ward • An unlabelled cleaning fluid in the cupboard of an individual's home • Hot cooking oil left unattended in the kitchen of an after-school club
Psychological hazards, such as stress and violence that can affect people's physical and emotional wellbeing	• Stress caused by people in a dentist's waiting room behaving in a challenging way • Tiredness caused by a high workload due to staff absence in a supported living scheme • Stress caused by children not wanting to participate in the activities that have been planned for them
Working conditions, such as poor lighting and environments that are too hot or too cold that can cause harm and ill-health	• Noise and disruption to the reception area of an opticians due to maintenance works • A senior homecare worker that travels long distances in between individuals' homes • A child's bedroom that is very cold and has poor lighting
Working practices that are unsafe, such as lack of fire training or long working hours that can cause injuries, fatalities and illnesses.	• Long working hours due to staff absence on a mental health community unit • Lack of supervision for new volunteers working in a support group for adults who have **dementia** • Lack of training for staff in a children's residential home on the procedures to follow when a faulty hoist is identified
Lack of security systems, such as window locks and alarm systems that can cause security and fire risks	• Faulty smoke alarm systems in a clinic • A broken security chain on an individual's front door • Lack of interlocking doors in a school

Hazard finding (45 minutes)

Work in small groups to find as many examples of types of potential hazards that you can see in the classroom. Award 2 points for each different type of hazard and 1 point for each example of a hazard that has been identified. Record and present your findings to the other groups.

1.2 Potential impacts of hazards for individuals who require care or support, employees and employers

Hazards can impact on the individuals who require care and support as well as on the employees and employers in health, social care and child care settings.

Injury or harm

Individuals who require care and support may be harmed if environmental hazards have not been identified. For example, an individual attending an appointment at their local GP surgery may fall if uneven steps at the front entrance are not repaired. Similarly, a support worker providing support to an individual in their own home may be prone to injuries or harm if the large and heavy items on top of the individual's wardrobe are not moved to a safer location.

Chemical hazards can cause injuries and harm to both individuals who require care and support and employees of organisations. For example, not using cleaning agents in line with the manufacturer's instructions by not wearing protective equipment such as aprons and gloves may lead to employees sustaining skin rashes and burns. Not storing medicines securely in a locked room and/or cupboard may lead to children swallowing them mistakenly thinking that they are sweets or them being accessed by unauthorised employees.

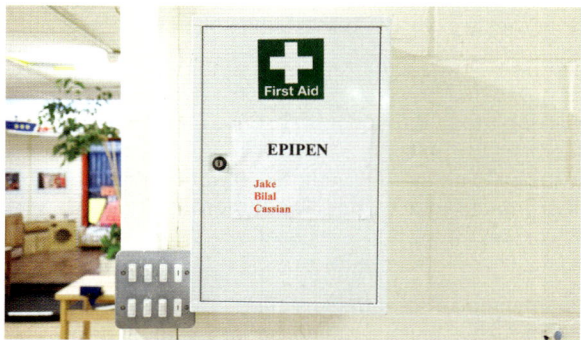

▲ **Figure 3.1** Safety is paramount

Illness

Biological and psychological hazards, if not identified and managed, can cause life-threatening and long-term illnesses. For example, used dressings need to be safely disposed of, dirty laundry needs to be washed separately and body fluid spillages need to be cleaned quickly using the correct protective equipment and cleaning agents. Not doing so may lead to the spread of infections and ultimately serious illnesses like **Clostridium difficile** that can prove fatal.

Psychological hazards, such as stress and tiredness, have the potential to impact on everyone. Employees will be more likely to make mistakes when carrying out their day-to-day working practices if they are tired and their interactions with others may also become strained if they are stressed. As a result, individuals who require care and support may receive a poor or even unsafe level of care. Biological and psychological hazards can also impact on employers, who may incur unplanned costs, in terms of having to recruit and train additional staff as a result of employees' absences from work due to stress and fatigue.

Poor standards of care

Unsafe working conditions and working practices can result in hazards not being identified, reduced or removed, which can impact directly on the standards and quality of care and support being provided. For example, a lack of properly maintained handwashing facilities can result in employees not maintaining a good level of personal hygiene which in turn can lead to the spread of infections like **Methicillin-resistant Staphylococcus aureus (MRSA)**. The buildings of health, social care and child care settings must also be properly maintained; water tanks and pipework, for example, must undergo regular checks to prevent the growth of **Legionella bacteria** that can cause serious diseases.

Poor working practices can also impact on the standards of care and support. For example, a lack of regular supervision for all employees can lead to poor communication within the team and with the individuals who require care and support, which can in turn cause conflicts and misunderstandings, employees and employers not being able to work in partnership and experiencing higher levels of stress. Similarly, if employees do not follow the organisation's health and safety procedure for reporting hazards such as slip and trip hazards or unsafe working practices, then this may cause injuries and harm to others; all of which could have been preventable.

Financial loss

Hazards can also have a devastating effect on employers and organisations as a whole. A lack of effective security systems, for example, may result in theft of personal belongings and damage to property. When a hazard results in an injury or fatality of an employee, the employee or their family may bring a lawsuit against the organisation which may result in the organisation having to pay for costs in relation to court fees and compensation. The organisation may also be subject to fines from regulatory agencies such as the **Health and Safety Executive (HSE)**. Lawsuits and fines can also damage the reputation of the organisation and future business may suffer as a result.

🔑 KEY TERMS

Clostridium difficile – a bacterium infectious agent that causes infections in the digestive system. It is also referred to as *C. difficile* or *C. diff.*

Methicillin-resistant *Staphylococcus aureus* (MRSA) – a bacterium infectious agent that causes infections in different parts of the body where the risk of it occurring is higher in people with open wounds, invasive devices and weakened immune systems.

Legionella bacteria – a type of bacteria that causes diseases such as Legionnaire's disease that affect the lungs.

Health and Safety Executive (HSE) – the national independent regulator or official supervisory body for the health safety and welfare of people in work settings in the UK.

1.3 Harm and abuse

Anyone in health social care and child care settings can be vulnerable to harm and abuse. Individuals who require care and support may be vulnerable to harm and abuse from a paid worker, manager or owner of a setting, from a family member, a friend or visitor and even from other individuals who access the same setting. Harm and abuse can also be carried out by individuals who require care and support who may be verbally or physically aggressive towards others. You will explore the topic of abuse and the different types of abuse that exist in more detail in Unit 7: Safeguarding.

Intentional abuse

Harm and abuse towards others can be deliberate. For example, a senior care assistant who supports an individual requiring care and support with their shopping and buys items for themselves with the individual's money is deliberately abusing that individual financially. An individual who is upset that their senior health worker has advised them to not smoke following their recent operation and hits them is deliberately abusing the worker physically. A child care worker who neglects the safety and comfort of a child in their care by not ensuring that the child eats or wears warm clothes when playing outside is deliberately abusing that child by neglecting their needs.

Unintentional abuse

Harm and abuse towards others can also be unintentional, through poor care. For example, a senior care worker who supports an older individual to move position in bed in a careless manner is unintentionally physically abusing that individual. An individual who has dementia and is anxious about visiting their GP and shouts out at all the individuals and staff in the immediate area is unintentionally abusing them. A play group volunteer who forgets to ask the children to wash their hands after using the toilet is unintentionally neglecting the children and putting them in danger of illnesses and infections.

Effects of abuse

Irrespective of whether harm and abuse is intentional or unintentional, it can have far reaching effects on the health and wellbeing of both individuals who require care and support and employees in health, social care and child care settings. Short-term effects can include:

- bruises, cuts and broken bones
- contracting a sexually transmitted infection (STI)
- low self-esteem
- poor self-image
- displaying challenging or needy behaviour
- feeling angry, anxious or tearful.

Long-term effects can include:

- low self-esteem
- feeling angry, anxious or tearful
- developing mental health issues, such as depression, self-harm and suicidal behaviour

- inability to sleep
- developing physical health conditions such as **hypertension**, anorexia and obesity
- difficulties with trusting others, forming relationships and friendships
- difficulties with addictions such as alcohol and drugs.

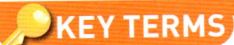

1.4 Types of settings

Hazards are everywhere and some types of settings may be more likely to contain hazards that are specific to the activities that take place in these and the people that use them. See Table 3.2.

Table 3.2 Potential hazards in different settings

Setting	Example	Potential risks
Health care environments	Intensive care unit in a hospital, a clinic, GP surgery or dentist	Health professionals carry out tasks such as surgical procedures that involve contact with body fluids that can contain pathogens and carry infectious diseases. Tasks that involve coming into contact with hazardous chemicals can lead to accidental spillages. Stress can be experienced by those who work in these types of environments.
Care environments	An individual's home, a residential care home or a nursing home	Vulnerable residents (those that are frail and or ill) may have vulnerable **immune systems** that can be damaged by illnesses such as leukaemia and therefore can make them more susceptible to infections. Individuals living in care environments may also have additional visual and/or mobility impairments that may mean that they are more susceptible to having falls.
Child care environments	Crèches or schools	Children's immune systems are immature and therefore are more susceptible to infections. Children may also not recognise potential hazards such as sharing toys that have been put in other children's mouths, choking on food, picking up food that has dropped on the floor, not washing hands after high risk activities such as coughing, sneezing and using the toilet.
Public environments	Shopping centres, parks, cinemas: places where large crowds of people gather	Slips, trips and falls. Food poisoning from food outlets. Harm and injuries can also occur from people that may be abusive or violent.
Transport	Centre minibus, ambulances	Slips and trips while getting on and off the minibus. Wheelchairs not secured properly. Faulty seatbelts may cause accidents. Individuals travelling in ambulances may experience sudden ill-health that requires first aid. Body fluids from medical equipment could lead to the spread of infections.

THINK ABOUT IT

Case study: Lions After-school Club

Lions After-school Club is registered for a maximum of 20 children, aged 5–11, at any given time and opens from 3.15 to 6.00 p.m. Monday to Friday.

Marie, the Club Leader, has come in to work even though she had been feeling unwell the night before, as she did not want to let the children or her colleagues down. As Marie is not feeling well, a new member of staff has offered to carry out the safety checks both indoors and outdoors; although she has not been trained to do so, she is confident that she is able to as she has observed Marie carry them out.

During the cooking activity in the afternoon, one of the electric cooker rings did not appear to be working. Marie and her colleague decided to use one of the other rings instead so that they could continue with the cooking activity as planned. All the children were supervised at all times while in the kitchen apart from when two of the children wanted to use the toilet.

Ten minutes before the out of school club closed one of the children spilt their drink on the floor. As it had been a long and busy afternoon the team decided to do the cleaning and tidying up the following day.

Analyse the potential hazards. Present your findings to the manager of the after-school club in the form of a report.

KNOW IT

1 Define the term hazard.
2 Identify two examples of chemical hazards.
3 What are the effects of poor working conditions?
4 What are the long-term effects of abuse?
5 What potential hazards may there be in a public environment?

LO2 Understand how legislation, policies and procedures promote health, safety and security in health, social care and child care environments

GETTING STARTED

Health and safety law (10 minutes)

In small groups, think about the importance of health and safety law. What could happen without it?

2.1 Legislation

Legislation is in place to ensure that everyone's health, safety and security is safeguarded. This includes all those who live in, work in and visit health, social care and child care settings. Table 3.3 provides you with additional information about the key pieces of relevant legislation.

Table 3.3 Key legislation promoting health, safety and security in care settings

Legislation	How it promotes health, safety and security in health, social care and child care settings
Health and Safety at Work Act (HASAWA) 1974	• An important Act that is the basis for other health and safety regulations and guidelines. • It established the Health & Safety Executive (HSE) as the **regulator** for the health, safety and welfare of people in work settings in the UK. • It established the key duties and responsibilities of all employers and employees in work settings.
Management of Health and Safety at Work Regulations (MHSWR) 1999	• This Act places duties on employers to carry out and implement **risk assessments** of the health, safety and security of their employees and others who live and work in these settings. • It requires work settings to have arrangements in place including appointing competent people to manage health, safety and security as well as procedures for emergency situations that may arise. • It requires employers to provide information, training and supervision so that work activities can be carried out safely.
Food Safety Act 1990	• This Act requires that good personal hygiene is maintained when working with food so that it is safe to eat. • It requires that records are kept of where food is from so that it can be traced if needed. • It requires that any food that is unsafe is removed and an incident report completed.

Legislation	How it promotes health, safety and security in health, social care and child care settings
Food Safety (General Food Hygiene) Regulations 1995 (amended 1999 and 2004)	• This Act requires that food safety hazards are identified. • It requires that food safety controls are in place, maintained and reviewed. • It requires that environments where food is prepared or cooked are kept clean and in good condition. • Raw meat and ready-to-eat products must be prepared on separate chopping boards to prevent cross-contamination.
Manual Handling Operations Regulations 1992	• This Act requires that employers avoid hazardous **manual handling** tasks where possible and assess those that cannot be avoided. • It requires that employers eliminate or reduce the risks associated with manual handling tasks. • It requires employers to provide information, training and supervision about safe moving and handling.
Reporting of Injuries, Diseases and Dangerous Occurrences Regulations (RIDDOR) 2013	• This Act requires employers to report and keep records for three years of work-related accidents that cause death and serious injuries (referred to as reportable injuries), diseases and dangerous occurrences (i.e. incidents with the potential to cause harm). • It requires work settings to have procedures in place for reporting injuries, diseases and incidents. • It requires employers to provide information and training on reporting injuries, diseases and incidents.
Data Protection Act 1998	• The main Act that protects the security of personal information. • It requires that information is accurate and up to date. • It requires that information is kept secure.
Control of Substances Hazardous to Health Regulations (COSHH) 2002	• This Act requires employers to carry out a risk assessment to prevent or control exposure to hazardous substances. • It requires employers to have procedures in place for safe working with hazardous substances. • It requires employers to provide information, training and supervision so that work activities can be carried out safely.
Civil Contingencies Act 2004	• This Act sets out how organisations must work together to plan and respond to local and national emergencies. • It establishes how organisations, such as emergency services, local authorities and health bodies, can work together and share information. • It requires that risk assessments are undertaken and emergency plans are put in place.
The Health and Social Care (Safety and Quality) Act 2015	• This Act sets out how health and adult social care providers must share information about a person's care with other health and care professionals so that safe and effective care can be provided. • It requires health and adult social care organisations to use a consistent **identifier** (the NHS number) when sharing information about a person's care • It reduces the risk of harm and abuse by making provision for removing people convicted of certain offences from the registers kept by the regulatory bodies for health and social care professions.

> ## 🔑 KEY TERMS
>
> **Manual handling** – the transporting or supporting of a person or object by hand or bodily force.
>
> **Identifier** – a tool that is used to match people to their records, e.g. to their health records.

2.2 Safeguarding

Safeguarding adults and children from harm and abuse is everyone's responsibility. The actions taken by professionals can help to ensure safe and effective care; this includes acting on any concerns they may have as quickly as possible. For example:

'Safeguarding referrals were opened for 104,050 individuals during the 2013-14 reporting year. 60 per cent of these individuals were female and 63 per cent were aged 65 or over. Just over half (51 per cent) of the individuals had a physical disability, frailty or sensory impairment.'

(Source: HSCIC, Safeguarding Adults Return, Annual Report, England 2013–14, Experimental Statistics, October 2014)

'In 2013–14 over 650,000 children in England were referred to local authority children's social care services by individuals who had concerns about their welfare.'

(Source: Working Together to Safeguard Children: A Guide to Inter-agency Working to Safeguard and Promote the Welfare of Children, March 2015)

The need for safeguarding

In April 2015 the Care Act 2014 established a new statutory framework for care and support, including adult safeguarding. Safeguarding adults is needed to ensure that individuals' rights to live free from abuse and neglect are protected and that working in partnership to prevent the risk of abuse or neglect takes place. Safeguarding is also needed for children. Safeguarding is defined in Working Together to Safeguard Children 2015 (a revised and updated version of the government's 2013 guidance) as necessary for:

● protecting children from maltreatment
● preventing impairment of children's health and development
● ensuring that children grow up in circumstances consistent with the provision of safe and effective care
● taking action to enable all children to have the best outcomes.

(Source: Working Together to Safeguard Children: A Guide to Inter-agency Working to Safeguard and Promote the Welfare of Children, March 2015)

You will explore this topic in more detail in Unit 7: Safeguarding (page 133).

Disclosure and Barring Service (DBS)

The Disclosure and Barring Service works closely with the police and helps to safeguard both adults and children from harm and abuse by preventing unsuitable people from working with vulnerable adults and children by:

● processing requests for criminal records checks by searching police records and **barred list** information
● deciding whether it is appropriate for a person to be placed on or removed from a barred list
● placing people on the DBS children's barred list and adults' barred list for England, Wales and Northern Ireland.

> 🔑 **KEY TERM**
>
> **Barred list** – a list of individuals held by the DBS who are unsuitable for working with children and/or adults.

Disclosure and Barring Service checks

An employer can request a DBS check for roles that may involve working or volunteering in health, social care and child care settings or when, for example, someone is applying to foster or adopt a child. DBS applicants must be aged 16 or over and it can take up to 8 weeks to have a DBS check completed. Figure 3.2 details the process to follow.

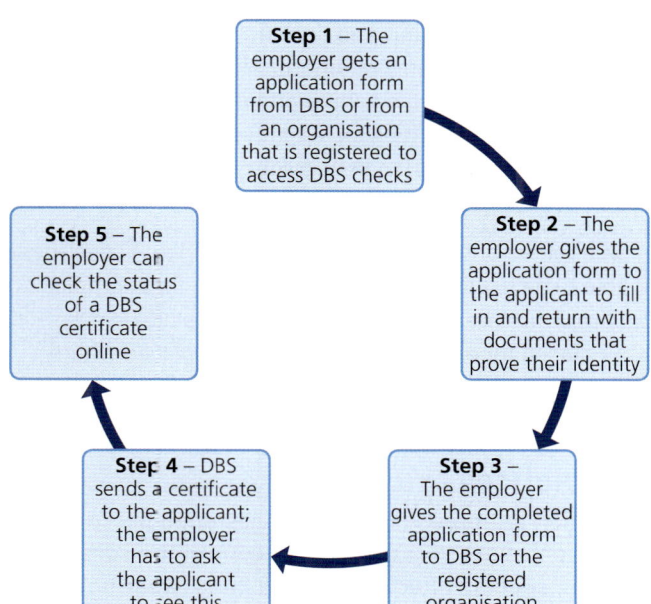

▲ **Figure 3.2** The DBS check process

DBS checks do not have an expiry date; they can be updated and checked as and when required by employers. There are three types of DBS checks.

1 Standard – this checks for spent and unspent convictions, cautions, reprimands and final warnings.
2 Enhanced – this includes the same as the standard check as well as any additional information held by local police that's considered relevant to the role being applied for.
3 Enhanced with list checks – this includes the same as the enhanced check as well as a check of the DBS barred lists.

2.3 Influences of legislation

On staff

Health, safety and security legislation promotes safe staffing levels as well as the provision of effective supervision, instruction and training of staff. Having safe staffing levels and correct staff-to-client ratios, with staff who have suitable levels of awareness, knowledge and skills, is essential for promoting wellbeing as well as safe and secure environments and working practices.

Legislation also gives staff a role in implementing and making changes to health, safety and security arrangements in these work settings.

On premises

Legislation also has a direct impact on how health, social care and child care premises are maintained in terms of ensuring that they are kept clean (for infection prevention and control) and in good condition (for security). Suitable and sufficient ventilation and lighting will ensure that employees work in safe conditions. Handwashing facilities, materials for cleaning and drying hands as well as changing facilities for employees that are kept in good condition must also be provided to ensure staff can maintain good levels of personal hygiene.

Escape routes and exits must also be provided. These must be able to be used at all times by ensuring, for example, that fire doors are not wedged open or exits blocked by items placed there. Signs must also be displayed where necessary to help people identify escape routes and find equipment such as fire alarms and extinguishers.

On practices

Legislation promotes and encourages good personal hygiene practices that can help to control the spread of infection, such as effective handwashing, wearing clean clothes, wearing protective equipment such as aprons and gloves when carrying out activities that may involve coming into contact with individuals' body fluids, as well as safe removal and storage of waste.

Recording and storing information correctly and securely is also encouraged through legislation requiring the development of workplace processes for reporting and recording accidents, illnesses and incidents.

2.4 Implementation of policies and procedures

As you have read in LO2.1, the health, safety and security legislation that exists requires employers to have in place policies and procedures that explain how people's health, safety and welfare will be safeguarded in their work setting. As all work settings are different, in terms of the nature of tasks carried out, specific job roles and the needs of individuals who require care and support, these policies and procedures will vary in terms of how they are implemented.

Table 3.4 is an extract from a senior support worker's completed task checklists for each of the three settings he works in: a mental health unit, an individual's home and a children's residential home. Note in particular how the policies and procedures in place are implemented in different ways.

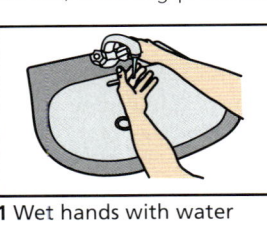

1 Wet hands with water

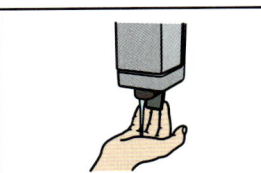

2 Apply enough soap to cover all hand surfaces

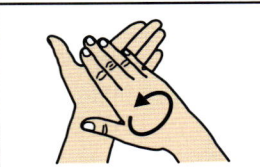

3 Rub hands palm to palm

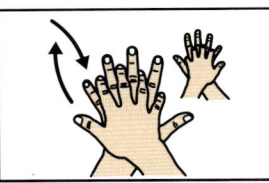

4 Right palm over back of left hand with interlaced fingers and vice versa

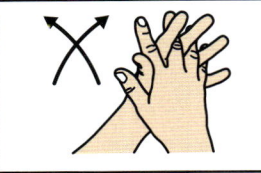

5 Palm to palm with fingers interlaced

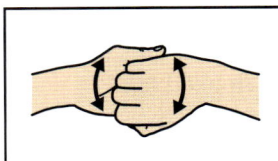

6 Backs of fingers to opposing palms with fingers interlocked

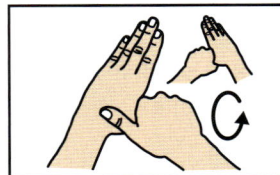

7 Rotational rubbing of left thumb clasped in right palm and vice versa

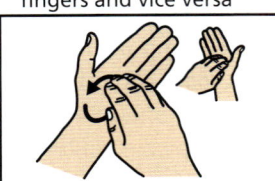

8 Rotational rubbing, backwards and forwards with clasped fingers of right hand in left palm and vice versa

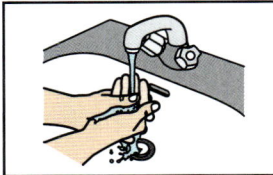

9 Rinse hands with water

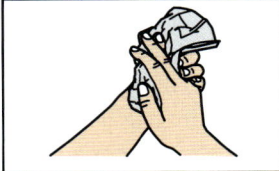

10 Dry hands thoroughly with a single-use towel

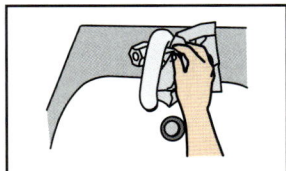

11 Use towel to turn off tap

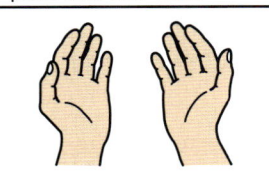

12 Your hands are now safe

▲ **Figure 3.3** The correct handwashing technique (Source: NHS)

Table 3.4 Bartosz's task checklist. An example of how to implement policies and procedures to promote health, safety and security

Policies and procedures	Birch Mental Health Unit	Shamila's home	Marshes Children's Residential Home
Health and safety	Removed bed linen from Rooms 2 and 3; wore a disposable apron and gloves, disposed of these in linen room waste bag. Completed health and safety checks of outdoor patio area, fences, and bins. No sharp objects found; all areas safe.	Completed health and safety checks of the kitchen and bathroom with Shamila. Discussed option of replacing the high bathroom cabinet with a lower one that Shamila can access more easily. Shamila to discuss this with her key worker.	Completed a check of CF's bedroom with his consent. Home Manager present. Incident form completed.
Risk assessment	Completed an individual risk assessment with respect to one individual who wanted his electronic swipe-card programmed to leave the building; this was agreed with the individual and the Unit Manager as no risk was posed by this individual.	Completed a risk assessment of back garden; slippery steps and rubbish at the bottom of the garden identified as hazards. Shamila to arrange for removal of rubbish. Steps to be looked at by Risk Manager; report made today.	Completed a risk assessment for a trip out to the cinema next week. Placed risk assessment in file; to be discussed at staff meeting on Monday.
Fire evacuation	Checked that both fire exits could be opened immediately and easily and that escape routes were clear. Checked assembly point outside unit; fences and bins.	Checked front door and hallway were not obstructed as this is the only fire escape route.	Checked lighting, signs, fire exits and fire doors; all in effective working order.
Safeguarding	Unexpected visit by an individual's son was refused by Ward Manager; after discussion with the team and the individual's mental health today. Agreed for another visit to be booked in for the following month.	Checked with Shamila that she has not given her keys to M; Shamila confirmed that she hasn't although she has asked her for them again. Recorded this on the alert form and reported this to the office. Discussed with Shamila how she feels about the situation with M; she confirmed that she is happy that she has not continued to have a relationship with M.	Individual MP reported being left out of morning activity this morning by the rest of the group. Listened carefully, reassured MP and recorded in the complaint book. Home Manager and Social Worker also informed.
Reporting of accidents	Minor cut to my right thumb when closing filing cabinet in the office. Accident form completed and passed on to Unit Manager.	None to report; confirmed this with Shamila	None to report. Accident Book and forms re-located to main staff office for ease of access; in staff procedures cabinet.
Food safety	Checked temperatures of fridge and freezer on unit and in the staff office. Recorded on daily check sheet.	Reminded Shamila to empty the waste bin in the kitchen that was close to being full; Shamila agreed to empty this tonight.	Checked with Home Manager the expiry dates of the food left in the fridge over the weekend. Convenience foods left in fridge have been disposed of.
Cleaning	Used neutral detergent for routine cleaning of main coffee area. Disposed of disposable cloth, aprons and gloves in allocated waste bag.	None required. Shamila confirmed that she hoovered yesterday downstairs as per her cleaning rota.	Checked downstairs areas; all clean, hygienic and tidy. Bathroom clean checks completed.

Policies and procedures	Birch Mental Health Unit	Shamila's home	Marshes Children's Residential Home
Disposal of hazardous wastes	Checked waste bags on unit emptied all three as all were 3/4 full. Reported to Unit Manager that more bags needed to be ordered. Checked sharps bins is only 1/3 full and not up to manufacturer's fill line.	Reminded Shamila to return the part-used antibiotics to her local chemist; Shamila confirmed that she will do this on Tuesday morning when she goes shopping with her support worker.	Small spill of saliva on floor by entrance to lounge; cleaned immediately with neutral detergent and hot water. Apron and gloves worn.
Lone working	Chaperoned one individual who left the unit at lunchtime to meet with a friend after completing risk assessment.	Signed and dated task sheet and Shamila countersigned. Phoned office before and after my visit to confirm time of arrival and departure.	Risk assessment completed and agreed with Home Manager to work with individual CS on my own this morning. No risks identified.
Storage and dispensing of medicines	Assisted Ward Manager in stock rotation of medicines and expiry dates checks.	No support required; Shamila continues to self-medicate.	Medication received at the home today was stored in the locked cabinet; completed form to indicate this, signed and dated it, in presence of Home Manager. Individual CF requested aspirin this morning for a headache. Aspirin not administered as per Home's procedure; referred request to Home Manager who met with CF.
Security of premises, possessions and individuals	**Protected time** completed between 2 and 4 p.m.; this worked well, all 4 individuals were engaged in one-to-one activities.	Reminded Shamila to close the downstairs bathroom window at nights as it was open upon arrival this morning; discussed security of house with Shamila.	Windows and door locks checked both upstairs and downstairs. Access and exit routes to and from the building checked.

KEY TERMS

Policies – clear statements of intent of how an organisation intends to conduct its services.

Procedures – the way in which the service or organisation expects its employees to put its policies into action.

Protected time – a period of time where staff spend one-to-one time with individuals.

2.5 Review of policies and procedures

Policies and **procedures** must be reviewed regularly to ensure that they reflect any changes that are made to legislation, an organisation's needs and aims, individuals' existing needs or the development of a new need. It is good practice to date and number policies and procedures once they are reviewed and updated; in addition there should be a system in place for regularly reviewing these, including planned review dates and how any changes will be communicated. This allows the updated versions to be easily accessible.

Policies and procedures will only be effective if they contain up-to-date information and reflect safe working practices that staff can follow and comply with. Not complying with these can have serious consequences for employees, employers and organisations. Employees may be asked to attend further training, closer monitoring and/or supervision of their activities or face disciplinary action. Employers may be liable to imprisonment and organisations may be liable to fines and closure

INDEPENDENT ACTIVITY

Policies and procedures (50 minutes)

Conduct some independent research in your local area on health and safety policies and procedures used in two different health, social care or child care settings. Think about the differences that exist between these as well as the consequences of not complying with them.

LO3 Understand the roles and responsibilities involved in health, safety and security in health, social care and child care environments

3.1 Roles

Employers

As you will have read in Section 2.1, key pieces of health, safety and security legislation such as the Health and Safety at Work Act (HASAWA) 1974 set out roles and responsibilities for employers and employees as well as others, such as individuals who require care and support. Figure 3.4 provides additional information about some of the key aspects of the roles or functions of specific employers in relation to promoting health, safety and security in health, social care and child care settings.

Employees

Legislation also requires that employees work together with their employers with respect to maintaining health, safety and security in health, social care and child care environments. Employees' roles include:

- maintaining their own and others' health, safety and security
- following employers' guidance and instruction
- attending health and safety training
- using equipment provided for health and safety purposes i.e. aprons, gloves
- reporting hazards observed in the work setting.

Individuals who require care and support

As you know, health and safety is everyone's responsibility so individuals who require care and support should be involved in maintaining safe, healthy and secure environments. They should follow health and safety guidance and instructions such as what to do in an emergency. They should comply with health and safety procedures such as those in relation to moving and handling and food safety, for example. They should also observe health and safety signs, such as those in relation to escape routes, those that indicate when cleaning is in progress and those indicating no smoking.

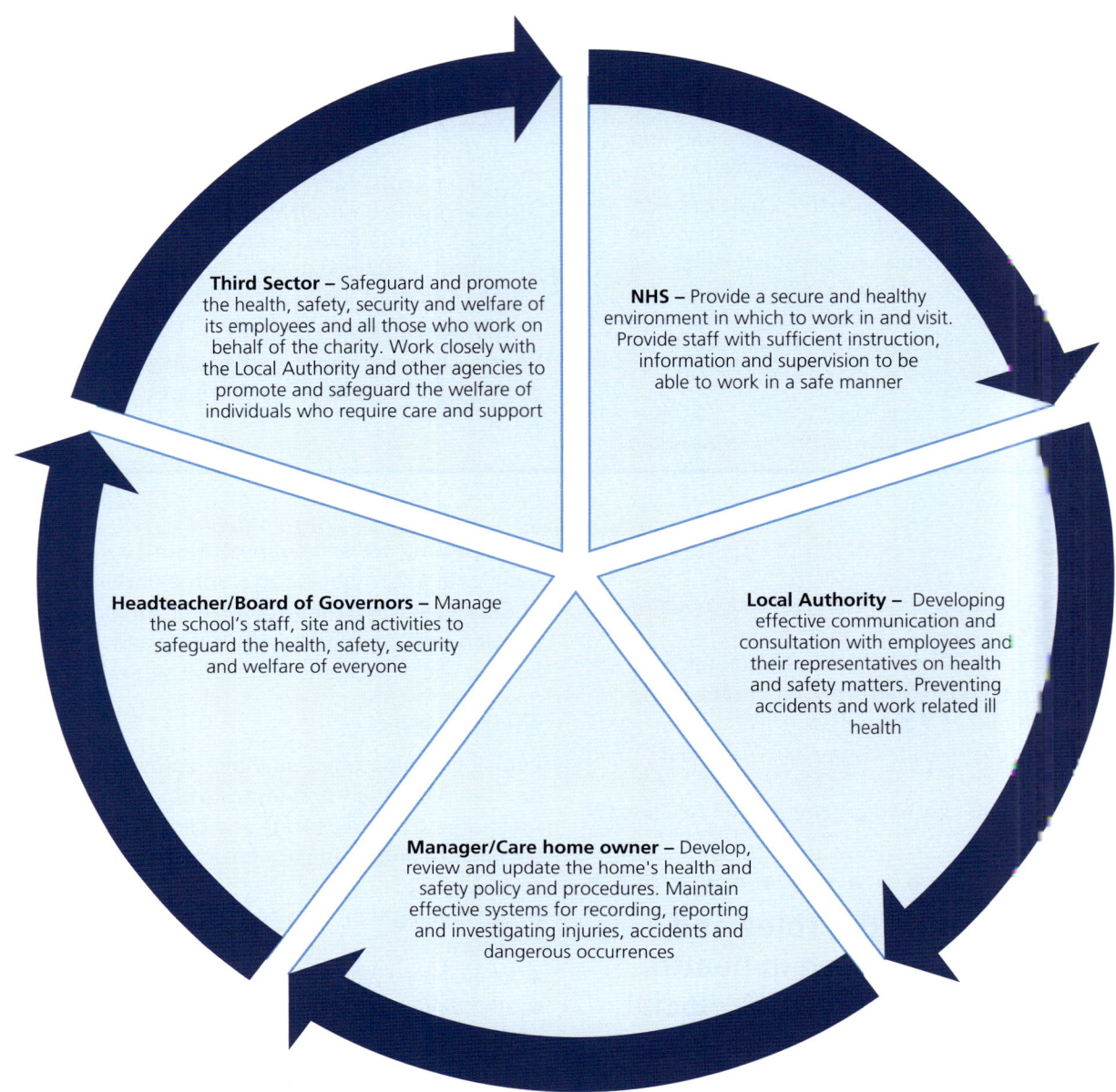

Third Sector – Safeguard and promote the health, safety, security and welfare of its employees and all those who work on behalf of the charity. Work closely with the Local Authority and other agencies to promote and safeguard the welfare of individuals who require care and support

NHS – Provide a secure and healthy environment in which to work in and visit. Provide staff with sufficient instruction, information and supervision to be able to work in a safe manner

Headteacher/Board of Governors – Manage the school's staff, site and activities to safeguard the health, safety, security and welfare of everyone

Local Authority – Developing effective communication and consultation with employees and their representatives on health and safety matters. Preventing accidents and work related ill health

Manager/Care home owner – Develop, review and update the home's health and safety policy and procedures. Maintain effective systems for recording, reporting and investigating injuries, accidents and dangerous occurrences

▲ **Figure 3.4** Employers' roles in ensuring health, safety and security

3.2 Responsibilities

Employers, employees and individuals are also responsible for carrying out day-to-day tasks to comply with legislation and organisational policies and procedures. The health and safety procedure extract in Table 3.5 is for Women Now, a small, local charity that provides support to young women with physical disabilities. Note how these responsibilities differ for the employer, the employees and the individuals who access the charity's services.

Table 3.5 Examples of how the employer, staff and individuals can fulfil their responsibilities for health, safety and security

Chief executive's responsibilities (employer)	Staff and volunteers' responsibilities (employees)	Members' responsibilities (young women who have physical disabilities)
Develop, maintain and review the charity's health and safety policy and procedures.	• Read through the charity's health and safety policies and procedures. • Sign and date the procedures, once read and understood. • Ask questions if information contained within these procedures is unclear.	Read through the members' welcome pack that includes the charity's health and safety policy and procedure.
Develop and deliver training and support on health and safety in line with the charity's training plan.	• Participate in **induction training** and **mandatory training**. • Attend additional training as requested by supervisor. • Attend supervisions and support groups for staff and volunteers.	Attend members' bi-monthly **briefings** on health and safety.
Conduct, review and update the organisational risk assessment for the charity's activities. Manage the charity's individual risk assessments for its staff, volunteers and members.	• Identify, review and record potential and actual health and safety risks. • Suggest options for eliminating and reducing risks identified. • Promote health and safety practices.	Co-operate with staff and volunteers who carry out risk assessments.

PAIRS ACTIVITY

Roles and responsibilities (10 minutes)

In pairs, work out the difference between a role and a responsibility and then provide a definition of each.

3.3 Consequences of not meeting responsibilities

Failing to meet legal and organisational health and safety responsibilities can have drastic consequences for employers, employees, individuals who require care and support as well as others who may visit health, social care and child care settings.

Disciplinary action

Employers can bring about formal disciplinary procedures, which may include a first written warning, a final written warning and dismissal. Before entering into any disciplinary action, the employer will carry out an investigation to establish all the relevant information and facts; during this period the employer may decide to suspend the employee who is being accused of misconduct.

If, after the investigation, the employer decides that there has been no misconduct, the employee will be asked to return to work and will resume their day-to-day duties and responsibilities. If the employer decides that there is a case, they will notify the employee in writing of the alleged misconduct as well as the time and venue of a disciplinary meeting. Any evidence related to the case, such as witness statements, may also be made available to the employee prior to the meeting as well as their right to be accompanied by a representative.

Criminal prosecution

Under the Health and Safety (Offences) Act 2008, the conviction of a director or other employee of failing to take reasonable care for the health and safety of themselves and others can result in either imprisonment for up to a two-year period or an unlimited fine.

The Health and Safety at Work Act (HASAWA) 1974 states that if a director or senior manager personally commits an offence and their actions are deemed grossly negligent and can cause a person's death, then a charge of gross negligence manslaughter could be brought.

The Corporate Manslaughter and Corporate Homicide Act 2007 states that a corporate manslaughter offence can be committed by an organisation. The offence is committed if the way in which an organisation's activities are managed by senior management causes a person's death.

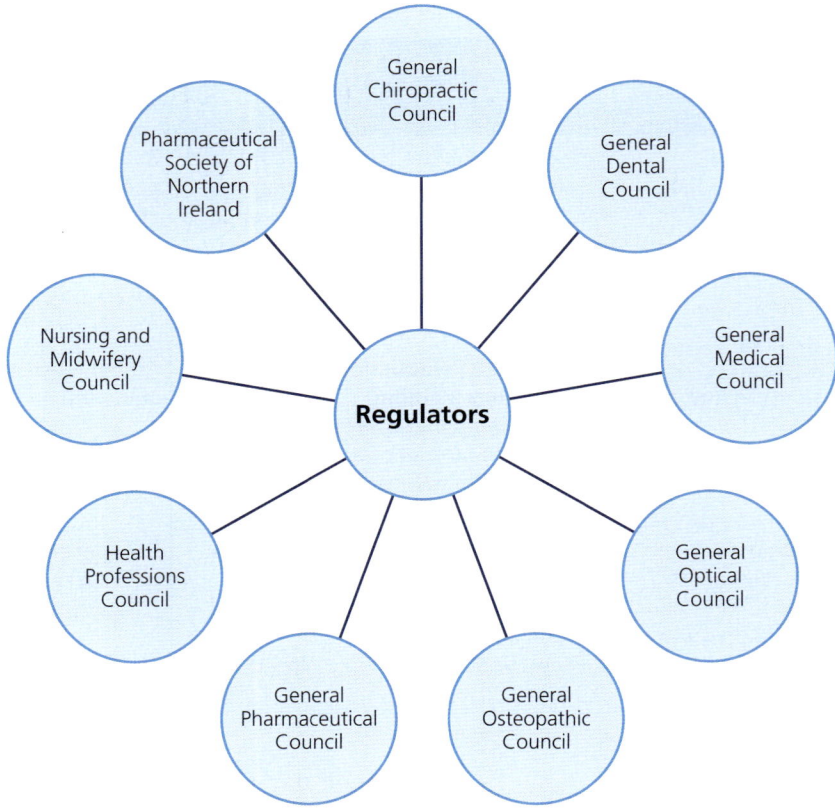

▲ **Figure 3.5** Health profession regulators

Fines imposed on individuals and organisations have ranged from hundreds of thousands to millions of pounds depending on whether there have been single or multiple fatalities.

Being removed from professional registers

Regulators of professions such as medicine and teaching hold registers of professionals because they have a duty to safeguard the public and ensure professionals provide high standards of care. For example, Figure 3.5 identifies the nine health profession regulators.

Professionals, such as nurses and midwives, must be registered to be able to practise in the UK; it is a criminal offence to practise without being registered. If a professional is not deemed fit to practise, for example due to poor health and safety, record-keeping or a failure to assess risks effectively, then the professional can be removed from the register or be suspended from the register for up to a period of two years or be subject to a 'conditions of practice' order which restricts their duties and responsibilities.

Causing injury or harm

Employers, employees and individuals who require care and support may cause injury or harm not only to themselves but to others too if they fail to carry out their responsibilities. Not having a clear procedure in place for carrying out risk assessments could mean that your employer cannot identify health and safety hazards.

Employees also have a responsibility to only carry out tasks that they are competent to do. If they are unsure about a task or have not received sufficient training they must inform their employer. Not doing so could lead to injury or harm to themselves, their colleagues or the individuals they provide care and support to.

Individuals are responsible for working with employers and employees in promoting their own and others' health, safety and welfare; not doing so may lead to putting themselves and others working in and visiting the setting in danger and could result in causing injuries or harm.

Being injured or harmed

A failure to meet health and safety responsibilities can lead to a range of injuries or harm, some minor, others more serious and some that could even result in fatalities.

Statistics available from the NHS Safety Thermometer, a measurement tool that records harms suffered by individuals (so that the safety of individuals can be improved) across a range of health care settings indicates that pressure ulcers and falls were two of the most common harms experienced by individuals that could be prevented through safe care. Between April 2014 and April 2015, out of a total of 2,716,837 patient assessments, 122,872 individuals were assessed for pressure sores and 18,497 for falls with harm.

(Source: HSCIC, NHS Safety Thermometer: Patient Harms and Harm Free Care England April 2014–April 2015, official statistics published 6 May 2015)

? THINK ABOUT IT

Case study: Kelly

Kelly is 12 years old and has learning disabilities. She receives weekly home visits from a community worker who provides both practical and emotional support to Kelly and her family. During her visit this morning, Kelly's mother explains that last night Kelly once again did not sleep throughout the night and kept on saying that she was thirsty and used the toilet more frequently than usual. The community worker records this information and advises her to make an appointment with Kelly's GP as soon as possible as these could be symptoms of an underlying condition. The community worker also noted that Kelly indicated several times that she had blurred vision and asked her mother to also pass this information on to the GP.

At the community worker's next home visit, Kelly's mother thanked her for her vigilance as she explained that the GP carried out a urine sample and a blood test which resulted in Kelly being diagnosed with Type I diabetes and receiving treatment for her condition.

Analyse the consequences if the community worker had not met her responsibilities.

KNOW IT

1 What is the role of the NHS with respect to health, safety and security?
2 What health, safety and security responsibilities do employees in child care settings have?
3 How can failing to meet health, safety and security responsibilities lead to criminal prosecution?

LO4 Know how to respond to incidents and emergencies in a health, social care or child care environment

GETTING STARTED 👤

Emergencies (10 minutes)

Think about an emergency in a health care or child care setting you have heard about. Where was it and what happened? Share with a partner.

4.1 Incidents and emergencies

Incidents and emergencies can occur unexpectedly in health, social care and child care settings.

Accidents

Accidents can be the result of poorly maintained areas, fittings or equipment. For example, a fractured limb can result from a slip on a wet bathroom floor, electrical injuries from faulty wiring or burns and scalds from hot water temperatures. Individuals in health, social care and child care settings may also be more susceptible to accidents due to their reduced abilities to mobilise and their lack of awareness of potential hazards. Poor working practices can also be the cause of accidents such as a slipped disc from positioning an individual on a bed without using safe moving and handling techniques.

Exposure to infections

Individuals in health, social care and child care settings may be more susceptible to bacterial infections such as gastroenteritis, MRSA, *C. difficile*, food poisoning and viral illnesses such as norovirus, chickenpox and influenza. Poor environmental conditions, such as inadequate ventilation and lack of running water, can create conditions where **pathogens** that cause infections can thrive. Poor working practices, such as inadequate cleaning of facilities and poor personal hygiene, can also encourage the growth and spread of pathogens.

Exposure to chemicals

Exposure to chemicals can occur if individuals are exposed to a **hazardous substance** when carrying out their day-to-day work tasks, such as when cleaning areas or **sterilising** equipment and aids. Hazardous substances are classified as very toxic, toxic, harmful, corrosive and irritant. Exposure to these can also occur unexpectedly if a spillage has occurred or safe practices as specified in the manufacturer's instructions for storing, handling and disposing of these have not been followed.

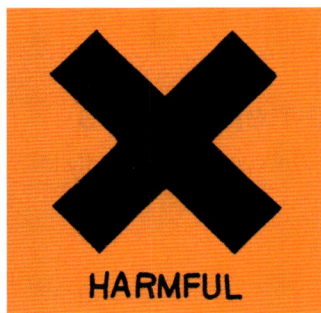
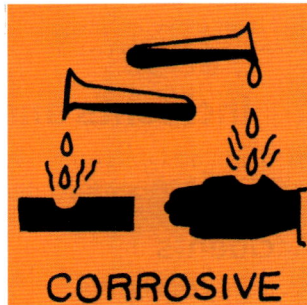
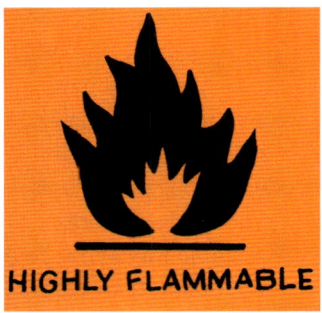
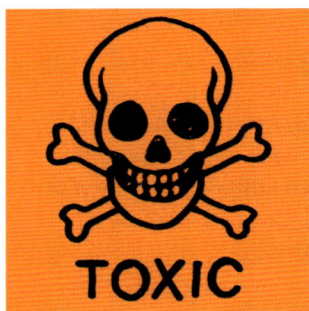

▲ **Figure 3.6** Hazard symbols

Spillages

Spillages of body fluids, such as blood, vomit, urine and faeces, can lead to outbreaks of infections and cause diseases if they are contaminated with pathogens. Spillages of waste and other hazardous substances also have the potential to have serious consequences for those who work, live in and visit health, social care and child care settings.

Intruders

When premises are poorly maintained there may be broken doors and/or inadequate window locks which could result in intruders entering the building. Intruders may also access premises due to poor working practices that fail to ensure that only those who are authorised have access. In order to protect the privacy of both electronic and paper-based information and records, guarding against intruders is essential. Intruders not only cause damage and loss but can also be the source of emotional upset and harm for those whose safety has been threatened.

Aggressive and dangerous encounters

Accidents can also result from aggressive and dangerous encounters, such as a bruised eye from an individual hitting out, a fall down the stairs by an individual who has abused alcohol or a bite to the arm from an aggressive individual who has abused drugs.

Fire

Fires can have devastating consequences for everyone. Fire safety in health, social care and child care settings includes knowing how to prevent fires from starting and spreading and is everyone's responsibility. Fires will only start if these components are present: oxygen (present in the air), fuel (solid, liquid or gas items that can burn) and heat (for example from heaters or a cigarette).

Floods

Floods in premises are usually caused by water escaping from an item inside the premises, such as a washing machine, bath, toilet, water tank or pipes. This can be due to the failure to carry out routine maintenance checks. This has the potential to cause long-term damage to the premises as well as raise the risk of the spread of diseases that can be carried in water.

Loss of water supply

A loss of water supply could indicate that there is a burst pipe somewhere in the premises or that there may be a leak in the mains system; again most commonly due to a failure of routine maintenance checks. This can have an impact on key care and support activities that involve cleaning, washing, cooking and drinking.

Other critical incidents

A faulty light switch or electrical appliance may cause the electricity to cut out; sometimes emergency power cuts also occur in the local area. A gas leak from faulty appliances and pipework can also lead to fires and explosions. A bomb threat should always be taken seriously.

💬 **CLASSROOM DISCUSSION**

(30 minutes)

Discuss the accidents and incidents that are most likely to take place in health, social care and child care settings. Share any personal experiences you have or news stories you have heard or read about that involve accidents and incidents that have occurred and have involved adults or children.

4.2 Responses to incidents and emergencies

Reporting of accidents

It is a legal requirement that records are kept of all accidents and incidents, including when an individual has refused treatment. The following information must also be recorded:

- the name of the person injured or taken ill
- the date, time and place of the accident/incident
- the details of the injury/illness
- the treatment given, including what happened to the injured/ill person afterwards.

All records must also be signed.

Evacuation procedures

Evacuation procedures and escape routes for emergencies such as fires, bomb scares and gas leaks will vary for different health, social care and child care settings; this is why it is important to familiarise yourself with these. Evacuation routes must be kept clear at all times, well lit and signposted where possible.

Below are some of the key actions to take when following evacuation procedures in the event of a fire, in the acronym **ACT FAST**.

- **A**ct fast, do not panic, sound the fire alarm.
- **C**ontrol and contain the fire only if you have been trained to do so and it is safe.
- **T**elephone the fire brigade and provide them with details about you, your location and the fire.
- **F**ollow your emergency procedure to ensure the safety of everyone.
- **A**ssist in ensuring everyone is in a place of safety, either inside or outside the building.
- **S**upport others to ensure that no one stops or returns for personal belongings.
- **T**ry to remain calm and wait until the fire brigade informs you that it is safe to re-enter the building.

Follow-up review of critical incidents and emergencies

Critical incidents and emergencies that cause death or serious injury usually occur suddenly and unexpectedly. Casualties, witnesses and those who respond to these will all be affected and so counselling and support services must be offered to everyone involved and their health and welfare monitored by employers on an ongoing basis as effects can be long lasting. Implementing actions and recommendations from the findings of reviews will also form part of the follow-up review process.

Report to relevant authorities

Depending on the nature of the incident or emergency, external agencies such as the Police, Fire and Social Services may also be involved in the reporting stage.

Employers have a responsibility to report suspected outbreaks of infection, changes in resistance to antibiotics and occurrences of notifiable diseases to the local health protection unit (HPU). The Reporting of Incidents, Diseases and Dangerous Occurrences (Amendment) Regulations (RIDDOR) 2013 require that certain work-related injuries, diseases and dangerous occurrences are reported to the HSE or local authority.

> **? THINK ABOUT IT**
>
> **Case study: Sabrina's home visit**
>
> Sabrina is an occupational therapist on a home visit to Stan who has recently been discharged from hospital following his recovery from a chest infection. Stan is upstairs in his bedroom and gives Sabrina access to his home using the door buzzer system. Upon entering the property, Sabrina calls out to Sam who asks her to come upstairs. As Sabrina closes the front door behind her she notices a faint smell of gas.
>
> 1 What actions should Sabrina take and why?
> 2 What are the consequences of Sabrina not taking any action?
> 3 What reporting requirements should Sabrina follow and why?

4.3 Responsibilities of a first aider

A trained and qualified first aider has many important responsibilities that include the 3 Ps.

- **P**reserving life by carrying out emergency first aid procedures that do not place anyone in any danger – this is why the first step should always be to assess for danger.
- **P**reventing deterioration by preventing further harm to the casualty or their condition worsening, e.g. by not moving the casualty's limb if it appears broken and by making the area safe from any further danger, for example by not allowing other people to enter into the area and by maintaining the casualty's respect and dignity such as by covering them with a blanket.
- **P**romoting recovery by getting medical help quickly. Staying with the individual until help arrives can be reassuring for the individual and can enable an effective handover of their condition to take place.

You may have also heard of the DR'S ABC acronym. It is also used by first aiders to help them to remember what to do when they come across an accident or sudden illness.

- **D**anger checks – look around you and check for any risks or signs of danger.
- **R**esponse assessment – assess all casualties and check whether or not they are conscious.
- **S**hout for help – call an ambulance or get someone else to do this for you, and ask them to come back and tell you when this is done.
- **A**irway checks – check that the casualty's airway is open and not blocked. Check that help is on its way.
- **B**reathing checks – check whether the casualty is breathing normally. If they are, place them in the recovery position. If the casualty is not breathing, start CPR only if you have been trained to do so. Check that help is on its way.
- **C**irculation checks – continue to monitor the casualty. Check that help is on its way.

KNOW IT

1 What actions should be taken in the event of a gas leak in a health, social care or child care environment?
2 What does RIDDOR stand for?
3 How can first aiders maintain casualties' respect and dignity?

? THINK ABOUT IT

Case study: Little Faces

Little Faces is a crèche that provides short-term child care for children aged up to 8 years of age.

This morning, crèche worker Angelika has slipped on a toy and while falling backwards has knocked herself unconscious on a table. Lidia and Jeremy, two of the children sitting at the table, have also sustained cuts to their hands and faces and are in shock and crying. Roberto, the first aider, is the first to arrive at the scene.

Describe the main responsibilities of Roberto, the first aider, including the actions he should take and why.

Read about it

Bateman, M. (2006) *Tolley's Practical Risk Assessment Handbook*, Taylor & Francis.

Health and Safety Executive (1997) *Successful Health and Safety Management* (guidance booklet), HSE Books.

Morris, C., Ferreiro Peteiro, M. and Collier, F. (2015) *Level 3 Health and Social Care Diploma*, Hodder Education.

Unit 3: Assessment practice

Below are practice questions for you to try.

1 a) Alecia is the manager of a children's centre and this morning will be carrying out a risk assessment of the building. Describe two examples of environmental hazards that Alecia may find. (4)
  b) Explain the impact psychological hazards may have on the individuals and staff who work in a residential care home. (6)
  c) Analyse the types of hazards that there may be in a hospital. (10)
2 a) Identify the act that sets out how organisations must work together to plan and respond to local and national emergencies. (1)
  b) Analyse how the Manual Handling Operations Regulations 1992 promote health and safety in an after-school club for children who have physical disabilities. (10)
  c) Afolabi is a community care worker who provides care and support to individuals who live in their own homes. Analyse the importance of lone working policies and procedures for Afolabi. (10)
3 a) Tulisa works for Age UK as a volunteer befriender to an older adult. Identify the role Age UK has in promoting health, safety and security. (2)
  b) Describe the health, safety and security responsibilities employees have. (3)
  c) Explain the consequences of the employees of a school not meeting their health, safety and security responsibilities. (6)
4 a) During busy Saturday morning surgery there is a flood in the local GP practice. Describe the procedures that must be followed. (4)
  b) Identify two pieces of information that must be recorded in an accident report. (2)
  c) Miriam is a school first aider. Explain her responsibilities. (6)

Total marks: 64

Unit 04

Anatomy and physiology for health and social care

ABOUT THIS UNIT

In this unit, you will learn about the structure and function of some of the tissues, organs and bodily systems that enable healthy bodily processes to take place in a co-ordinated way.

You will learn about the cardiovascular, respiratory and digestive systems, as well as the roles played by organs such as the pancreas, liver and kidney. You will learn that, in order to survive and stay healthy, we have to detect and respond to changes not only in our external environment but also in our bodies. You will investigate the systems and organs involved in detecting and responding to these changes and how they maintain a natural harmony.

You will learn about some of the conditions that are the result of body parts malfunctioning. You will discover how some are present from birth while others can develop at any time. You will learn that, as individuals grow older, they are more likely to be affected by malfunctions as a result of degeneration. You will understand the effects on individuals and what has to be done to enable them to lead as full and independent a life as possible.

LEARNING OUTCOMES

The topics, activities and suggested reading in this unit will help you to:

1 Understand the cardiovascular system, malfunctions and their impact on individuals
2 Understand the respiratory system, malfunctions and their impact on individuals
3 Understand the digestive system, malfunctions and their impact on individuals
4 Understand the musculoskeletal systems, malfunctions and their impact on individuals
5 Understand the control and regulatory systems, malfunctions and their impact on individuals
6 Understand the sensory systems, malfunctions and their impact on individuals

How will I be assessed?

You will be assessed through an external assessment set and marked by OCR.

LO1 Understand the cardiovascular system, malfunctions and their impact on individuals

1.1 Composition of blood

If a small sample of blood is spun very fast in a machine called a centrifuge, the red colour disappears and a clear pale yellow liquid is seen, accounting for over half the original volume. The red colour appears as a pellet at the bottom.

The yellow liquid is **plasma** and makes up 55 per cent of the blood. It is mostly water but has substances dissolved in it including proteins, glucose, amino acids, various salts, carbon dioxide and other poisonous wastes such as urea.

The remaining 45 per cent is made up of cells – mostly red blood cells (**erythrocytes**). Other cells include white blood cells (**leucocytes**) and tiny fragments of special cells known as **platelets**.

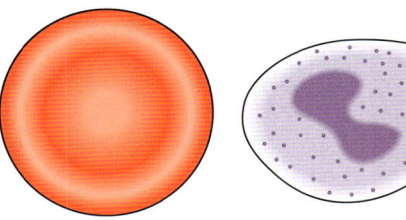
An erythrocyte

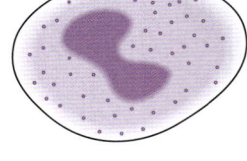
A leucocyte

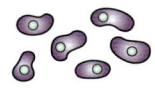
A thrombocyte

▲ **Figure 4.1** The components of blood

1.2 Functions of blood

Transport

One of the main functions of blood is to transport elements required for life around the body. Many are transported from the digestive system to the tissues or to storage areas such as the liver. Those that cannot dissolve in water, for example fats, are carried by blood proteins called **lipoproteins**.

There are two main forms of lipoprotein – high density lipoprotein (HDL) and low density lipoprotein (LDL). While both transport fat to the tissues where it is needed for energy, LDL appears to deposit fat and cholesterol in the walls of arteries while HDL appears to prevent or even reverse these harmful deposits. This has led to HDL and LDL sometimes being called good and bad cholesterol.

Blood also transports gases such as oxygen and carbon dioxide between the tissues and the lungs. Red blood cells contain an iron-containing protein called **haemoglobin**. This combines with oxygen to produce a bright red substance called **oxyhaemoglobin**. In the tissues, oxygen is released and the darker haemoglobin is reformed.

To increase the space for carrying the maximum amount of haemoglobin, erythrocytes have no cell nucleus. They also have a special disc shape to help the exchange of oxygen. The haemoglobin on the return trip to the lungs will also carry a small amount of carbon dioxide.

Table 4.1 Composition of blood

Component	Function
Plasma – 90% water	Transports dissolved substances
Glucose	Nutrient needed for energy
Amino acids	Nutrient needed to make proteins
Vitamins	Nutrients needed for essential processes
Minerals	Nutrients needed for essential processes
Albumin	Blood protein needed to maintain fluid levels
Fibrinogen	Blood protein involved in clotting
Antibodies	Proteins made by the immune system
Lipoproteins	Proteins that carry fats/cholesterol
Carbon dioxide	A poisonous waste gas
Urea	A poisonous waste product from protein
Electrolytes	For example, sodium, needed to help maintain correct concentration of the blood
Erythrocytes	Carry oxygen and some carbon dioxide
Leucocytes – consist of many types, e.g.	Helps destroy bacteria
Neutrophils	B-type cells produce antibodies
Lymphocytes	T-type cells destroy viruses and cancer cells
Monocytes	Removes dead cells and bacteria
Platelets	Triggers blood clotting

Blood also transports **hormones**, for example insulin and adrenalin, which are chemicals produced in glands. They travel in the blood to target organs where they trigger a response or initiate a particular process, e.g. fertility or growth.

Temperature regulation

As mammals, we are endothermic. This means we generate our own internal temperature and maintain it. Life is maintained by millions of chemical reactions that are all affected by heat. We operate best at an internal temperature of 37 degrees centigrade – this is our optimal temperature.

All our chemical reactions are regulated by proteins called enzymes, which are determined by our genes. These enzymes, like all proteins, become unusable or denatured at high temperatures and chemical reactions slow down at low temperatures. Thus, for life and good health to continue, our optimal temperature must be maintained. Heat is generated in all our cells but especially in tissues such as the muscles. Blood removes this heat and circulates it around the body.

Exchange of materials in body tissues

See the sections on capillaries and the respiratory system in LO6 and LO7.

Preventing infection

Combating infection, a complex process that is not fully understood, is the role of the immune system. Leucocytes are white blood cells involved in the **immune response**.

The body is under threat from disease-causing organisms, generally called **pathogens**, like bacteria, parasites and viruses. Bacteria and parasites will be recognised as threats by cells such as the neutrophils and B-type lymphocytes, which act as **antigens** – they form special proteins called **antibodies**. These lock onto specific chemicals in the walls of the bacteria and parasites, immobilising them and making them targets for the monocytes that then kill them and break them down. Special lymphocytes 'remember' these particular pathogens and will respond quickly if there is a re-infection. This is the principle behind vaccination.

Viruses, however, pose a different threat. These simple organisms cannot live independently and need to hijack cells to survive and reproduce. They change the outside of the infected cell, but T-lymphocytes recognise this and latch onto the cell and destroy it along with the virus. It is this cell destruction that causes many symptoms of viral infections.

Blood clotting

Women have 4–5 litres and men 5–6 litres of blood. Losing 2 litres will lead to serious issues or even death. Also, if the skin is broken, pathogens can gain access and blood poisoning or sepsis can quickly cause organ damage.

When exposed to air or foreign material such as glass or plastic, tiny cell fragments from the bone marrow, called platelets, activate a chain reaction known as **coagulation** that converts the soluble blood protein (**fibrinogen**) into an insoluble form (**fibrin**) that forms a net-like structure, trapping both platelets and erythrocytes to form a clot. Individuals with haemophilia lack one or more of these factors and so have longer clotting times, leading to chronic blood loss.

The platelets also help activate the immune response, minimising the threat of a pathogenic invasion.

If, during operations or kidney dialysis, blood is passed outside of the body to machines in tubes, anticoagulants have to be added to stop the blood from clotting.

1.3 Structure of the heart

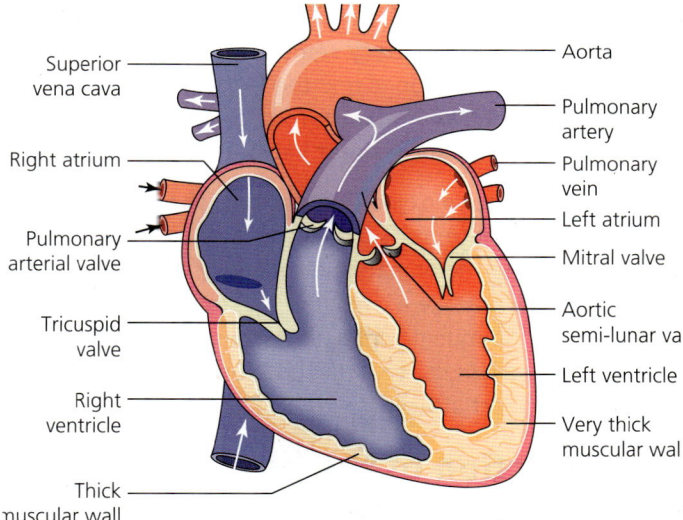

Superior vena cava
Right atrium
Pulmonary arterial valve
Tricuspid valve
Right ventricle
Thick muscular wall
Aorta
Pulmonary artery
Pulmonary vein
Left atrium
Mitral valve
Aortic semi-lunar va
Left ventricle
Very thick muscular wal

▲ **Figure 4.2** Blood flow through the heart

The cardiovascular system is also called the circulatory system because the majority of blood flows in a circuit around the body, pumped by the heart, a muscular organ located in the chest. More accurately, it is a **double circulatory system** as there are two distinct circuits – the **systemic** (around the body) and **pulmonary** (to and from the lungs).

The right side receives blood returning from the tissues and sends it to the lungs to drop off carbon dioxide and pick up oxygen. The left side receives oxygenated blood from the lungs and sends it off round the body again to the tissues.

The heart muscle is unusual in that it is **myogenic** – it can beat automatically without stimulation by nerves and is co-ordinated by a region at the top of the right side known as the **pacemaker**. It is also unusual in that it does not become fatigued even over a lifetime.

Each side of the heart consists of two chambers – the upper thin-walled **atria** and the lower, thicker-walled **ventricles**. An opening between the atria and the ventricles with a one-way valve allows blood to move down but not back up. On the right side, this valve is called the **tricuspid**; on the left it is the **bicuspid** or **mitral** valve.

Attached to the right atrium are two large veins that bring the blood back from the tissues – the **superior vena cava** that leads from the arms and head and the **inferior vena cava** that brings blood from the lower body and legs. Leading out from the top of the right ventricle is the **pulmonary artery** which has a branch going to each lung.

Another valve is located in the entrance to the pulmonary artery which allows blood to flow out of the heart but not back in again. This valve is called a **semi-lunar valve** or **pulmonary arterial valve**.

On the left side, **pulmonary veins** return blood to the left atrium from the lungs and the largest artery of the body – the **aorta** – takes it from the left ventricle through the **aortic semi-lunar valve** around the body.

All muscles require oxygen to function. The heart muscle gets this from its own intricate blood supply branching from the aorta – the **coronary arteries**. These branch out like a tree, getting smaller as they burrow into the muscle cells. Disturbances to these small arteries can cause heart problems such as angina and heart attacks.

1.4 Function of the heart

The heart acts as a double pump. Blood enters the two atria simultaneously and each atrium, once full, contracts, pushing the blood down into the ventricles through the tricuspid and bicuspid valves.

Once the ventricles have filled, they too contract in a squeezing action from the bottom of the heart upwards. This forces blood up against the tricuspid and bicuspid valves, closing them. Blood can only leave the heart through the semilunar valves and the pulmonary arteries and aorta. Once the blood has left the ventricles

they relax and start to open up again. Backflow of blood is prevented by the semi-lunar valves snapping shut. This results in the characteristic heart sounds – the 'lub' sound is the synchronised shutting of the tricuspid and bicuspid valves and the 'dup' sound is the synchronised semilunar valves shutting.

This co-ordinated flow of blood through the heart is called the **cardiac cycle** and takes place on average 70 times a minute. The part of the cycle when the ventricles are contracting is known as **systole**; when they are relaxing and the atria are filling it is called **diastole**.

The left ventricle wall is much thicker than the right. The right side is less muscular to prevent blood from entering the lungs under too much pressure. If it did, water from the blood would be forced into the airspaces of the lungs, effectively drowning us.

1.5 Control and regulation of the cardiac cycle

The heart's co-ordinated pumping and filling is brought about by a specialised form of 'electrical' control. The SA node (**sino-atrial node**) passes a wave of electrical current through the atria, making them contract.

A special layer of fibrous tissues spans the heart between the atria and the ventricles, preventing this wave of current passing through. However, at the top of the wall separating the two ventricles is a patch of tissue that does allow this current through – the **atrial ventricular** or **AV node**. This acts like a turnstile at a station, slowing the passage of current down to allow the ventricles to fill with blood. **Purkyne fibres** carry the current down the middle of the ventricles to the base or apex of the heart. This allows the bottom of the heart to contract first, resulting in an upwards squeezing action, forcing the blood out into the arteries.

This complicated electrical co-ordination can be observed by using an electrocardiogram (ECG) monitor. Electrodes are attached to the chest and fed to a computer linked to a screen or printer. The activity of the heart can then be represented as a trace consisting of a number of waves or spikes. These are the characteristic patterns we see in hospital dramas.

A small blip known as the P wave shows the moment when the atria are both contracting. A fraction of a second later is a bigger spike (the QRS wave). This shows the ventricles contracting (systole). A smaller T wave shows the period the ventricles are relaxing (diastole). The whole **ECG trace** represents the cardiac cycle and lasts on average 0.85 seconds – a heartbeat. To a trained eye, ECG traces can show issues affecting the heart.

1.6 Types, structure and function of blood vessels

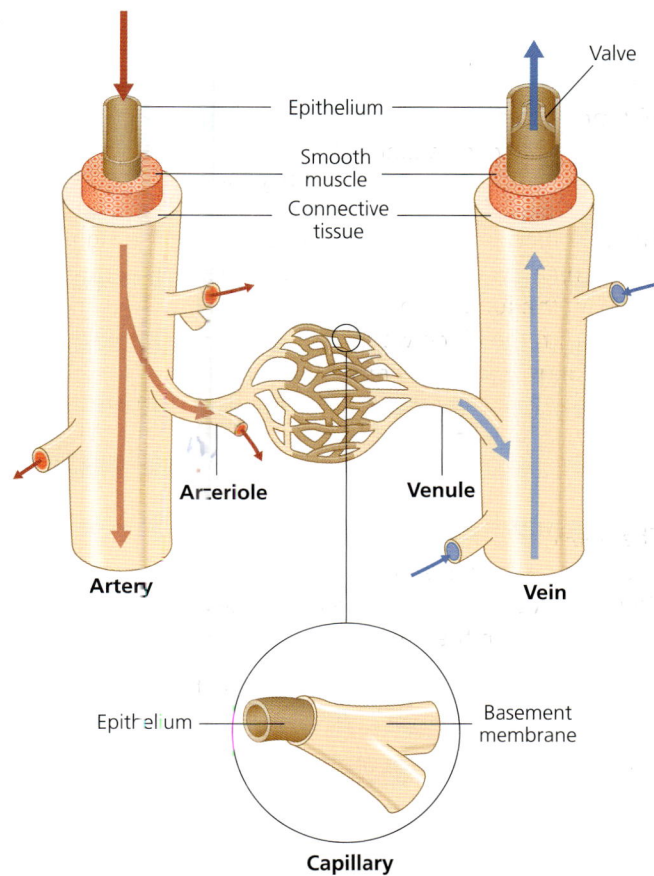

▲ **Figure 4.3** Structure of the blood vessels

Arteries

These are the blood vessels that carry blood away from the heart. With the exception of the pulmonary arteries, they carry oxygen-rich blood. Their walls contain several layers of thick elastic fibres and muscle. The aorta is the largest and its thick elastic walls deal with the surge of blood leaving the heart. Other large arteries leading to the head, arms and legs have a similar structure. As blood enters, they expand and recoil, helping to maintain the flow of blood. This is the pulse that we detect in the neck or the wrist, where these large arteries are close to the surface.

Arteries branch into smaller distributive arteries and eventually arterioles, which are very small arteries that lead to capillary beds in the tissues. The distributive

arteries have muscular walls so that they can regulate blood flow to where it is needed, for example the skin if we are hot, leg muscles if we are running and the reproductive organs during sex. If these muscles contract too much too frequently, blood pressure can harmfully increase. Sensors in the walls normally keep blood pressure under control.

Capillaries

Arteries take blood with oxygen and nutrients to capillary beds. There are masses of interconnected capillaries that surround and interweave between cells and tissues. A capillary is a microscopic tube with walls only one cell thick covered by a sieve-like basement membrane.

Capillaries supply the tissues with oxygen and nutrients whilst removing waste products such as carbon dioxide.

Veins

Plasma leaves the capillaries and enters small blood vessels known as **venules** that join together to form larger tubes or veins. Veins have large internal diameters or lumens with walls much thinner than arteries that contain less muscle and elastic tissue. Blood flowing in veins is not under pressure and, with the exception of the pulmonary veins, veins carry deoxygenated blood back to the heart. Because of the low pressure of blood in them they are often buried between our body muscles so that movements of the body help squeeze blood along. To ensure blood flows in the right direction, veins have valves throughout their length that prevent backflow. Blockages can cause varicose veins.

1.7 Formation of tissue fluid and lymph

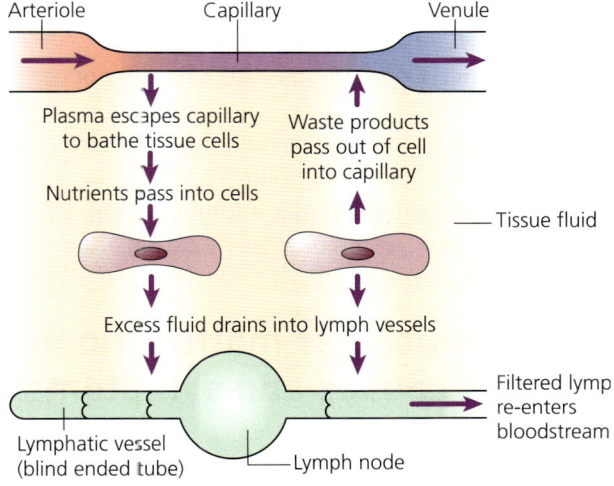

▲ **Figure 4.4** The formation of tissue fluid

Capillaries allow materials to pass in and out of cells. Water in the plasma is forced out of the cells by the pressure of the heart's contraction (**hydrostatic pressure**), taking with it dissolved nutrients and oxygen from the oxyhaemoglobin in the red cells. Blood cells and blood proteins such as albumin cannot pass through the basement membrane and so remain behind. The tissue fluid must return to the circulatory system, otherwise our bodies would swell with the accumulating tissue fluid. This is a condition known as oedema which, if not treated, can kill.

Tissue fluid is mostly returned to the capillaries by a process called **osmosis**. This is the movement of water through a semi-permeable membrane from a less concentrated solution to a more concentrated one. As plasma is forced out by the hydrostatic pressure, more water surrounds the tissues, creating an imbalance resulting in water being drawn back into the capillaries by osmosis due in particular to the presence of albumin in the capillaries. This is referred to as an **osmotic pressure**.

As water returns to the capillaries it takes with it the dissolved carbon dioxide and other waste products.

About 10 per cent of the fluid (now known as **lymph**) drains into another type of transport system – the **lymphatic system**. It drains into lymph capillaries, which lead to lymph vessels, which have a similar structure to veins. This transport system is one way, leading from the lymph capillaries in the tissues through the lymph vessels to join the circulatory system at the top of the chest. There, the lymph drains into the main veins leading from the arms to the superior vena cava. This maintains the correct blood volume.

The lymphatic system serves a number of other purposes. Along it are swellings called **lymph nodes** – particularly in our neck, under our arms and in our groin. These nodes store and develop lymphocytes that screen the returning tissue fluid or lymph for pathogens, destroying any that are found. When fighting an infection these nodes swell so we often refer to our 'glands' swelling.

1.8 Cardiovascular malfunctions – possible causes and symptoms

Hypertension

Blood pumped from the heart exerts **systolic pressure** on the walls of arteries. Less pressure is exerted on the walls when the heart is relaxing – this is **diastolic pressure**. Both pressure readings can be obtained with an inflatable cuff attached to an arm and connected to a recording device called a **sphygmomanometer**.

Readings are recorded as a systolic value written over a diastolic one.

Table 4.2 The meanings of blood pressure values

Values	Blood pressure	Medical notes
70–90/40–60 mmHg	Low	Dizziness and fainting
90–120/60–80 mmHg	Ideal	Healthy
120–140/80–90 mmHg	Pre-high	Monitored and lifestyle changes implemented
140/90 mmHg and above	**Hypertension** or high	Increased risk of strokes, heart attacks and kidney damage

Coronary heart disease

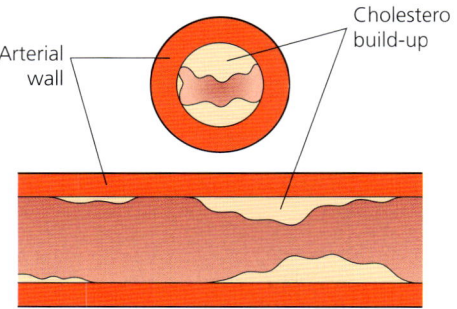

▲ **Figure 4.5** Build-up of cholesterol in a new artery

Coronary heart or arterial disease is a blanket term that relates to issues concerning the coronary arteries that supply the heart muscle itself with nutrients and oxygen.

While age, genes and gender can influence the likelihood of developing this condition, most causes relate to lifestyle. A healthy artery has a normal wall and the inner surface is protected by a smooth layer called the **endothelium**. This allows smooth and uninterrupted blood flow to the heart muscle. However, components in cigarettes that enter the blood via the lungs affect this protective layer. So too does high blood pressure, which is linked to excessive alcohol and obesity. Once damaged, the wall of the artery is easily 'invaded' by the fat/cholesterol-carrying lipoproteins LDL which deposit their fats into the wall of the artery.

These deposits are targeted by white blood cells that die and get trapped with mineral deposits. The resulting gunge is known as **atheroma**, which gradually distends the wall, reducing the space inside and obstructing blood flow to the heart. This could lead to **angina**, a condition arising when the cells beyond the obstruction get less oxygen, resulting in pain on exertion – even when climbing a few steps.

If the atheroma completely blocks the lumen or breaks up to form a clot, no oxygen and nutrients can reach the cells beyond and that part of the heart is damaged. If left untreated, this could result in a **heart attack** or **myocardial infarction**.

Disruption to the electrical activity of the heart can result in a chaotic beating of the ventricles called **ventricular fibrillation**. This can lead to a **cardiac arrest**.

> ## 🔑 KEY TERMS
>
> **Angiogram** – a type of X-ray that involves a dye visible in X-ray photographs that is injected into the blood system so that narrowing of coronary arteries can be seen.
>
> **Angioplasty** – a microscopic deflated balloon is passed into a narrowed artery and inflated, pushing the artery open. Sometimes a microscopic mesh tube or stent is inserted at the same time, keeping the artery open for longer.
>
> **Coronary bypass** – using a piece of artery from the chest to bypass or bridge a blocked region of coronary artery, allowing blood to flow beyond the blockage.

1.9 Monitoring, treatment and care needs for cardiovascular malfunctions

> ### ❓ THINK ABOUT IT
>
> #### Case study: Daniel
>
> Daniel is in his 40s and has a deskbound job with responsibility for a large team and budget. He has to work to strict deadlines. He smokes to help deal with the stress. He also relaxes by joining friends for a drink while watching televised sport. When at home he enjoys watching television and playing computer games and he eats a lot of takeaway and microwave meals.
>
> At a recent company medical his blood pressure was found to be 155/95 mmHg and his body mass index (BMI) was 34.
>
> 1 Comment on Daniel's blood pressure and BMI.
> 2 Explain how these measurements were made.
> 3 Analyse how his lifestyle has contributed to these measurements.
> 4 Provide Daniel with information on what the possible consequences of his current lifestyle might be.
> 5 Produce an advice sheet or presentation on how Daniel might change his lifestyle to improve his health.
>
> #### Case study: Robert
>
> Robert is in his 60s and has suffered from angina for a number of years. He is regularly monitored by his GP for his high blood pressure and cholesterol levels and is on appropriate medication. Despite this close supervision he suffered a suspected heart attack and was admitted to hospital. He was attached to an ECG monitor and given an **angiogram**. As a result, he received a **coronary bypass** which was successful.
>
> 1 Explain why Robert is displaying the signs of angina. Research the medication used to treat angina.
> 2 What medication is Robert likely to be given for his high cholesterol levels?
> 3 Recent research has shown that individuals such as Robert are likely to benefit from a daily dose of aspirin. Why?
> 4 What evidence might his ECG have supplied?
> 5 What is an angiogram and what information does this supply?
> 6 What happens during a coronary bypass? Why is it carried out?
> 7 A less invasive procedure might have been an **angioplasty**. What is the point of this medical intervention?
> 8 Produce an information leaflet or presentation on how Robert should minimise any likelihood of a repeat heart attack.

LO2 Understand the respiratory system, malfunctions and their impact on individuals

2.1 Structure of the respiratory system

Our respiratory system takes in air containing oxygen, which is needed by all cells and body tissues, and enables poisonous carbon dioxide to be removed from the body.

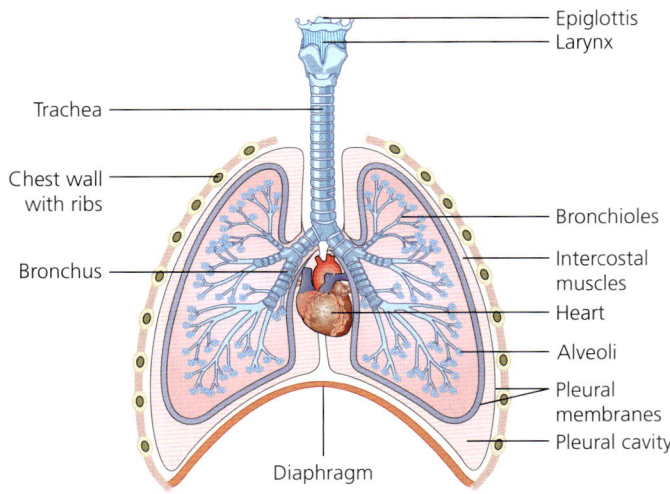

▲ **Figure 4.6** Structure of the respiratory system

The lungs consist of millions of tiny elasticated cavities called **alveoli**. These are closely surrounded by capillaries and are the site of oxygen uptake and carbon dioxide removal.

The **trachea** or windpipe leads from the throat, where its opening is protected from food particles by a flap called the **epiglottis** which should close whenever we swallow. At the top of the trachea is an enlarged area – the **larynx** – containing muscles and ligaments. These are our vocal cords which enable us to speak.

The trachea branches into two further large tubes – the **bronchii**. Each bronchus leads into one of our lungs. Between the bronchii and the alveoli are thousands of smaller branching tubes – **bronchioles**.

The trachea, bronchii and larger bronchioles are kept open by incomplete rings of cartilage. Without these, upon breathing the tubes might collapse like a drinking straw sucked too hard. These tubes also have muscles in their walls that allow them to widen (dilate) or narrow (constrict) to vary the amount of air that enters or leaves the lungs. These muscles can cause the symptoms of asthma.

The inside lining of these tubes has two specialised forms of cell. One is glandular – they produce and release a sticky, slimy fluid called **mucus** that traps dirt particles and bacteria breathed in. The second has microscopic hair-like extensions called **cilia** that beat backwards and forwards. These work together like a conveyer belt to move the mucus and trapped particles back up to the throat where we swallow them. These cilia are paralysed by the chemicals in cigarette smoke, which is why smokers' lungs tend to be dirtier and why smokers often have a cough, as this is the only way they can clean their lungs.

The lungs are in a cavity called the **thorax**. Along the sides and at the top are the ribcage and two sets of **intercostal muscles** – internal and external – which are located between and attached to the ribs. At the bottom, the lungs are separated from the digestive organs by a domed sheet of muscle – the **diaphragm**. Around each lung is a double set of coverings – the **pleural membranes**. Between the membranes is a narrow space filled with **pleural fluid**. This causes the membranes to stick to each other. One membrane is attached directly to the lung itself; the other is attached to the rib cage and diaphragm. The pleural membrane causes the lungs to be indirectly attached to both the ribcage and the diaphragm. As we will, see these membranes play an important part in breathing.

2.2 Inspiration and expiration

Breathing refers to the movement of air in and out of the lungs. Inspiration is breathing in and expiration is breathing out.

Most air is nitrogen, which we do not need or use. It passes harmlessly in and out of our lungs.

Role of intercostal muscles

To draw air into the lungs, the brain sends nerve messages to the external intercostal muscles and the diaphragm. Because the ribcage is hinged to the spine, the contraction of the external muscles causes the ribcage to swing up and out. Nerve impulses to the diaphragm make it contract and flatten, pressing on the digestive organs below. As the pleural membranes attach the lungs to both the ribcage and diaphragm, movement of these structures means the lungs have to follow and so the lungs are stretched, opening the microscopic alveoli. This increases the internal volume of the lungs, which means that the pressure of the air in the lungs decreases below that of the atmosphere and so air rushes into the lungs, inflating the alveoli. This is **inspiration**.

Role of the diaphragm

To carry out **expiration** the brain stops sending nerve messages to the ribs and diaphragm and so they stop contracting. The diaphragm recoils upwards into its domed position and gravity causes the ribcage to drop back and downwards. This decreases the volume of the lungs, and air pressure in the lungs increases above the pressure of atmospheric air and so air is forced out.

If we wish to force the air out more quickly, for example when coughing, the internal intercostal muscles contract to pull the ribcage back down with more force.

Role of the pleural membranes

The pleural membranes are crucial to the lungs inflating and deflating as well as preventing friction as the lungs move. If the space between the membranes is punctured, the lung on that side will not inflate.

2.3 Gaseous exchange

Role and structure of alveoli walls

The alveoli are the site of gaseous exchange – oxygen enters the blood and carbon dioxide is removed from it. The alveoli have a number of adaptations that increase the efficiency of this vital process.

1 The vast number of these air sacs, with the capillaries surrounding them, make a large surface area – the equivalent of two tennis courts. This means that a large amount of gaseous exchange can occur.
2 The walls of the alveoli are very thin – just one flattened cell thick, as with capillaries. This means there is a minimal distance for gases to pass through.
3 The inner surfaces of the alveoli are coated with a thin layer of water that allows oxygen to dissolve before travelling through the walls of the alveoli and capillaries.

Diffusion gradient

There is a higher concentration of oxygen in inhaled air than there is in the blood. Oxygen diffuses into the blood and combines with the haemoglobin in the **erythrocytes**, forming oxyhaemoglobin.

Carbon dioxide in the blood diffuses in the opposite direction, as there are higher levels of this gas in the blood than there is in the alveoli. Exhaled air has higher levels of carbon dioxide and lower levels of oxygen than inhaled air.

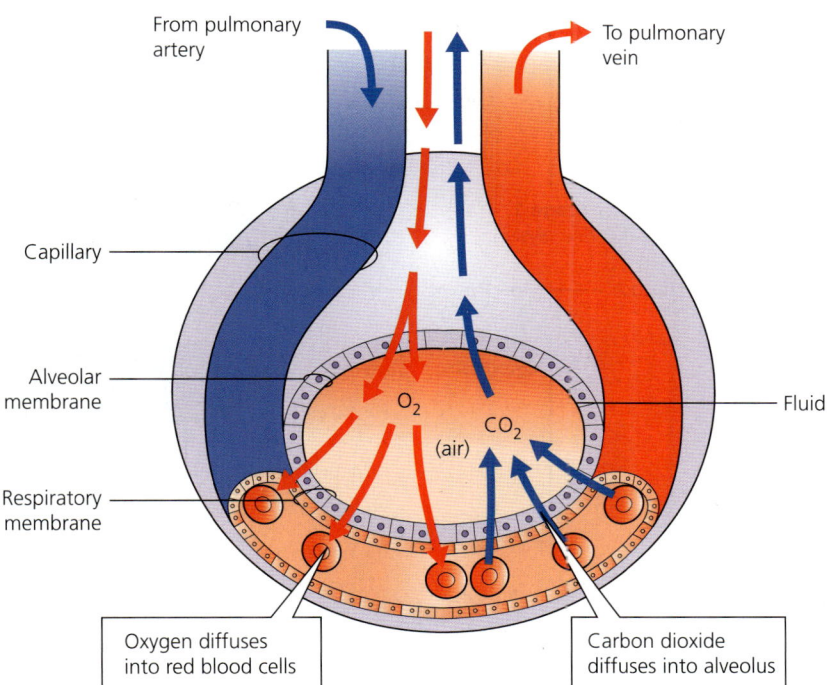

From pulmonary artery

To pulmonary vein

Capillary

Alveolar membrane

Respiratory membrane

O_2 (air)

CO_2

Fluid

Oxygen diffuses into red blood cells

Carbon dioxide diffuses into alveolus

▲ **Figure 4.7** Gas exchange between alveoli and capillaries

2.4 Cellular respiration

Cellular respiration is why we need oxygen to live. It occurs in the **cytoplasm** and **mitochondria** of all living cells.

Food supplies the energy we need, in particular a sugar called **glucose**. This is broken down into simpler substances – water and carbon dioxide – and the energy that was holding the glucose molecule together is released. This energy needs to be captured in a useable form in a chemical called **adenosine triphosphate (ATP)**. This is formed from a molecule called **adenosine diphosphate (ADP)** using the energy released from the breakdown of the glucose. ATP can then be quickly broken down again to ADP, so releasing the energy. This simple reaction is used to power every process in the body. ATP is the cell's equivalent of cash being used to provide energy in every chemical transaction.

Cellular respiration is a complex series of reactions with several stages that release enough energy to turn ADP into ATP. Any energy released that is not enough to generate ATP is given off as heat, which we use to maintain our optimal temperature of 37 degrees centigrade.

There are three stages to cellular respiration. **Glycolysis** occurs in the cytoplasm of a cell. This involves the breakdown of glucose into pyruvic acid with some energy. This chemical passes into the mitochondria of the cell and enters a complex series of reactions involving two further stages that result in much more energy being released and more ATP being generated. The third and last stage, which takes place in the walls of the mitochondria, needs oxygen. The reaction in the mitochondria is called **aerobic respiration**. Carbon dioxide is a by-product.

During intense exercise, some pyruvic acid is converted to another molecule called **lactic acid**. This stage is known as **anaerobic respiration** as oxygen is not required. We use it when we need extra supplies of ATP; for example, when exercising. It occurs as an additional process to supplement the energy provided by aerobic respiration, not as an alternative. We would not get enough energy from only anaerobic respiration.

Lactic acid is poisonous and its build-up in our muscles causes **fatigue**. If we have had to use anaerobic respiration to gain some extra ATP then we develop an **oxygen debt**. This means that once exercise is finished we need to get rid of the lactic acid by breaking it down in the mitochondria using oxygen. This is why we continue to breathe deeply after exercise.

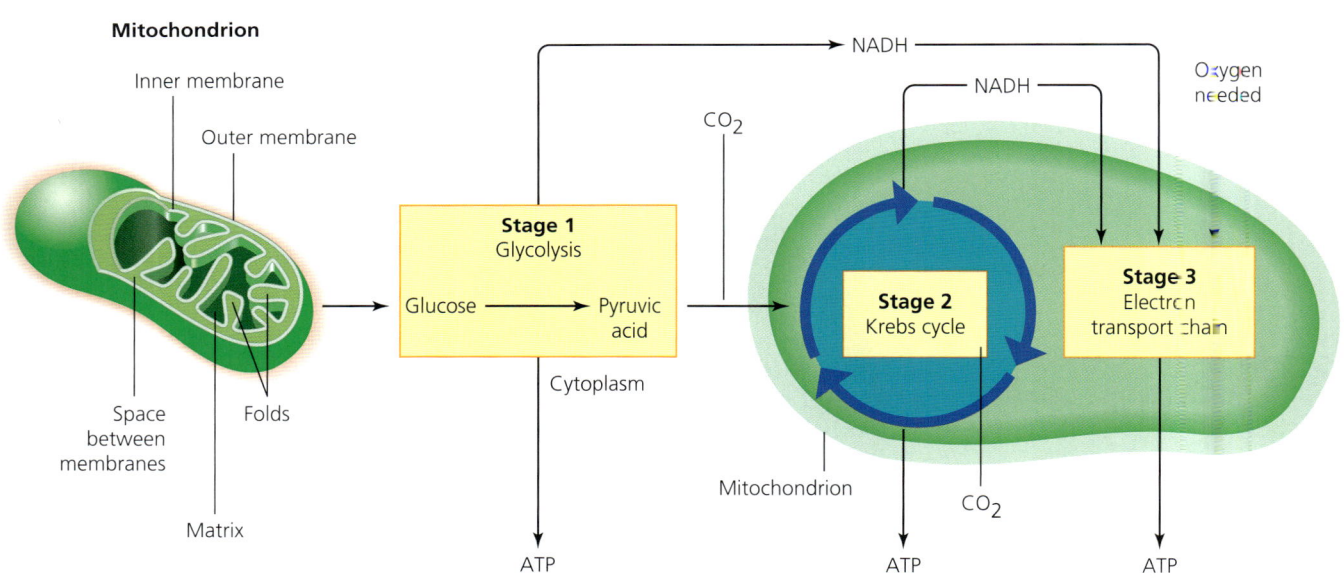

▲ **Figure 4.8** Cellular respiration

2.5 Respiratory malfunctions – possible causes and effects

Asthma

In individuals susceptible to asthma, certain triggers cause the bronchii of the lungs to become inflamed and narrow as the muscles contract. There is also an increase in the production of mucus. As a result, the individual begins to wheeze, is short of breath, has a tight chest and will cough a lot. If these symptoms become severe and the episode prolonged they are having an **asthma attack**. A severe attack will reduce the amount of air reaching the lungs and their lips and finger tips may go blue, showing a lack of oxygen. A cardiac arrest or death can result from a prolonged, untreated attack.

Factors that can act as triggers vary but include cigarette smoke, atmospheric pollution, cold air, dust, animal fur, dust mites, pollen, exercise, stress and even laughter.

Emphysema

Emphysema is a condition within a group of respiratory illnesses called **COPD** (chronic obstructive pulmonary disease). It is mainly caused by long-term smoking. Chemicals in the smoke paralyse the lung-cleaning cilia and eventually kill them, leading to a build-up of mucus and, with pathogens trapped in the lungs, increasing infections. Continued exposure to chemicals, inflammation and infections damages the alveoli and smaller terminal bronchioles. This in turn decreases the efficiency of the lungs as these tissues collapse. It becomes increasingly difficult to obtain oxygen and so exertion results in breathlessness and coughing.

Cystic fibrosis

Cystic fibrosis (CF) is present from birth and is caused by a defective gene on one of our chromosomes, which come in pairs. CF is caused by having one defective gene on each pair of chromosomes. This means that individuals' parents each carried one copy of the defective gene, giving a 1 in 4 chance of a child being born with the condition. In Europe about 1 in 20 people carry a defective copy.

The **CFTR gene** makes a defective form of a protein that should move water and salt in and out of cells. As it doesn't work properly, individuals with CF produce unusually thick and sticky mucus which blocks the bronchioles and prevents efficient movement of respiratory gases in and out of the lungs. As with emphysema, this sticky mucus also traps bacteria and so coughing and repeated chest infections result.

Mucus is also produced in the digestive and reproductive systems, impairing their function and resulting in poor weight gain, abnormal stools and reduced fertility.

A symptom of CF is increased salt in sweat and this is used to diagnose the condition.

There is no cure but advances in treatment have lengthened the lives of sufferers.

2.6 Monitoring, treatment and care needs for cardiovascular malfunctions

> ### 🔑 KEY TERMS
>
> **Peak flow** – the rate of expired air, measured on a hand-held device.
>
> **Inhaler** – a method of getting medication directly into the lungs. May be pressurised. Two types – relievers (blue) that dilate the bronchii during an attack and preventers (red, brown or orange) that reduce sensitivity and inflammation of the bronchii.

> ### ❓ THINK ABOUT IT
>
> #### Case study: Jackie
>
> Jackie has asthma. She regularly monitors her condition using a **peak flow** test. She has been supplied with two types of **inhaler**.
>
> 1 Explain how a peak flow test provides useful information on Jackie's condition.
> 2 Describe the role of inhalers in treating asthma.
> 3 Produce an advice sheet or presentation on how Jackie might adapt her lifestyle to avoid aggravating her asthma.
>
> #### Case study: Mohammed
>
> Mohammed is in his late 60s and has been a heavy smoker for 40 years. He built car engines in a factory where most of the workers also smoked. Until recently they could smoke on the factory floor. He has been diagnosed with emphysema. He uses a wheelchair and has to rely on a portable cylinder of oxygen to help his breathing. He still lives in his own home but is restricted to the ground floor.

KEY TERMS

Nebuliser – a mouthpiece or facemask that introduces medication to the lungs as a fine spray.

Spirometer – equipment that measures the volume of the lungs and how much air can be exchanged per breath.

LO3 Understand the digestive system, malfunctions and their impact on individuals

3.1 Gross structure of digestive system and functions of component parts

Our digestive system is a long tube that begins at the mouth and ends at the anus. Along its length are specialised regions to help break food down until it can pass into our blood and then be transported by it to the cells and tissues. The liver and pancreas assist with the process and both have tubes connecting them to the gut.

We put food into our mouths or **buccal cavity** (sometimes known as the oral cavity) and use our jaws, teeth and tongue to make the food small enough to swallow. Saliva from our **salivary glands**, located under the tongue and in the cheeks, helps moisten the food and make it easier to swallow. The food slides past the **epiglottis** and enters the **oesophagus** or gullet. This is a muscular tube down which food is squeezed by muscles in an action called **peristalsis**.

The **stomach** is a muscular sack that churns our food around and starts to chemically alter the protein in our diet. After leaving the stomach, food, or **chyme**, as it is now called, enters the **small intestine** – initially the **duodenum**. Here, further chemical alteration takes place aided by fluids provided by the **liver** and **pancreas**. **Bile**, made by the liver and stored temporarily in a small sack called the **gallbladder**, passes down the **bile duct** to the gut. Another fluid containing digestive enzymes and alkaline salts passes down the **pancreatic duct** – a tube leading from the pancreas.

The altered nutrients now pass into a further region of the small intestine, the **ileum**. It is covered with small finger-like projections (**villi**), containing blood vessels, like a thick carpet. The nutrients are now in a small enough form to be picked up by the blood

Remaining in the gut are water and food substances we are unable to break down chemically. These move into the **large intestine** or **colon** where much of the water is taken back into the blood.

Living in the colon are trillions of mostly beneficial bacteria. They feed off undigested food, providing us with vital vitamins such as folic acid and vitamin K. They also produce intestinal gases that we either find hilarious or embarrassing!

The dried out remains of our food and dead bacteria form faeces which is stored in the **rectum** – a muscular tube that eventually expels the waste from the **anus**.

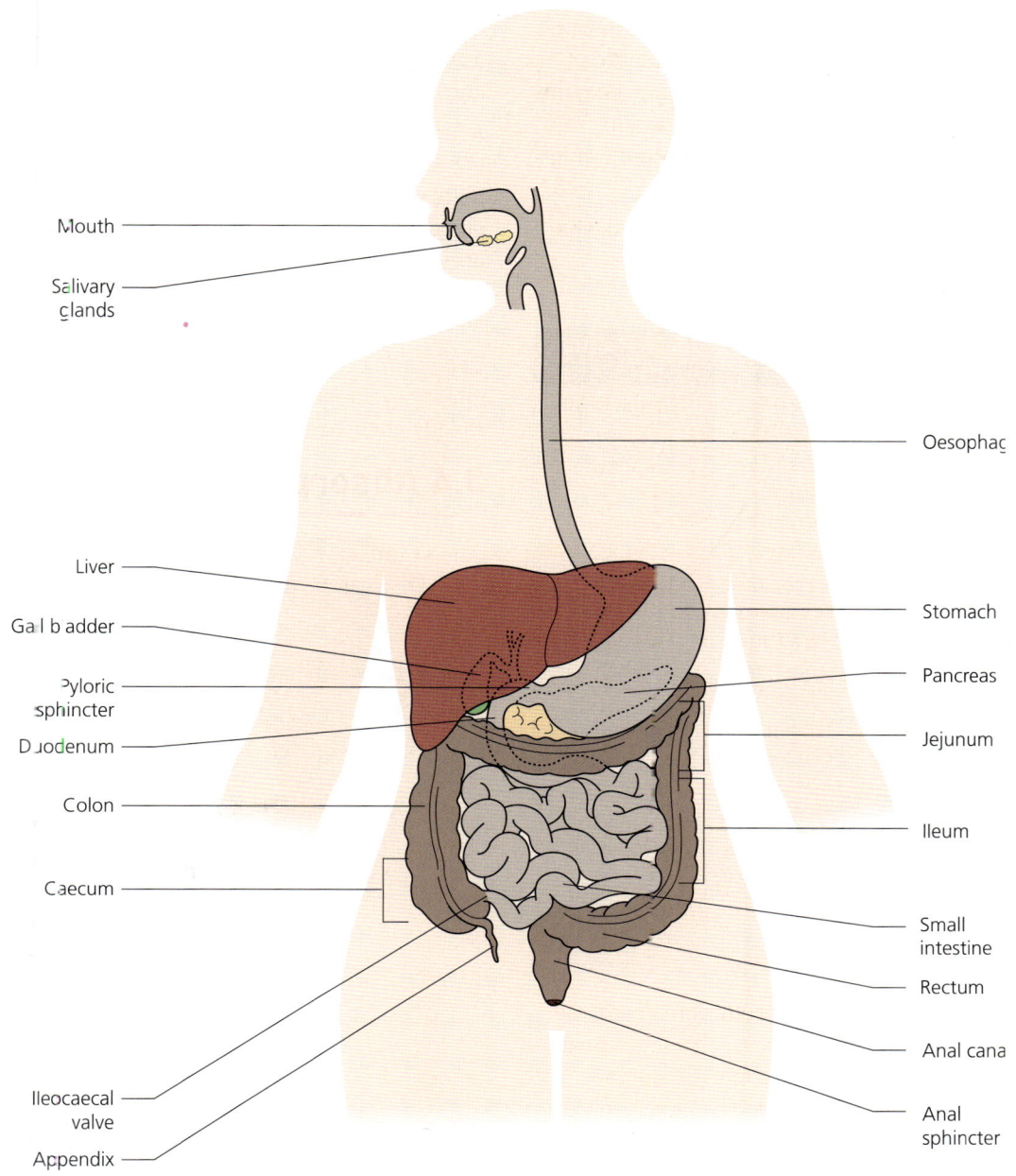

Mouth

Salivary glands

Oesophagus

Liver

Gall bladder

Pyloric sphincter

Duodenum

Colon

Caecum

Ileocaecal valve

Appendix

Stomach

Pancreas

Jejunum

Ileum

Small intestine

Rectum

Anal canal

Anal sphincter

▲ **Figure 4.9** The digestive system

3.2 Mechanical and chemical digestion and 3.3 Digestive roles of the liver and pancreas

Essential nutrients from food have to be changed into forms that can be absorbed by the blood and can dissolve in the water of the plasma. Our digestive system uses specialised proteins, **enzymes**, to chemically change these nutrients into smaller, soluble units. This is known as **chemical digestion**. However, the food must be small enough for the millions of enzyme molecules to get at the nutrients, so food must also be physically broken down by **mechanical digestion**.

Mechanical digestion

This starts when we chew our food, making it small enough to swallow; however, the most important form of mechanical digestion takes place in the stomach.

Muscles in the wall of the stomach churn our food around, breaking it up into small pieces. This chyme is what we see when we vomit. This pulverised food provides our digestive enzymes with much easier access to the nutrients.

Chemical digestion

Proteins, carbohydrates and fats are large chemical nutrients that are too big to pass through the wall of our gut into the blood and then be carried by it. They must be dismantled into smaller molecules. This usually involves breaking the chemical bonds that hold them together. Each type of action is carried out by a particular **enzyme** that has the precise shape to carry out its function. This shape, as we have already seen, can be distorted by high temperatures and extremes of pH.

Table 4.3 shows some enzymes, what they do and where they do it.

Table 4.3 Enzymes in the digestive system

Substrate	Enzyme	Result of action	Site of action
Carbohydrate (starch)	Salivary amylase	Starch to maltose	Buccal cavity
Carbohydrate (starch)	Amylase	Starch to maltose	Duodenum
Carbohydrate (maltose)	Maltase	Maltose to glucose	Duodenum
Carbohydrate (sucrose)	Sucrase	Sucrose to fructose and glucose	Duodenum
Protein	Pepsin	Protein to polypeptides	Stomach
Polypeptides	Peptidases, e.g. trypsin	Polypeptides to peptides	Duodenum
Peptides	Peptidases	Peptides to amino acids	Duodenum
Fats	Lipases	Fats to fatty acids and glycerol	Duodenum
DNA/ chromosomes	Nucleases	DNA to nucleotides	Duodenum

This chemical change starts in the mouth with an enzyme found in saliva starting to break down starch into a simpler sugar called maltose. As soon as food hits the stomach this reaction stops because the stomach has a very low pH – it is acidic. This acidity destroys the shape of the salivary amylase and prevents it from working. The stomach produces **hydrochloric acid** from pits in its walls to activate an enzyme called **pepsin**. This unique enzyme will only work in acidic conditions, starting the breakdown of proteins into smaller but still large molecules called polypeptides.

This acidity in the stomach means that the chyme now has a low pH and this will prevent any further chemical digestion as other enzymes will be distorted or denatured. The chyme as it enters the duodenum has to be **neutralised**. This means **alkaline salts** must be added to make the gut contents slightly alkaline. These salts are supplied by the **bile** from the **liver** and the **pancreatic juice** from the **pancreas**.

The pancreas and the walls of the duodenum also supply further digestive enzymes that bring about the

necessary changes to carbohydrates, proteins, fats as well as to the DNA that makes up the genes and chromosomes found in the cells of the food we eat.

A further problem for successful chemical digestion is the presence of water in the gut. Fats and water don't mix! Salts in bile act as a detergent, breaking fats up into tiny globules that form an **emulsion**, allowing the fat-digesting enzymes to reach the fat molecules. The **gallbladder** stores bile which it releases when fat is eaten. The more fat we eat in a meal, the more bile is produced.

By the time the chyme reaches the ileum of the small intestine, the bulk of the nutrients are in a form that is readily absorbed.

3.4 Absorption and assimilation

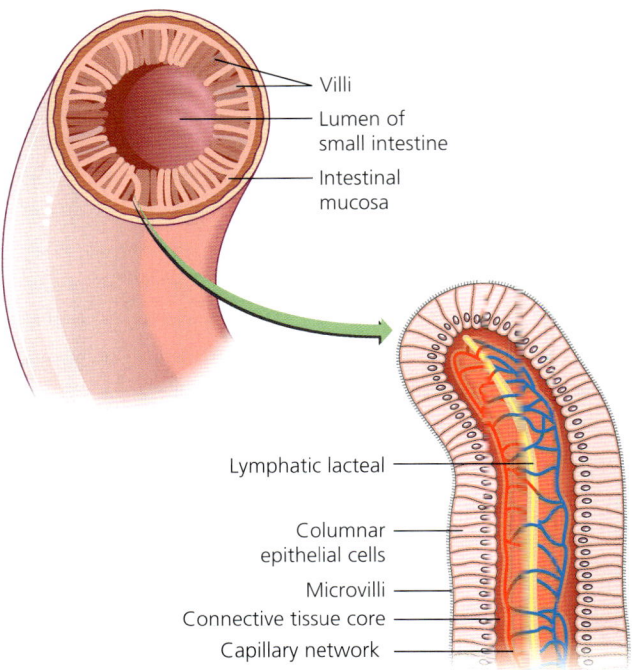

▲ **Figure 4.10** A cross-section of a villus

The **villi** of the ileum wall increase the surface area so that as many nutrients as possible are absorbed. Each villus contains blood capillaries and a central vessel – the **lacteal** – which is connected to the lymph system. Sugars, amino acids, minerals and water soluble vitamins (B and C) enter the blood by diffusion. Fatty acids and glycerol recombine as fats once absorbed by the villus and pass into the lacteal together with fat-soluble vitamins such as A, D, E and K.

When the products of digestion enter the blood, they are not taken off around the body via the heart. Instead, they travel along the **hepatic portal vein** that carries them to the **liver**.

The liver carries out over 500 different functions within the body. One is to act as a storage/distribution centre, much like giant warehouses located near motorways. The liver stores excess glucose as a carbohydrate called **glycogen**. It also stores fats, fat-soluble vitamins and minerals such as iron. The liver distributes the nutrients to cells when they are required. This role of the liver in sorting, utilising and distributing necessary metabolic chemicals is known as **assimilation**.

3.5 Digestive malfunctions – possible causes and effects

Irritable bowel syndrome (IBS)

The symptoms of IBS occur when the muscles of the gut and especially the colon alter their normal rhythms. The result can be alternating bouts of constipation and diarrhoea. Other symptoms are abdominal pain, a bloated feeling, indigestion and increased flatulence or wind.

The cause of IBS is not yet understood, though there may be dietary triggers including alcohol, carbonated drinks, caffeine, chocolate, fried food and processed food. Stress is also considered a contributory factor.

Gallstones

Gallstones form in the gallbladder due to an imbalance in the composition of bile. High levels of cholesterol and bilirubin (produced by the liver) result in the formation of crystals that grow to form gallstones ranging in size from specks to pebbles. These stick in the bile duct causing pain and discomfort. Pain is most intense as more bile is released after a fatty meal. Some individuals will feel sweaty and nauseous and may vomit.

There is no specific reason for getting gallstones but a number of risk factors have been identified. These include being female, overweight, over 40 years old, having existing liver damage, IBS and a family history of gallstones.

Coeliac disease

Coeliac disease is an autoimmune disease. This is when our immune system mistakes our own body tissues as being harmful and is activated to destroy them. In coeliacs, a protein from wheat called gluten triggers an immune response that results in the villi of the ileum wall being destroyed. The flattening of the villi and associated inflammation results in reduced absorption of nutrients.

Gluten is found in bread, pasta, cereals, cakes and biscuits, and is used as a thickening agent in processed food. Vigilance and accurate food labelling is required for coeliacs to avoid ingesting gluten.

The effects of coeliac disease are abdominal pain, bloating, flatulence, diarrhoea, fatty stools and weight loss due to the poor absorption of nutrients. This can also lead to secondary conditions such as anaemia and osteoporosis.

As with IBS the causes are not fully understood. The condition tends to run in families and a childhood infection of the gut may trigger the condition later.

3.6 Monitoring, treatment and care needs for digestive malfunctions

> ### 🔑 KEY TERMS
>
> **Ultrasound** – using high-frequency sound to generate internal images of structures within the body. Echoes from the objects are interpreted by a computer.
>
> **Lithotripsy** – using high-frequency sound waves to vibrate apart solid objects like gall stones.
>
> **Endoscopy** – inserting a microscopic light source and video camera at the end of a long flexible tube through either end of the gut. Images are relayed to a screen.
>
> **Biopsy** – a sample of tissue that is taken from the body for examination under a microscope.

> ### ❓ THINK ABOUT IT
>
> #### Case study: Eva
>
> Eva has been diagnosed with IBS. She enjoys meeting her friends for coffee and at fast food outlets after a busy working day. She is also studying in the evenings. Once a week she goes clubbing. She has been advised by her GP to keep a food diary and to examine her lifestyle. It has also been suggested that she take up yoga. He also prescribed some medication.
>
> 1 Why should Eva keep a food diary?
> 2 Suggest how Eva might change her lifestyle.
>
> #### Case study: Lisa
>
> Lisa has been diagnosed with gallstones, as were her mother and aunt. She has a BMI of 36 and is in her 50s. Her gallstones were diagnosed by using **ultrasound** and she was treated using **lithotripsy**. She has been advised to lose weight.
>
> 1 What factors support the likelihood of Lisa having gallstones?
> 2 What is lithotripsy and how does it work?

Case study: Anjie

Anjie developed acute abdominal pains in her 20s. She noticed she was losing weight. Her GP referred her to a specialist who arranged for an **endoscopy** examination and **biopsy**. The results showed that her intestinal wall had damaged and flattened villi. Blood tests confirmed that she had coeliac disease. She was referred to a dietician and given mineral and vitamin supplements.

1 What is endoscopy? How would it have been used on Anjie?
2 What advice would the dietician give to Anjie? What are the difficulties in following this advice?

LO4 Understand the musculoskeletal systems, malfunctions and their impact on individuals

4.1 Structure of bone

Bone is a living, growing and developing tissue requiring supplies of oxygen and nutrients. The **musculoskeletal system** provides us with the means of support and movement.

A typical bone has a shaft of **compact bone** with enlarged spongy ends arranged in thin irregular sheets or **trabeculae**. Underneath lie **growth plates** which, until we reach late adolescence, are responsible for bone growth in terms of our height. However, bone growth and activity continue throughout life. Within the centre of the bone shaft is the **bone marrow** which is the site of blood cell production and where stem cells can be found. These cells can develop into any type of cell. The ends of bones that articulate with a neighbouring bone are covered in a protective layer of **cartilage**.

While developing in the womb our skeletons are made of this tough but springy cartilage. Proteins called **collagen** and **chondrin** remain in our bones after birth, helping to give them a little elasticity. Cells called **osteoblasts** gradually invade the cartilage of the early skeleton, depositing mineral salts such as **calcium phosphate**.

Once they have deposited their minerals the osteoblasts become known as **osteocytes** and help maintain the bone as it forms and increases in size.

Another type of cell – the **osteoclast** – removes bone by using enzymes to dissolve the bone salts. This occurs when we take up a new physical activity: osteoclasts work with osteoblasts to re-sculpt our skeleton.

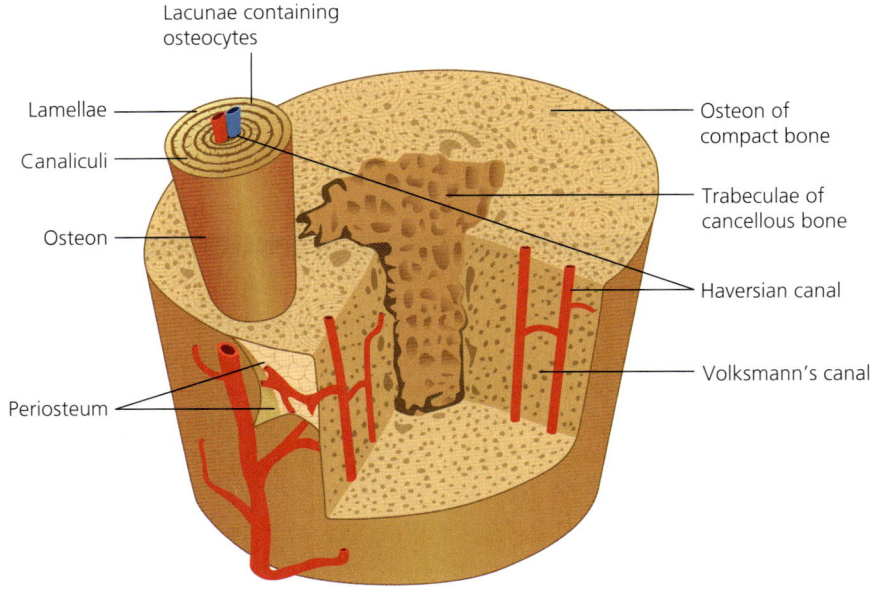

▲ **Figure 4.11** Structure of bone

Normally these two bone-forming and bone-removing cells work in harmony, but the osteoblasts are influenced by **oestrogen** levels. This female hormone promotes the activity of osteoblasts but after the menopause in women levels of this hormone drop and the balance swings in favour of the osteoclasts, so bone becomes thinner and more like a honeycomb. Thus in older age bone becomes more brittle and can result in the condition **osteoporosis**. While osteoporosis can occur in men it is more common in women because of the oestrogen effect.

4.2 Types of joint

Table 4.4 Types of joint

Joint type	Example/location
Ball and socket	Hip, shoulder
Hinge	Knee, elbow
Pivot	Skull on vertebral column
Sliding/gliding	Wrist, ankle
Saddle	Thumb
Fixed	Cranium, pelvis

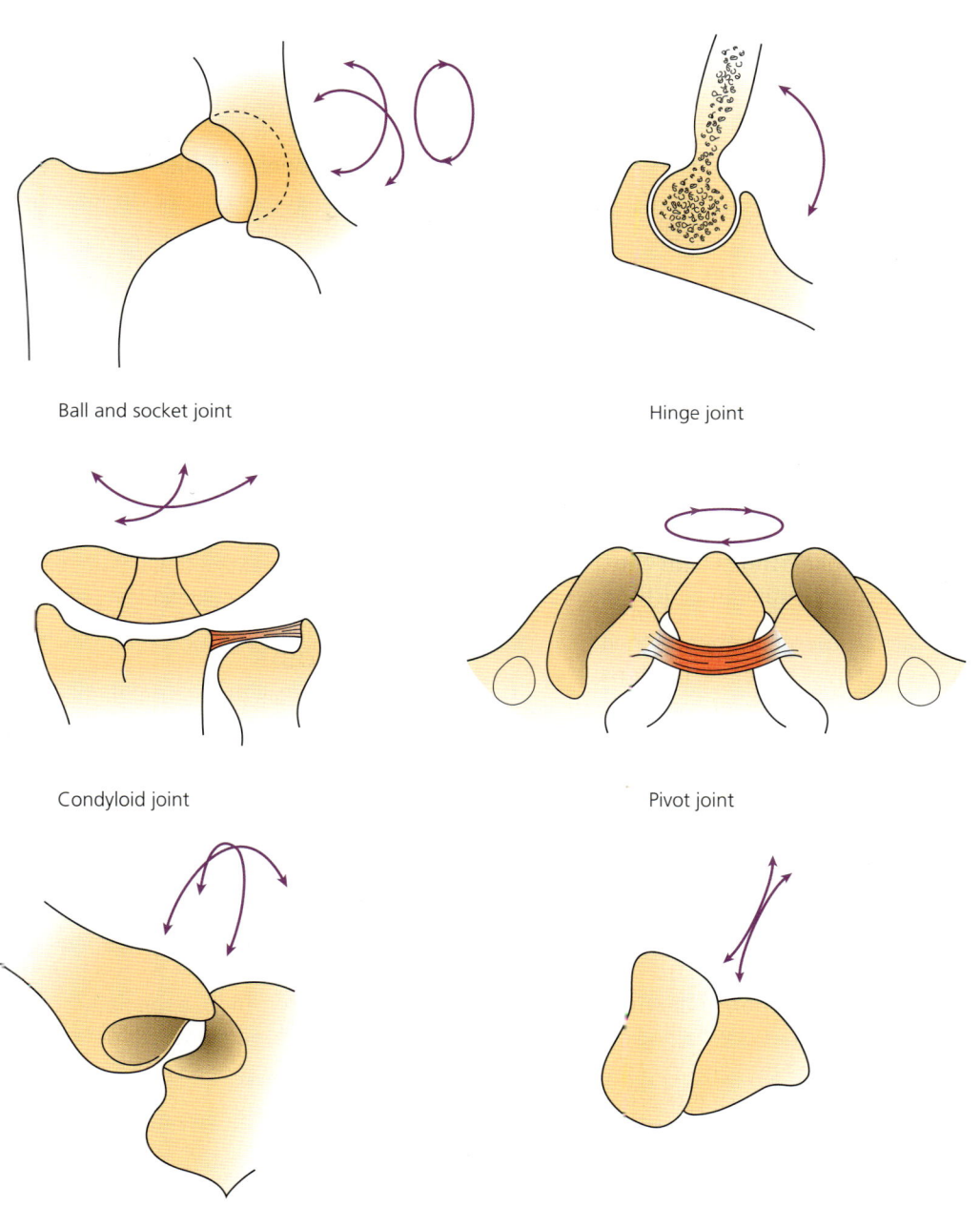

Ball and socket joint

Hinge joint

Condyloid joint

Pivot joint

Saddle joint

Gliding joint

▲ **Figure 4.12** Types of synovial joint

4.3 Components of a synovial joint

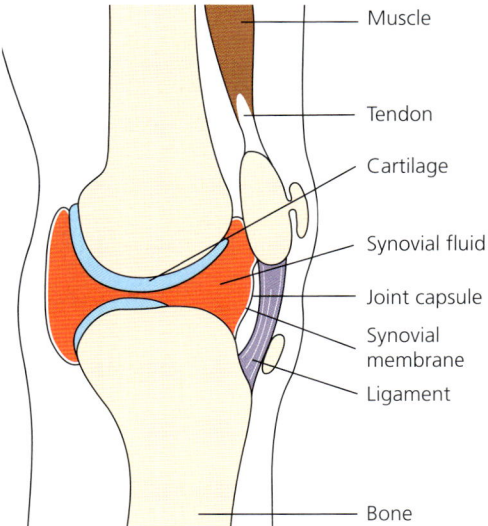

- Muscle
- Tendon
- Cartilage
- Synovial fluid
- Joint capsule
- Synovial membrane
- Ligament
- Bone

▲ Figure 4.13 The knee joint is a synovial joint

A typical synovial joint is the hinge joint of the elbow. The two bones of the lower arm articulate with the humerus bone of the upper arm. Tough cords called **ligaments** hold the bones in position with tough membranes known as the **synovial capsule**. This capsule produces and contains a thick slippery **synovial fluid** that acts as both a lubricant and shock absorber. The ends of each bone are further protected by tough smooth **cartilage**. It is the erosion of this cartilage and decrease in synovial fluid that allows the bones to make contact with one another, resulting in the pain and inflammation of arthritis.

Muscles that allow arm movement are attached to the humerus, radius and ulna bones by **tendons** – another type of fibrous tissue made of connective tissue.

4.4 Muscle action around a joint

Skeletal muscles are made up of muscle cells or fibres consisting of two types of protein that can slide past each other using energy supplied by ATP. The sliding makes the muscle fibres shorten, contracting the muscle. These proteins cannot slide back in the opposite direction to increase the muscle length again. Instead they must be pulled out by the action of another muscle as it **contracts**. The original muscle is said to be in a state of **relaxation**. This means muscles can pull but not push. Skeletal muscles therefore have to work in pairs that bring about opposite actions (**antagonistic** pairs).

We can relate this to elbow joints. To raise the forearm, the biceps muscle contracts while its antagonist – the triceps – relax. To straighten the arm, the opposite occurs – the biceps relax while the triceps contract.

Tendons allow muscles to operate at a distance from a bone. Waggle your fingers and you will observe 'lines' moving beneath your skin – these are the tendons allowing your fingers to move. After a while, fatigue in your wrist will confirm that this where the muscles operating your fingers are located – not in your hand.

4.5 Musculoskeletal malfunctions – possible causes and effects

Arthritis

There are two main forms of arthritis – osteoarthritis and rheumatoid arthritis.

Osteoarthritis affects the smooth cartilage usually of the hands, spine, knees and hips. The cartilage erodes, allowing the bones to make contact, resulting in pain, inflammation and restricted movement. Repeated movement throughout life can increase the development of this condition and so is often the result of sports such as athletics, rugby and rowing, and manual occupations such as building, farming and roofing.

Rheumatoid arthritis is an autoimmune disease where antibodies produced by the immune system attack the linings of joints such as those found in the hands, wrists and feet, causing pain and swelling. This inflammation causes further damage, resulting in a breakdown of both bone and cartilage. The exact cause is not known but risks factors are being female (suggesting that oestrogen levels are involved), a family history of the condition and being a smoker.

Osteoporosis

In some individuals the natural thinning of bones as we age is accelerated and results in the symptoms of osteoporosis. As bone loss is linked to falling levels of oestrogen, the condition is associated with post-menopausal women, but men can develop this condition, particularly those with lower levels of testosterone, and young people can develop it, especially if they are anorexic.

As there is no pain, unless it is tested for, often the only warning is a fracture. As the bone thins, fractures become more common, especially of the wrist, hip, ribs and vertebrae of the spine. Sometimes a sudden cough or sneeze can fracture a rib.

This pronounced thinning of bone can be linked to rheumatoid arthritis, COPD, the long-term use of steroids, a family history and poor absorption in the gut, as a consequence of coeliac disease for example. Smoking and high alcohol consumption also increase the risk of developing osteoporosis.

4.6 Monitoring, treatment and care needs for musculoskeletal malfunctions

❓ **THINK ABOUT IT**

Case study: Ahmed

Ahmed is a retired builder in his 60s. His passion is gardening on his allotment but severe osteoarthritis in his knees and hands is making bending, kneeling, walking and carrying difficult. His GP has prescribed medication and has referred him to a specialist for possible knee surgery.

1 Suggest the medication that the GP may have prescribed.
2 How could the extent of the arthritis in Ahmed's knees be diagnosed?
3 What surgical intervention could be carried out on Ahmed? How will this affect him in both the short and long term?
4 Research the aids and support available to those with arthritis. Produce an advice leaflet for Ahmed and those like him.

Case study: Preya

Preya is in her late 60s and has a BMI of 28. After a fall that resulted in her fracturing her hip she has been diagnosed with osteoporosis. Her GP has prescribed her medication and has made some lifestyle suggestions.

Mya, her daughter, who is in her 30s, is concerned that she too may develop the condition in later life.

1 Suggest the medication that the GP may have prescribed. What is its role?
2 What suggestions might the GP have made regarding her diet and lifestyle?
3 How might Mya minimise the possibility of also developing the condition later in life?
4 Some doctors recommend putting post-menopausal women on **hormone replacement therapy (HRT)** partly to prevent osteoporosis. What are the risks of this strategy?

LO5 Understand the control and regulatory systems, malfunctions and their impact on individuals

5.1 Components of nerve systems

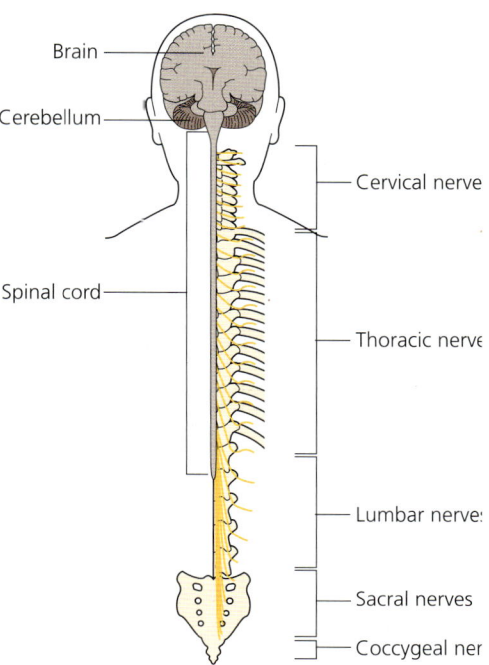

▲ **Figure 4.14** Major nerves of the spinal cord

Our nerve system consists of two integrated systems or networks – the voluntary and involuntary systems.

The voluntary system consists of **peripheral** nerves spreading out from the **brain and spinal cord** – known together as the **central nervous system** or CNS. The peripheral nerves travel, for example, to and from our skin and muscles. These nerves contain two types of nerve cell – **sensory neurons** that carry messages from sense organs such as pain receptors in the skin to the CNS, and **motor neurons** that carry messages from the CNS to tissues such as muscles.

The involuntary or **autonomic** system is made up of two further networks of nerves – the **sympathetic** and the **parasympathetic** systems. Normally we are not aware of using these nerves but they play a vital role. The sympathetic system prepares us for action by activating functions needed for survival and suppressing less important activities. The parasympathetic system is an antagonist – it does the opposite – damping down the sympathetic and restoring the body to its normal 'resting' state.

Table 4.5 The autonomic nerve system

Parasympathetic nerves: rest and digest	Sympathetic nerves: fight or flight
Constrict pupils	Dilate pupils
Stimulate saliva	Inhibit salivation
Slow heartbeat	Increase heartbeat
Constrict airways	Relax airways
Stimulate stomach	Inhibit activity of stomach
Inhibit release of glucose; stimulate gallbladder	Stimulate release of glucose; inhibit gallbladder
Stimulate intestines	Inhibit intestines
Contract bladder	Relax bladder
Promote erection of genitals	Promote ejaculation and vaginal contraction

Some of these nerves have their origins in the brain and are referred to as cranial nerves; many others branch out from the spinal cord and are known as spinal nerves.

5.2 Structure and function of the brain

Our brain has many areas yet to be fully understood. It is made up of two halves – the **cerebral hemispheres** – that are connected by a bridge of nerve tissue known as the **corpus callosum**.

The left side of the brain connects with the right side of the body and vice versa. This swapping over by the nerve cells occurs in the corpus callosum. Individuals tend to have one side of the brain more dominant.

The cerebral hemispheres are folded with deep crevices that increase the size of the brain but allow it to fit into the cranium of the skull. The outside of the brain is protected by a triple layer of tough membranes called the **meninges**.

The outer few millimetres of the upper cerebral hemispheres form the **cerebral cortex**. This area has been extensively mapped with precise functions allocated to various areas. Essentially this area is where sensory information is received from various areas of the body and corresponding actions are sent to the muscles of the body. These areas can become damaged as a result of a head injury or a stroke, resulting in the loss of specific senses or actions.

The **frontal lobe** has many functions including emotions, decision making, speech, language, conscience and memory. Being at the front of the brain, it can be damaged relatively easily, altering ability and personality.

The **cerebellum** sits at the back, tucked beneath the cerebral hemispheres. This relays signals to the muscles allowing us accuracy and dexterity of movement.

It also acts as a memory of muscle actions and allows the rapid repetition of learnt actions such as playing a musical instrument. It is also involved in balance as that is maintained by many precise muscle actions. This region is affected by alcohol which explains the loss of co-ordination and balance of someone who is drunk.

Between the frontal lobes and the cerebellum lies a small area called the **hypothalamus** which detects changes in blood chemistry and temperature, regulates our appetite and controls a number of hormones including those which prompt our sexual development and reproduction. Associated with the hypothalamus is a glandular area called the **pituitary body** which releases a number of important hormones.

At the base of the brain as it merges with the spinal cord is a swollen area known as the medulla oblongata or **medulla**. This is the most basic part of the brain controlling vital processes such as swallowing, heart rhythm and breathing.

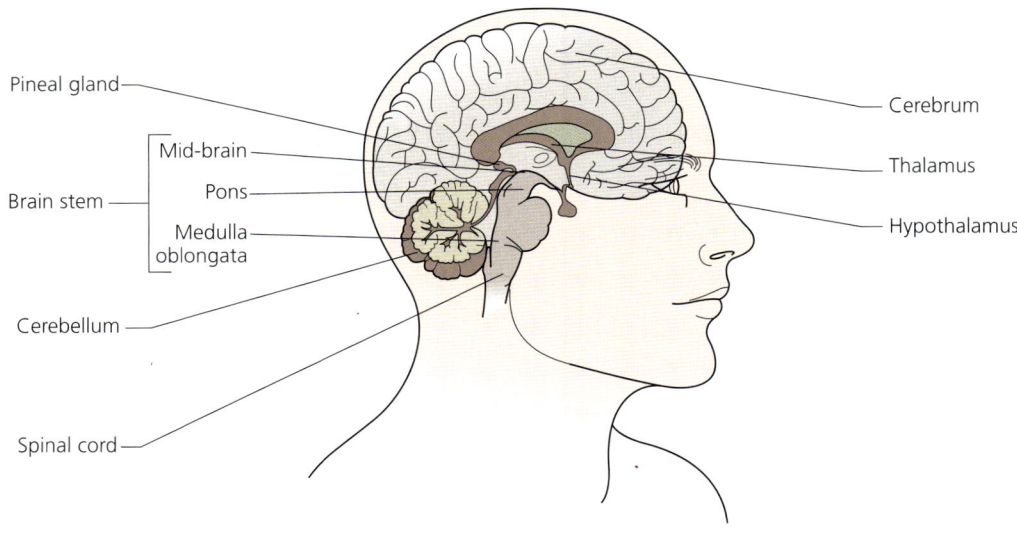

▲ **Figure 4.15** Structure of the brain

5.3 Nerve action

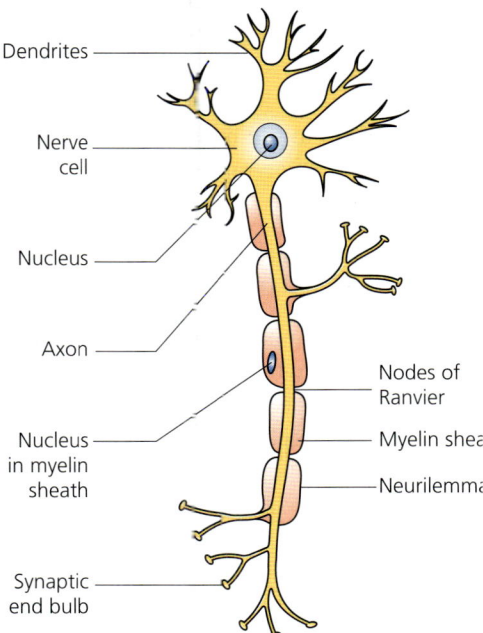

Dendrites

Nerve cell

Nucleus

Axon

Nucleus in myelin sheath

Nodes of Ranvier

Myelin sheath

Neurilemma

Synaptic end bulb

▲ **Figure 4.16** Structure of a neuron

Nerve cells or neurons transmit messages or impulses around the body. The most common types are the motor and sensory neurons. They differ slightly in structure, but their purpose is the same.

A **stimulus** sets off an exchange of chemicals from within and outside a nerve cell across the neuron's cell membrane. This swapping of chemicals sets off a further exchange in the neighbouring area of cytoplasm setting in motion a chain reaction. This can be visualised as a falling line of upright dominoes, where one falls against the next and so on.

Myelin sheath

Most nerve cells have special cells called **Schwann cells** wrapped around them. Collectively these cells make up the **myelin sheath** which can be compared to the plastic insulating layer around an electrical cable.

The myelin sheath speeds up nerve transmission and makes it more effective. Certain conditions, like multiple sclerosis, destroy the myelin sheath and this can have a major impact on the speed and effectiveness of the neural system.

Synapse

There is a microscopic gap called a **synapse** between neighbouring neurons and between neurons and muscle cells. A nerve impulse arriving at a synapse will produce a chemical called a **neurotransmitter** which diffuses across the gap and sets off a new nerve impulse or muscle contraction. Many drugs act on synapses and their neurotransmitters. Some common painkillers work by blocking the synapses of pain-detecting nerve cells.

5.4 Organisation and function of the endocrine system

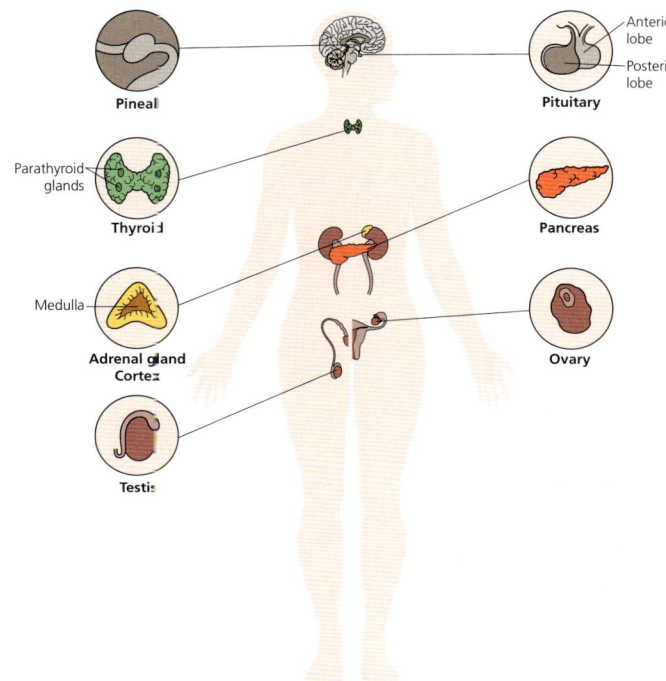

Pineal

Pituitary
Anterior lobe
Posterior lobe

Parathyroid glands

Thyroid

Pancreas

Medulla

Adrenal gland
Cortex

Ovary

Testis

▲ **Figure 4.17** Principal components of the endocrine system

The endocrine system consists of glands that produce **hormones**. Some glands, for example the pancreas, have non-endocrine functions as well.

Hormones are sometimes called chemical messengers. There are many types but they are all carried by the blood from the gland that secretes them to their target organ. They travel throughout the body but only carry out their action when they are 'caught' by specific receptor molecules in the target cell's membrane. In this way each hormone will have a particular effect on a specific tissue.

Some hormones and the glands that produce them are shown Table 4.6.

Table 4.6 Types of glands and their hormones

Endocrine gland	Hormone produced	Action of hormone
Adrenal gland	Adrenalin	Prepares body for action, e.g. increases heart and breathing rates
Pancreas	Insulin	Promotes uptake of glucose by cells so lowering blood sugar levels
	Glucagon	Raises blood sugar levels by converting a carbohydrate store (glycogen) in muscles and the liver into glucose
Thyroid	Thyroxine	Regulates cell metabolism
	Calcitonin	Regulates calcium absorption and use
Pituitary	Somatotrophin	Growth hormone – promotes bone growth
	Prolactin	Initiates production of breast milk
	LH	Both involved in controlling the menstrual cycle
	FSH	
	Oxytocin	Initiates contractions of uterus
	ADH	Triggers uptake of water from the urine in the kidney

5.5 Structure of the kidney

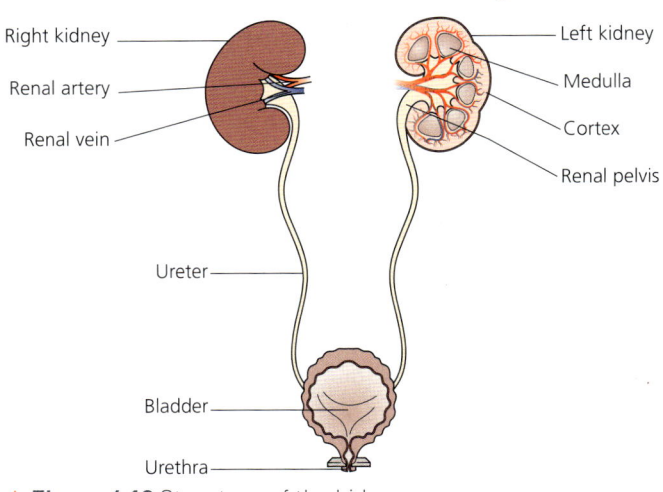

▲ **Figure 4.18** Structure of the kidney

We have two kidneys beneath our digestive system, on each side at the base of our back. Each kidney is connected to the aorta by the **renal artery** that branches many times within the kidney, supplying the working units of the kidney – the **kidney nephrons** – with blood. Blood is returned to the body via the **renal vein** which drains into the inferior vena cava.

Below the kidneys is the **bladder** which stores urine produced by the kidneys. Urine drains from each kidney to the bladder by a tube called the **ureter**.

An outer **cortex** lies above the inner **medulla**. In the centre of the kidney is a fibrous white region called the **calyx**. This collects urine from the nephrons and passes it onto the ureters. The kidney nephron is a complicated twisting tube, divided into special regions that help remove poisonous wastes from the blood as well as helping to control water, salt, pH and blood pressure levels. There are approximately a million nephrons per kidney.

5.6 Functions of the kidney

The kidney has two main functions both carried out by the kidney nephrons.

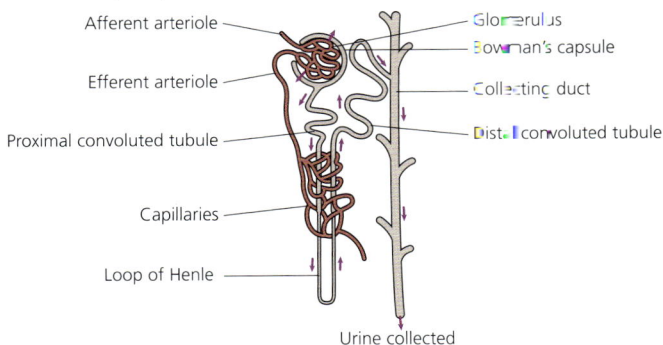

▲ **Figure 4.19** Structure of a kidney nephron

Removal of urea

When we digest proteins, they become amino acids used to build our own proteins. Generally, we have more amino acids than we can use and as we cannot store this excess, they are taken to the liver where they are stripped of a nitrogen-containing portion of the acid. This forms toxic ammonia, which is converted by the liver to a less toxic, but still poisonous, chemical called urea. This passes into the blood and eventually travels to the kidney. One of the vital functions of the kidney is the **removal of urea** from the blood and the body. Parts of each kidney nephron called the glomerulus and Bowman's capsule act like a filter.

The blood vessel draining from the glomerulus is narrower than the one entering it and the result is like putting a thumb over the end of a hose pipe. Blood enters the glomerulus at high pressure and the plasma is forced out through the capillary walls, into the Bowman's capsule. This rapid exit of the plasma is known as **ultrafiltration** and removes wastes, nutrients and water from the plasma, leaving blood proteins and cells behind. Much of what is in this filtrate is needed by the body and so must be taken back into the blood.

This **reabsorption** occurs in the proximal tubule. Here, 95 per cent of the water from the former plasma is reabsorbed, along with glucose, amino acids, vitamins and most mineral salts.

What happens next depends on circumstances. If we need to balance our salt and pH levels, then various elements and compounds may be exchanged or secreted. The main task of the remaining nephron sections is water regulation or **osmoregulation**.

Regulation of water levels

As land animals we have to conserve water, yet we are continually losing it in our urine, faeces, sweat and tears. This loss of water increases the concentration of the blood and if left uncorrected could result in our cells losing water by osmosis, as water diffuses into the now concentrated plasma. This could be lethal. The **hypothalamus** of the brain detects this rise in blood concentration and sends impulses to the neighbouring **pituitary gland**, resulting in the release of a hormone known as **ADH**. This hormone travels all over the body but its target cells lie in the walls of the kidneys' **collecting ducts**.

A specialised blood supply keeps the medulla region of the kidney salty by removing salt from the urine in the loop of Henle. The collecting ducts are also located in this salty medulla. In the presence of ADH, water can pass through the walls of the collecting ducts so water in the urine diffuses out of the ducts, into the salty medulla and from there back into the blood. The result is a return to the correct blood concentration and the production of a concentrated urine.

If we have drunk a lot of water and it is a cool day our blood can become too diluted, which risks our blood and cells taking up water by osmosis, swelling and possibly bursting. Under these circumstances the hypothalamus is not stimulated, the pituitary does not produce ADH and water remains in the urine and is passed to the bladder, making us urinate more.

5.7 Breakdown functions of the liver

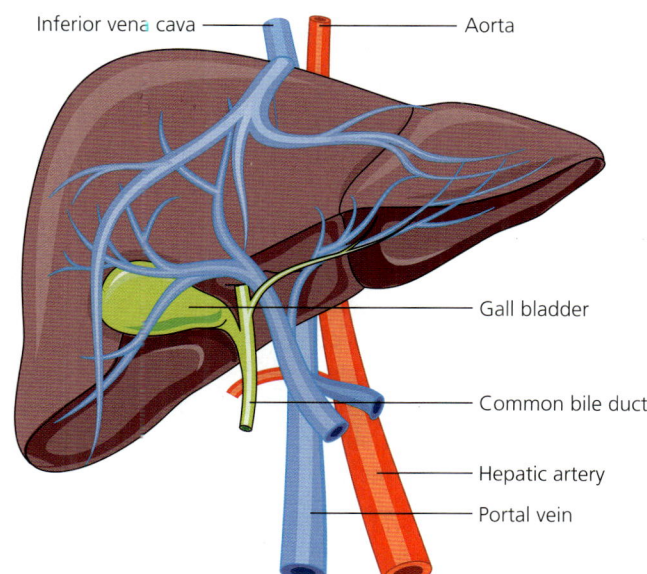

▲ **Figure 4.20** Structure of the liver

The liver performs hundreds of different functions, mostly by just one type of cell.

We have seen that liver cells remove surplus amino acids, resulting in the production of urea. This process is called **deamination**. The remaining amino acid is fed into cellular respiration within the mitochondria of the liver cell, resulting in the production of ATP and heat energy.

Liver cells also remove poisons like alcohol by breaking them down into harmless components. This is a process known as **detoxification**. Drugs such as **paracetamol** are also broken down and if overused will result in liver failure. This is why dosage instructions must be followed exactly.

We have referred to the **production of bile** by the liver and its role in digestion. Bile also allows the liver to remove some poisonous by-products from metabolism. Liver cells **break down and recycle red blood cells**. As these cells lack a nucleus, they have a limited life span of about three months after which the liver breaks them down. As the haemoglobin from the red blood cells is recycled, two poisonous, coloured chemicals are produced – **biliverdin** and **bilirubin** – that pass into the bile and out of the body. They give the characteristic colour to our faeces, which would otherwise be pale. With some forms of liver disease or with obstructions such as gallstones these chemicals cannot pass out in the bile and so pass into the blood instead. This results in a yellow tinge to the skin and the whites of our eyes known as **jaundice**. If not treated, rising levels of biliverdin and bilirubin will cause brain damage and even death.

5.8 The concept of homeostasis

The maintenance of ideal or optimal conditions in the body, as discussed throughout this unit, is known as **homeostasis** and is vital for life.

To maintain homeostasis there has to be some means of **monitoring** to detect any deviation from the optimum and allowing for correction. This is done through **effectors** and **feedback mechanisms**.

An example is the regulation of glucose. Too little glucose results in fainting, coma and death. Too much or wildly fluctuating levels results in glucose being lost in the urine and damage to blood vessels leading to heart and kidney disease, blindness, strokes and amputations as a result of tissue damage, especially in the limbs. A homeostatic mechanism maintains the correct levels.

Within the pancreas and the cells that produce the pancreatic fluids (including the digestive enzymes) are special groups of cells – the **islets of Langerhans**. These contain two types of cell that produce the hormones **insulin** and **glucagon**.

The islet cells detect rises in blood glucose levels after a meal and release insulin. This enables cells to take up glucose from the blood so dropping the level again. Within muscle and liver cells, the absorbed glucose is built up by specific enzymes into a carbohydrate storage molecule called **glycogen**. The resulting decrease in blood sugar level is monitored by the pancreas, and insulin production reduces and stops.

If as a result of normal metabolism and cellular respiration glucose levels drop significantly, the islet cells again detect this change but this time release glucagon. This hormone enters liver and muscle cells and activates enzymes that break glycogen back down into glucose, which exits the cells so raising blood sugar levels again. Upon detecting the rise the pancreas stops the production of glucagon.

5.9 Malfunctions of control and regulatory systems – possible causes and effects

Brain: stroke

Strictly speaking, a stroke is not a malfunction of either the control or regulatory systems but of the cardiovascular system; however, its effects are directed at the brain.

There are two main types of stroke – **ischaemic** and **haemorrhagic**. In the former, clots block a blood vessel in the brain, depriving an area of brain tissue of valuable oxygen and nutrients, causing the cells to die. In the latter, a blood vessel leading to the brain ruptures, cutting off the blood supply. The escaping blood confined by the skull presses down on brain tissue, damaging the cells. Sometimes a blockage can be temporary and clears itself – this is referred to as a **transient ischaemic attack** or TIA.

The symptoms of a stroke include numbness and weakness on one side of the body, one side of the face drooping, speech problems, blurred vision and loss of consciousness. A stroke can occur during sleep so an individual could wake up with the symptoms.

Long-term effects can include difficulties in swallowing, incontinence, memory loss, depression, angry outbursts, mobility issues and fatigue.

CNS: multiple sclerosis

This is an autoimmune disease, where the immune system attacks and destroys the **myelin sheath** of nerve cells, especially within the **central nervous system**. It is not known what triggers this response, but viral, genetic and environmental factors are all thought to play a part. The attacked sections of nerve tissue are replaced by scar tissue that prevents effective nerve transmission. This results in a variety of effects, from tingling sensations and numbness to affected vision and incontinence. Mobility can become difficult and simple tasks become impossible, with fatigue and depression often occurring.

Multiple sclerosis is a complex condition with different forms and severity, and periods of remission followed by relapses. Some individuals continue to lead normal lives for 20 or so years after diagnosis while others are affected more quickly and rely on a wheelchair and external care within a couple of years.

Endocrine: diabetes

There are two types of diabetes – **Type I (early onset)** and **Type II (late onset)**. Type I is thought to be autoimmune, with the **islets of Langerhans** in the **pancreas** being destroyed during childhood or early adulthood. **Insulin** is not produced and so affected individuals have to rely on insulin injections to control their blood sugar levels.

Type II is becoming increasingly common at all ages. This is thought to be linked with our intake of carbohydrates and fats and the resulting weight gain. Either the pancreas stops producing enough insulin or the body's cells lose their ability to recognise and respond to insulin, with the result that glucose remains in the blood. Insulin injections will therefore make no difference.

When blood sugar levels rise, more glucose is passed through the kidney than the proximal tubule can reabsorb, and glucose passes out in the urine and is lost from the body. This leads to sudden drops of blood sugar that can result in **hypoglycaemia** which can cause fainting, coma and death.

These fluctuating blood sugar levels damage and kill blood vessels, resulting in strokes, cardiovascular problems, kidney disease, **retinopathy** (where the blood supply to the retina of the eye is affected, resulting in gradual blindness) and loss of sensitivity in the skin as blood supplies to nerve endings are disrupted. This last effect can result in damage not being noticed and lead to serious infections. These infected areas may become rotten and require limb amputations, often of the lower leg, but some individuals may lose all four limbs.

Kidney: nephrotic syndrome

This rare form of kidney disease is usually a childhood condition that affects both kidneys. It normally responds to treatment but in some cases results in a kidney transplant and lifelong health issues.

In this condition, the immune system overreacts to a common infection, for example a sore throat, and begins to attack parts of the kidney such as the **glomerulus** and the **Bowman's capsule**. In particular, the **basement membrane** of the glomerular capillaries is damaged so blood proteins normally retained in the blood escape into the urine. There is no mechanism within the kidney tubule to reabsorb these and so they are lost in the urine.

Among the blood proteins lost is **albumin**, which is responsible for getting tissue fluid back into veins from capillary beds. As a result, more and more fluid collects in the tissues, causing the body to swell up, straining the heart and lungs.

Other proteins lost are **antibodies** so an individual's ability to ward off infections, for example chickenpox, is compromised. Many of the benefits of childhood vaccinations are lost.

Blood clotting proteins also end up in the urine, resulting in easy bruising and slower blood clotting times.

Cirrhosis of the liver

Liver tissue normally has amazing powers of regeneration. Over two-thirds of the liver can be removed and it will grow back to its original size. This is the only part of the body that can do this. However, as the liver is made up mainly of just one type of cell that carries out most of the liver's functions, it can easily become overloaded. This can be the situation if the cells have to continuously break down alcohol. In these conditions the cells die and do not regrow but are replaced by scar tissue. This is called cirrhosis of the liver and is a sign of long-term abuse of the liver. Eventually the scar tissue becomes so extensive that the liver fails and only an immediate transplant will prevent death.

As the liver cells become affected and replaced, many of the liver's functions become disrupted, resulting in a number of symptoms aside from pain and abdominal aches. Bile begins to build up and passes into the blood instead of into the gut. The bile pigments bilirubin and biliverdin accumulate in the skin and whites of the eyes, turning them yellow (jaundice).

The liver cells make albumin and so when this is disrupted swelling of the tissues or oedaema occurs, as with nephrotic syndrome.

The cells also make some of the blood clotting proteins and the failure of this action results in bruising and vomiting blood from internal haemorrhages, and bleeding onto the brain.

5.10 Monitoring, treatment and care needs for malfunctions of control and regulatory systems

> **? THINK ABOUT IT**
>
> ### Case study: Angela
>
> Angela, who is 72, went into her kitchen to make a cup of tea for her daughter who was visiting. Her daughter heard a crash and found her mother lying on the floor displaying the symptoms of a stroke. An ambulance was summoned and Angela was admitted to hospital.
>
> Three weeks later, Angela still has limited movement on her left side and has difficulties with her speech.
>
> 1 What symptoms might Angela have been displaying when her daughter found her?
> 2 What tests may have been carried out on her arrival at hospital?
> 3 What are Angela's care needs likely to be? How could these be met and by whom?

Case study: Nikita

Nikita, a teacher, suffered bouts of clumsiness, pins and needles in her hands, blurred vision and fatigue. After several months of consultations with her GP and consultants she was diagnosed with multiple sclerosis. Over the next two years her vision and speech deteriorated and she found it increasingly difficult to both stand for long periods and to walk without crutches. She found herself easily confused and her memory became muddled.

1 Why does it often take a long time to diagnose multiple sclerosis?
2 Outline some of the methods used to diagnose or monitor multiple sclerosis.
3 Assess how Nikita's lifestyle may be impacted by her condition.
4 Part of her care plan is physiotherapy. Why?
5 Evaluate possible forms of treatment that may be available for Nikita.

Case study: Anita

Anita has a BMI of 34 and has been diagnosed with Type II diabetes. She has been issued with equipment to allow her to monitor her condition at home. She has been put on medication, has been referred to the diabetic eye clinic and also to a dietician.

1 What lifestyle changes should Anita adopt if she is to avoid being adversely affected by this condition?
2 How will Anita monitor her condition?
3 What is the point of her medication?
4 Why is it so important to attend the eye clinic?
5 Suggest a diet plan that Anita could follow.
6 What might be the impact on her and her lifestyle if she does not take dealing with her condition seriously?

Case study: Tristan

When he was 8 years old, Tristan was diagnosed with nephrotic syndrome. He was put on **steroids**, **diuretics** and **immuno-suppressants**. The steroids made him appear fat. When there were outbreaks of infections such as chickenpox at his primary school he was sent home. Despite taking the medication for two years the condition did not improve and his kidneys failed. He was put on **dialysis** at his nearest renal unit, which was 30 miles from where he lived. He was also placed on the transplant list.

1 What tests would be carried out to identify and monitor his condition? What information would they show?
2 Explain the action of the medication given to Tristan.
3 What might be the impact of taking steroids on his time at school?
4 Why was Tristan sent home from school?
5 What does dialysis involve? How might being on dialysis affect Tristan's lifestyle and that of his family?
6 What are the issues concerned with having a kidney transplant?

Case study: Sergio

Sergio has drunk a lot of high alcohol vodka over many years. Now in his early 40s he has become aware of abdominal pain on his right side. He has noticed the whites of his eyes and skin have become yellow. He also seems to bruise easily. His GP referred him to a liver specialist and he underwent various tests and scans. It was confirmed that he had the beginnings of liver cirrhosis and was recommended to make changes to his lifestyle.

1 What possible tests and scans could be used to diagnose and monitor his condition?
2 Make suggestions as to how Sergio could change his lifestyle to prevent further cirrhosis.

🔑 KEY TERMS

Diuretics – drugs that flush out excess water from the body by increasing urination.

Steroids – drugs used to reduce inflammation brought about by overactive immune systems.

Immuno-suppressants – medication that suppresses the types of white blood cell involved in rejection, slowing down or preventing the destruction of the donated organ. Also suppresses the response to viruses and cancers.

Dialysis – devices used to clean blood of impurities such as urea.

L06 Understand the sensory systems, malfunctions and their impact on individuals

6.1 Structure of the eye

Light is reflected by objects we look at and it travels as rays into our eyes. When we view distant objects, the rays enter our eyes in almost parallel lines and so need little **refraction** or 'bending' to focus them as an image on the light-sensitive surface at the back of the eye – the **retina**. Light from close objects, however, spreads or diverges as it enters the eye and so needs to be refracted more. The eye focuses rays of light onto the retina, which sends nerve messages along the optic nerve to the brain where the images are interpreted.

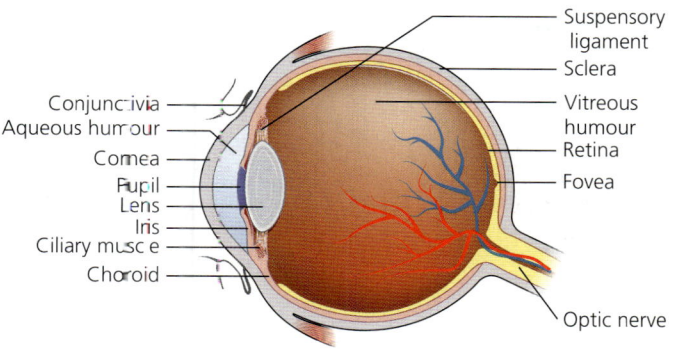

▲ Figure 4.21 Structure of the eye

The eye is a tough capsule filled with both watery and jelly like fluids – the **humours** – that keep the eye in shape and help nourish it. The outside is protected by a tough layer called the **sclerotic coat**. This is the part we see – the 'white' of the eye. At the front of the eye the outer layer is transparent to allow the light to enter. This is the **cornea** and is itself protected by a membrane – the **conjunctiva**. This outer layer is kept moist by tears produced by the tear glands. Tears contain salts, lubricants and ant bodies to defend against infection.

The amount of light that enters the eye is controlled by the **iris** – a pigmented ring of muscles. The opening in the middle through which light passes is the **pupil**. The iris causes the pupil to constrict (dilate) in bright light or open up to allow maximum light through in dim light.

Behind the pupil is the **lens**. Almost spherical and crystalline, it is attached to a ring of **ciliary muscles** by the **suspensory ligaments**. The ciliary muscles can contract to stretch the lens, making it flatter and thinner. Relaxing the muscles allows the elastic lens to return to its fatter, more spherical shape.

Light entering the eye is refracted by the conjunctiva and cornea and then further refracted and focused by the lens. When viewing far objects, the lens is stretched into a thinner shape that will refract less. However, if reading or working at a close distance, the light needs more refraction and so the lens relaxes into its spherical form. Unfortunately, as we age we lose elasticity throughout our bodies so the lens may not fully return to its original shape, affecting our eyesight. This is why it is common to require reading glasses as we grow older.

The retina contains the light-sensitive cells – the **rods** and **cones**. These are connected to nerve cells which exit the eye by the **optic nerve**. Where the optic nerve leaves the eye there are no rods or cones and we cannot detect light if it falls on this region – the **blind spot**.

Rods are more sensitive to light and so we use them in darker conditions and to give us early warning – when we see something 'out of the corner of our eye'. They are distributed around the sides of the retina and share nerve cells.

Cones work in bright light, allowing us to view colours. They connect to individual nerve cells to provide us with precise vision. They are concentrated at the back of the eye in the **macula** and in one small region directly in the centre of the retina – the **fovea** – where there are only cones. When we look closely at something, this is where the light is focused.

6.2 Structure of the ear

The ear's function is not just to hear sound but also to detect motion, orientation and to maintain balance.

Sound waves passing through the air are channelled into the ear by the outside parts of our ears – the **pinnae**. The waves pass down the **external ear** passage and cause the **ear drum** at the end to vibrate. This is allowed to happen as the drum separates another air-filled chamber – the **middle ear** – from the external ear. A small passageway – the **Eustachian tube** – connects the middle ear to the throat and allows the middle ear to be at the same pressure as atmospheric air. This equalising of pressure causes the popping sensation when we change height suddenly; for example, when in an aeroplane. If these two chambers were not at the same pressure the eardrum would not vibrate correctly and could even burst.

Air does not carry sound very well so sound waves have to be amplified by the body's smallest bones, located in the middle ear. These three bones, the **malleus**, **incus** and **stapes**, transmit the vibrations of the eardrum across the middle ear before striking a further membrane – the **oval window**. This is 22 times smaller than the eardrum and so magnifies the intensity of the vibrations.

On the other side of the oval window is the **inner ear** and in particular the **cochlea**. The cochlea contains a jelly-like fluid, the **perilymph**, contained in a coiled tube spiralled like a snail's shell.

Membranes lined with sensitive hair-like structures called the **organ of Corti** are located within the perilymph. A further drum-like membrane – the **round window** – allows vibrations from the oval window to pass through the fluid, rippling the membranes and stimulating the sensitive hairs. These fire impulses to the brain along the **auditory nerve** and are registered by the brain as sounds.

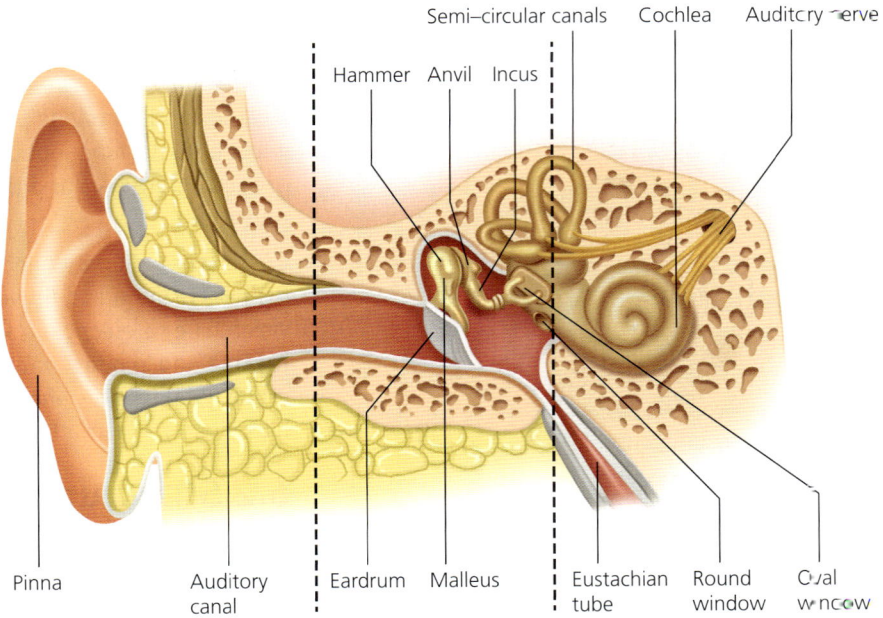

▶ **Figure 4.22** The structure of the ear

Semi–circular canals   Cochlea   Auditory nerve

Hammer   Anvil   Incus

Pinna   Auditory canal   Eardrum   Malleus   Eustachian tube   Round window   Oval window

Further fluid filled tubes (**semi-circular canals**) and swellings (**ampullae**) are connected to the cochlea but are not involved in hearing. In these tubes, movement of the fluid results in messages being sent to the brain that give us information on orientation and movement. To help this, microscopic granules called otoliths press against the sensitive hairs if we alter our position or rate of movement. This is vital in helping us maintain balance both when stationary and when moving.

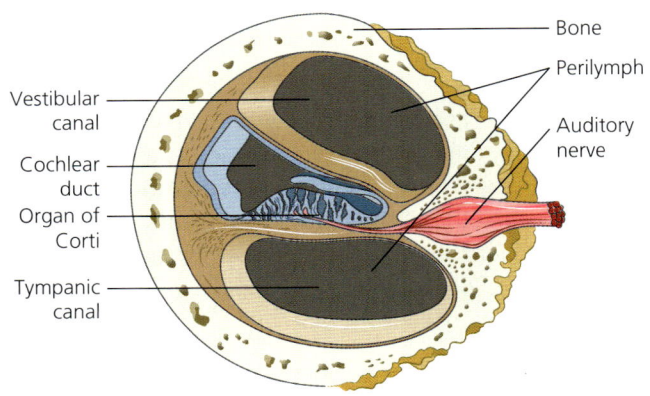

Bone
Perilymph
Vestibular canal
Auditory nerve
Cochlear duct
Organ of Corti
Tympanic canal

▲ **Figure 4.23** Structure of the inner ear

6.3 Malfunctions of eye and ear – possible causes and effects

The eye

Cataracts

Cataracts are very common. They are cloudy patches that develop in the lens of the eye and can cause blurred or misty vision as they stop some of the light from reaching the retina. Over time, the cataracts start affecting vision. Many people with cataracts will eventually need surgery to remove and replace the affected lens. While there are a number of causes for cataracts, most are linked to lifestyle choices, for example smoking, although changes in the lens appear to be more common as people age.

Glaucoma

Glaucoma can affect sight, usually due to build-up of pressure within both eyes. Glaucoma develops when the aqueous humour fluid cannot drain properly and so the pressure inside the eyeball increases. This can damage the optic nerve by pressing down on the nerve fibres of the retina.

There are a number of contributing factors, for example genetics and high blood pressure, but age is the most common. A progressive deterioration of vision will result if not treated.

Age-related macular degeneration (AMD)

AMD is a painless eye condition that results in the loss of central vision, usually in both eyes. Vision becomes increasingly blurred, so reading becomes difficult colours appear dull and faces are difficult to recognise. AMD doesn't affect peripheral vision so it will not cause complete blindness.

There are two main types of macular degeneration – dry AMD and wet AMD. Dry AMD develops when the cells of the macula become damaged by a build-up of deposits called drusen. It is the most common and least serious type of AMD. Vision loss takes many years to develop. However, some people with dry AMD will develop wet AMD when abnormal blood vessels form underneath the macula and damage its cells. This form is more serious than dry AMD and faster to develop. Without treatment, vision can deteriorate within days.

Retinopathy

Diabetic retinopathy is a common complication of diabetes. It occurs when high blood sugar levels, an effect of diabetes, damage the cells of the retina. To work effectively, the retina needs a constant supply of blood from tiny blood vessels. Over time, a continuously high blood sugar level can cause the blood vessels to narrow and leak. This damages the retina and stops it from working. If it isn't treated, it can cause blindness. With increasing numbers of people being diagnosed with Type II diabetes each year this is a problem that can easily be avoided by close monitoring and maintaining a healthy lifestyle to manage the diabetes.

The ear

Deafness

Some people are born without hearing but most cases of deafness are the result of an illness, for example meningitis or an injury to the head, repeated exposure to loud noises or simply growing older.

Hearing loss can occur suddenly but usually develops gradually. It is the result of sound signals not reaching the brain along the auditory nerve. There are two main types of hearing loss, depending on where the problem lies.

- **Conductive hearing loss** – when sounds are unable to pass from the outer ear to the inner ear usually because of a blockage, such as earwax or a build-up of fluid from an ear infection, or because of a perforated ear drum or disorder of the hearing bones. These can become fused and so cannot pass the sound across the middle ear.
- **Sensorineural hearing loss** – caused by damage to the sensitive hair cells of the organ of Corti in the inner ear or damage to the auditory nerve.

It is possible to have both types of hearing loss, known as mixed hearing loss.

6.4 Monitoring, treatment and care needs for malfunctions of the eye and the ear

> **? THINK ABOUT IT**
>
> **Case study: Pendy**
>
> Pendy has regular eye tests and it was at one of these that cataracts were identified in each eye. She was monitored until she reached a point where her vision was deteriorating. She had an operation on one eye and then a week later on the other eye. She had to apply eye drops for several weeks to reduce the chance of infection. She noticed an improvement in vision almost immediately.
>
> 1 What happens during a cataract operation?
> 2 What effect might cataracts have on an individual's life before and after the operation?
>
> As well as cataracts being detected as a result of her regular eye tests, Pendy was also diagnosed as having the early signs of glaucoma. She was found to have an eye pressure twice that of normal. Her peripheral vision was examined by flashing random pin pricks of light into the eye and asking her to press a button when she saw a flash. Her optic nerve was examined and photographs taken of her retina. She has to use eye drops each evening, which over time dilate the tiny drainage channels of the eye.
>
> 3 How is eye pressure determined?
> 4 Why are photographs taken of the retina?
> 5 Pendy's children, all in their 40s, can have free eye tests. Why is this?
>
> 6 Why should regular use of eye drop medication reduce the likelihood of developing glaucoma?
> 7 If an individual with glaucoma does not have it diagnosed early, how may their life be affected and what aids and support may they then benefit from?
>
> **Case study: Roy**
>
> Roy is now in his 70s. When he was 55 he noticed that his central vision was deteriorating – objects that he was looking at directly were initially blurred, but after a number of months started to disappear. At first only his left eye was affected but within a few years his right eye was also affected and he had to stop driving and rely on his wife and friends to get around. By the time he was 60 the condition had progressed rapidly and he had to give up many of his interests and reading became difficult. He often didn't recognise people he knew. Eventually he had to use a white stick which he found embarrassing at first. Two years later his wife died, leaving him to live and manage alone.
>
> His dry AMD progressed to wet AMD and his vision worsened. He uses medication in the form of eye drops and has received laser surgery. He has given up smoking, eats a healthy diet rich in green vegetables and has reduced his alcohol intake.

With the help of his eye specialist, Roy registered himself as severely sight impaired. This enabled him to access support through charities and from social services.

1 What is the point of the laser surgery and Roy's lifestyle changes?
2 Identify appropriate charities that can support individuals with impaired eyesight.
3 Produce a presentation package on the support Roy could receive from relevant charities and social services, indicating any aids or strategies that might help maintain Roy's independence.

Case study: Hardeep

Hardeep is in his early 40s and is overweight. His job involves long hours sitting at a desk and he enjoys takeaways, fast food and fizzy drinks. A routine visit to his doctor showed that he had high blood pressure, high cholesterol and his blood sugar levels indicated signs of early diabetes.

He was told to lose weight, take exercise and eat a healthy diet. The doctor told him he would be contacted by the diabetic eye clinic and that it was very important to attend. He was told that the NHS Diabetic Eye Screening Programme aims to reduce the risk of vision loss in people with diabetes due to retinopathy. Anyone diagnosed with diabetes is invited for screening once a year.

1 What is retinopathy and how is it diagnosed?
2 Why are regular eye examinations so important?
3 How might retinopathy impact on Hardeep's life?
4 What is the significance of the lifestyle changes suggested to Hardeep?

Case study: Megan

Megan, now aged 27, contracted meningitis at 3 years old. This left her with almost total hearing loss. She wore **hearing aids** as a child and when at secondary school her teachers used radio microphones that transmitted to an amplifier with earphones that Megan wore. Megan did not like using this system as she said it emphasised her condition. She learnt to lip read and, with those equally proficient in its use, sign language. At the age of 16 she had **cochlear implants** fitted and this revolutionised her life.

1 What are cochlear implants?
2 What sort of deafness is Megan most likely to have?
3 Produce a leaflet or information pack for individuals with impaired hearing, outlining the aids and support available for them.

🔑 KEY TERMS

Hearing aid – small digital or analogue amplification device worn in or behind the ear(s) to magnify sounds.

Cochlear implant – a small electronic device that detects sounds and sends impulses to the brain.

Read about it

BMA (2004) *A–Z Family Medical Encyclopaedia*, Dorling Kindersley.

Fermie, P. and Shepherd, S. (2013) *Family Health Encyclopaedia*, Anness Publishing.

Useful websites

Heart: www.bhf.org.uk

Coeliac: www.coeliac.org.uk

IBS: www.theibsnetwork.org

www.diabetes.org.uk

Multiple sclerosis: www.mssociety.org.uk

Asthma: www.asthma.org.uk

Cystic fibrosis: www.cysticfibrosis.org.uk

Kidney: www.kidney.org.uk

Liver: www.britishlivertrust.org.uk

Arthritis: www.arthritis.org.uk

Osteoporosis: www.nos.org.uk

Visual impairment: www.rnib.org.uk

Hearing loss: www.actionhearingloss.org.uk

Unit 4: Assessment practice

Below are practice questions for you to try.

1

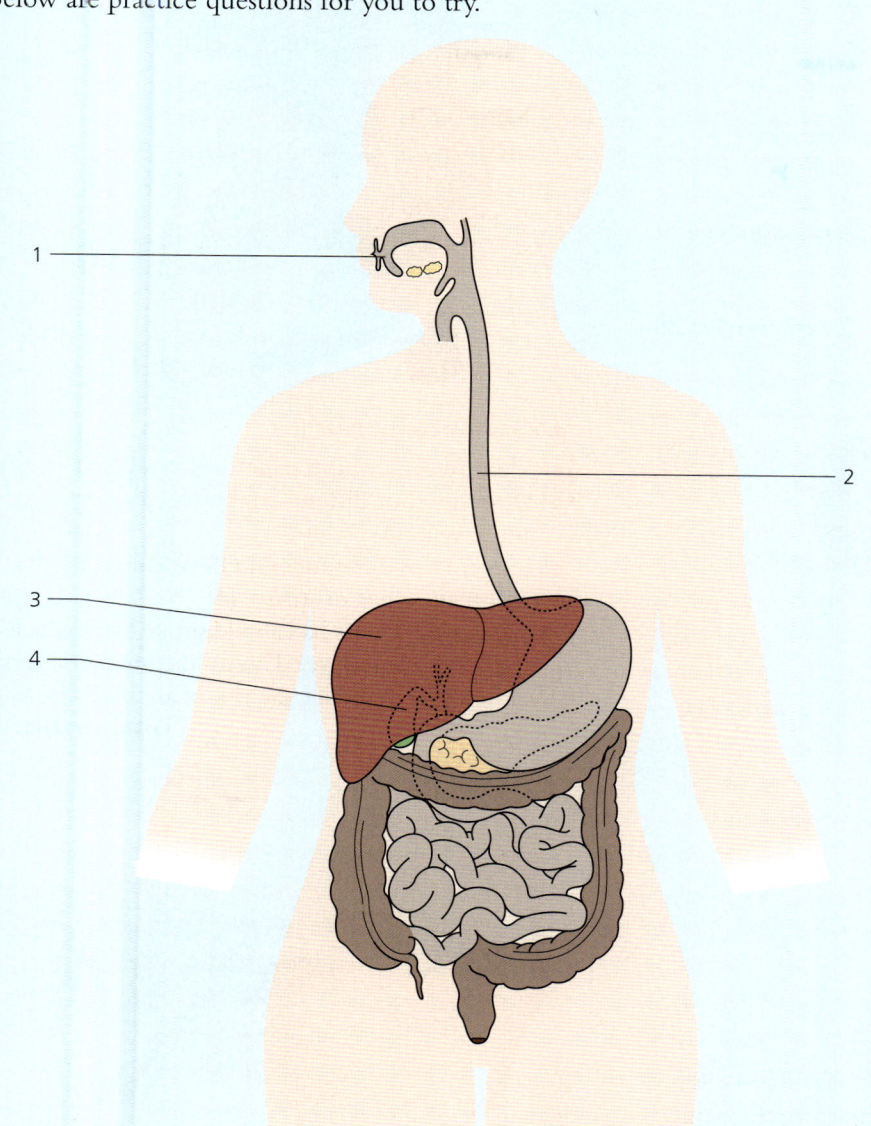

▲ **Figure 4.24** The digestive system

a) Identify the structures labelled 1–4. (4)

b) Describe **two** functions of each part of the digestive system given below. (8)
  i) Stomach
  ii) Pancreas
  iii) Small intestine
  iv) Rectum

c) Lily has been diagnosed with irritable bowel syndrome (IBS). Discuss actions she could carry out to minimise the effects of this condition. (8)

Total marks: 20

2
a) Describe **one** function of each of the following structures.
  i) Pituitary gland
  ii) Motor neuron
  iii) Synapse
  iv) Myelin sheath (4)
b) Trevor, aged 72, has severe osteoarthritis. Explain how Trevor's arthritis could be monitored and treated. (6)
c) Analyse how Trevor's everyday life could be affected by his arthritis. (10)

Total marks: 20

3

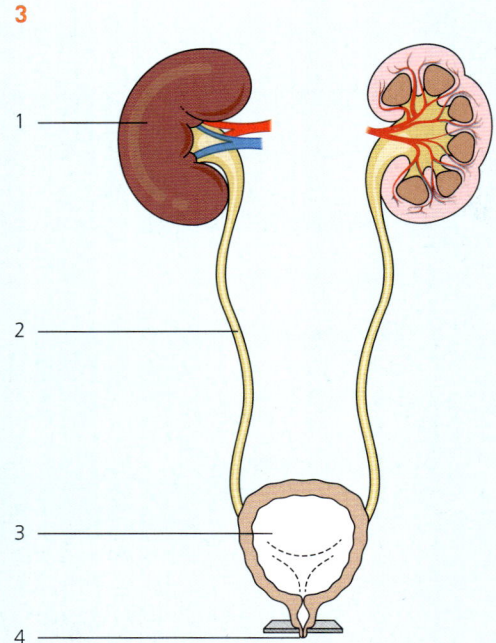

a) Name each of the structures labelled 1–4. (4)
b) Explain the role of the following structures in the production of urine by the kidney.
  i) Glomerulus
  ii) Bowman's capsule
  iii) Proximal tubules (6)
c) Piers, 14, has had nephrotic syndrome for five years. Medication has not worked and he is now on dialysis awaiting a possible transplant. Evaluate the use of dialysis and transplants for someone like Piers. (10)

Total marks: 20

4

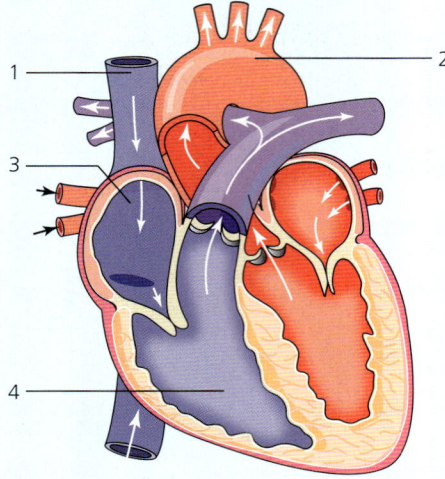

▲ **Figure 4.26** The heart

a) Identify each of the structures labelled 1–4. (4)
b) Describe four differences between an artery and a vein. (4)
c) Explain the difference in effect caused by the two main types of stroke. (4)
d) Silvia, aged 73, has had a mild stroke from which she has recovered well. Discuss the measures Silvia should take to reduce the risk of another stroke. (8)

Total marks: 20

5

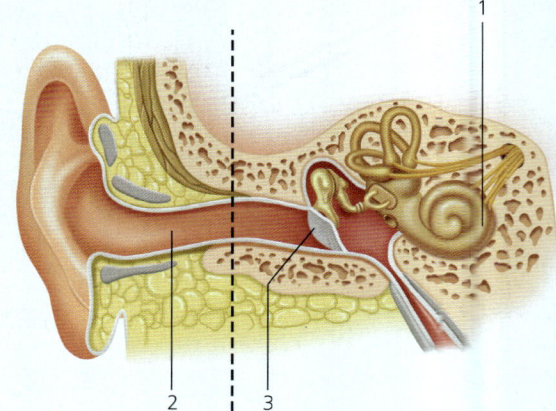

▲ **Figure 4.27** The ear

a) Identify each of the structures labelled 1–3. (3)
b) What is the function of part X? (1)
c) Veronica is severely visually impaired and has to rely heavily on her sense of hearing. Explain the roles played by parts 3, A, B, C and X from the diagram in allowing Veronica to hear. (5)
d) The reason for Veronica's impaired vision is that she has had diabetes for many years and has developed retinopathy as a result. Explain the link between diabetes and retinopathy. (2)
e) Summarise Veronica's possible care need. (8)

Total marks: 20

Unit 05
Infection control

ABOUT THIS UNIT

Infection control is very important for good health, especially in large organisations such as hospitals, schools and residential homes where an outbreak of an infectious disease can affect hundreds of people, sometimes causing death.

In this unit you will learn about the risks associated with poor infection control and the legislation that aims to keep the public free from infections. You will examine the chain of infection and the methods for controlling its spread. You will also learn about the importance of the health and social care worker in keeping the spread of infection to a minimum.

LEARNING OUTCOMES

The topics, activities and suggested reading in this chapter will help you to:

1 Understand infection control in health and social care
2 Know the chain of infection
3 Be able to control the spread of infection
4 Understand the role of the health and social care worker in controlling infection

How will I be assessed?
You will be assessed through a series of assignments and tasks set and marked by your tutor.

How will I be graded?

You will be graded using the following criteria.

Learning outcome	Pass assessment criteria	Merit assessment criteria	Distinction assessment criteria
You will:	To achieve a **pass** you must demonstrate that you have met all the pass assessment criteria	To achieve a **merit** you must demonstrate that you have met all the pass and merit assessment criteria	To achieve a **distinction** you must demonstrate that you have met all the pass, merit and distinction assessment criteria
1 Understand infection control in health and social care	**P1** Describe common terms in relation to infection control and their meanings	**M1** Evaluate the effectiveness of legislation in supporting infection control in health and social care	
	P2 Explain how risks associated with poor infection control are different for different health and social care environments		
2 Know the chain of infection	**P3** Describe sources of infection		
	P4 Outline the ways in which infection can be transmitted from one body to another		
3 Be able to control the spread of infection	**P5** Demonstrate methods used to prevent the spread of infection	**M2** Explain why a number of methods of preventing the spread of infection might be required in health and social care settings	**D1** Analyse the effectiveness of immunisation in controlling infection
	P6 Describe why standard precautions for infection control should be maintained at all times	**M3** Explain why infection control remains important when caring for the deceased	
	P7 Explain the purpose of protective clothing in controlling the spread of infection		
4 Understand the role of the health and social care worker in controlling infection	**P8** State a range of methods of monitoring to ensure adequate cleaning		**D2** Analyse the role of the health and social care worker in infection control where the individual refuses to comply
	P9 Describe how a health and social care worker should manage themselves to prevent the spread of infection		
	P10 Explain the importance of following policies and procedures to ensure effective infection control	**M4** Explain the purpose of policies and procedures in promoting good standards of infection control	

LO1 Understand infection control in health and social care *P1 P2 M1*

(15 minutes)

Jayne has been on a cruise and has just returned home. While she was away her father had a heart attack and is now in hospital. Since she returned, Jayne has been vomiting and has had diarrhoea and she thinks she may have norovirus as some of the other passengers were confined to their cabins with this complaint.

Should Jayne go to the hospital to visit her father? What advice would you give her?

1.1 Definition of infection control

The World Health Organization (WHO) defines infection control as:

'Infection prevention and control measures [that] aim to ensure the protection of those who might be vulnerable to acquiring an infection both in the general community and while receiving care due to health problems, in a range of settings. The basic principle of infection prevention and control is hygiene.'

(Source: www.who.int)

Epidemiology is the study of public health; that is, determining frequency, patterns, sources and other aspects of health of populations – for example, the number of cases of meningitis or diabetes in a population, but also the relationship of that number to the size of the population. The resulting rate allows epidemiologists to compare disease occurrence across different populations. This can be related to microbiology (the study of bacterial, viral, fungal and parasitic organisms) that cause infections in bacterial epidemics like the measles outbreak due to fewer people vaccinating their children in the UK, or determining the factors involved in the Ebola outbreaks in Africa in 2015. It also involves working on plans to control the spread of the outbreak, and prevent exposure to minimise the risk of spreading.

1.2 Common terms and their meanings in relation to infection control

> **KEY TERM**
>
> **Infection** – the process of bacteria or viruses invading the body and making someone ill or diseased.

1.3 Health and social care environments where infection control is important

Patients receiving health and social care are at risk of developing **infections** as a result of their compromised state of health, underlying medical conditions, or as a result of contact with health care interventions such as surgery, diagnostic testing or invasive (using instruments inside the body) devices.

One of the key clinical priorities for hospitals and residential care is to protect their patients, visitors and staff from the risk of health care-associated infections (HCAIs) caused by bacteria (germs). This is in accordance with the requirements of the Code of Practice on the prevention and control of infections and related guidance under the Health and Social Care Act 2008 ('the hygiene code').

In March 2012, NICE produced guidelines, Healthcare Associated Infections: Prevention and Control in Primary and Community Care, laying out infection prevention and control measures that should be taken by all health care workers. It applies to care in the community, such as in general practices (GP surgeries) or residential care settings, as well as in patients' homes or domiciliary care.

The guidelines state that, as a minimum, any health care workers in these settings should be educated about standard principles of infection prevention and control. They must also be trained in hand decontamination, the use of personal protective equipment, and the safe use and disposal of sharps.

The Public Health Agency Guidance on Infection Control in Schools and other Childcare Settings advises these settings to prevent the spread of infections by ensuring routine immunisation, high standards of personal hygiene and practice, particularly handwashing, and maintaining a clean environment.

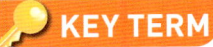

KEY TERM

Hygiene – conditions or practices that help to maintain health and prevent disease, especially through cleanliness to reduce the spread of germs.

The best way of preventing infection spreading in the home or anywhere is to keep the hands clean by washing frequently with warm water and soap. Hands can pass an infection on and can pick up germs from one place and transfer them to another.

You can read more about keeping health and social care settings safe and healthy in Unit 3.

1.4 Risks associated with poor infection control

The spread of disease

Poor infection control is responsible for health care-associated infections (HCAIs) that can develop either as a direct result of health care interventions, such as medical or surgical treatment, or from being in contact with a health care setting. The term HCAI covers a wide range of infections including those caused by methicillin-resistant *Staphylococcus aureus* (MRSA) and *Clostridium difficile* (*C. difficile*). HCAIs pose a serious risk to patients, staff and visitors as they are easily spread from one person to another. They can incur significant costs for the NHS and cause morbidity (likelihood of **disease**) to those infected. As a result, infection prevention and control is a key priority.

KEY TERM

Disease – a disorder or incorrectly functioning organ, part or body system in a human especially one that produces specific symptoms or that affects a specific location and is not simply a direct result of physical injury.

INDEPENDENT RESEARCH ACTIVITY

Go to:

www.cruisecritic.co.uk/articles.cfm?ID=71

Read the information about the outbreak of norovirus on board a cruise ship. What advice is given about how to avoid coming down with the virus? Norovirus is sometimes called the 'cruise ship' **virus**, explain why.

KEY TERM

Virus – tiny organisms that may cause illnesses in humans ranging from flu or a cold to life-threatening conditions like HIV/AIDS. They cannot grow or multiply on their own and need to take over a human or animal cell to help them multiply.

Ill-health

HCAIs are infections that are acquired as a result of health care and directly affect patients, carers and employers in several ways, such as severe or chronic illness, pain, anxiety, depression, ill-health, longer stays in hospital, reduced quality of life, loss of earnings, even permanent disability and death.

High rates of absenteeism through sickness

It is in the interests of employers to cut the spread of infection by ensuring that the workplace is clean and safe. In hospitals and residential care homes it is particularly important to keep staff free from sickness, as related bed and ward closures and postponed admissions may add to the overall burden. Antibiotic costs may increase if the infection is also due to a resistant micro-organism, as it is more expensive to treat these types of infection.

Death and legal action

Sometimes, poor infection control can lead to patients dying from conditions that are unrelated to the original reason they are in the health care setting. For example, an elderly person may break a hip in a fall but get food poisoning while in hospital and subsequently die. Their family may take legal action against the hospital trust if they believe this death could have been prevented.

1.5 Relevant legislation in relation to infection control

Health and Social Care Act 2012 (and 2008)

The Health and Social Care Act 2008, Revised 2010, introduced a statutory duty on health care providers to observe the provisions of the Code of Practice on Healthcare Associated Infections (see Figure 5.1). The purpose of the Code of Practice was to help NHS bodies plan and implement how they can prevent and control HCAIs.

The Health and Social Care Act 2012 reinforces the 2008 Act but also sets out a clear expectation that the care system should consider NICE quality standards for infection prevention and control, as part of a duty to secure continuous quality improvement.

All providers of health care and adult social care must demonstrate the following measures under the Health and Social Care Act 2008.

Table 5.1 The Code of Practice on healthcare-associated infections (HCAIs) from the Health and Social Care Act

What the registered provider will need to demonstrate
Systems to manage and monitor the prevention and control of infection. These systems use risk assessments and consider how susceptible service users are and any risks that their environment and other users may pose to them.
Provide and maintain a clean and appropriate environment in managed premises that facilitates the prevention and control of infections.
Provide suitable accurate information on infections to service users and their visitors
Provide suitable accurate information on infections to any person concerned with providing further support or nursing/medical care in a timely fashion.
Ensure that people who have or develop an infection are identified promptly and receive the appropriate treatment and care to reduce the risk of passing on the infection to other people.
Ensure that all staff and those employed to provide care in all settings are fully involved in the process of preventing and controlling infection.
Provide or secure adequate isolation facilities.
Secure adequate access to laboratory support as appropriate.
Have and adhere to policies, designed for the individual's care and provider organisations that will help to prevent and control infections.
Ensure, so far as is reasonably practicable, that care workers are free of and are protected from exposure to infections that can be caught at work and that all staff are suitably educated in the prevention and control of infection associated with the provision of health and social care.

Health and Safety at Work Act 1974

This places responsibility on the employer and individual employees to do what is reasonable to adequately control the risks of infection. Under this legislation all employees have the responsibility to co-operate with the employer on matters of health and safety, for example regarding the reduction of risks from HCAIs. Instructions are given on the use of appropriate personal protective clothing (PPE).

Control of Substances Hazardous to Health Regulations (COSHH) 2002

These regulations require employers to prevent or control exposure of employees, service users, visitors, etc. to biological hazardous substances such as micro-organisms at work.

In hospitals and residential care homes, hazards arise from handling clinical waste and soiled laundry, which can be contaminated with **pathogenic bacteria**. Such hazards should be identified and assessed under the provisions of COSHH. Procedures for safe handling, segregation, storage, spillage control and disposal should be laid down and staff trained accordingly. Staff should be protected against hazardous substances they may use in their work activities. Staff in residential care homes and hospitals are particularly at risk from clinical waste, including soiled laundry, so should be trained in safe working procedures and hygiene standards, as well as being provided with appropriate PPE.

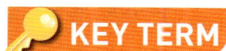

KEY TERM

Pathogenic bacteria – bacteria that can cause infection.

Public Health (Control of Disease) Act 1984

Under this legislation, doctors in England and Wales have a statutory duty to notify a 'Proper Officer' of the local authority if they are aware that, or have cause to suspect that, a patient is suffering from one of the notifiable diseases. The doctor must complete a certificate stating:

- the name, age and sex of the patient and the patient's address
- the notifiable condition that the patient is suspected to be suffering from
- the date, or approximate date, of the onset of the condition
- if the premises is a hospital, the day the patient was admitted, the address of the premises from which they came and whether or not, in the opinion of the person giving the certificate, the condition was contracted in the hospital.

Health Protection (Notification) Regulations 2010

The regulations cover requirements for notification of disease caused by infection or **contamination** by substances including chemicals or radiation, and allow for prompt investigation and response. Some powers, relating to specific circumstances, can be exercised directly by local authorities. In other circumstances, local authorities can apply to a justice of the peace (JP) to impose restrictions or requirements to protect human health.

> ### 🔑 KEY TERM
>
> **Contamination** – to have made something dirty, polluted or poisonous by adding a chemical, waste or infection.

The JP can make an order requiring a person to:

- undergo medical examination (NOT treatment or vaccination)
- be taken to hospital or other suitable establishment
- be detained in hospital or other suitable establishment
- be kept in isolation or quarantine
- be disinfected or decontaminated
- wear protective clothing
- provide information or answer questions about their health or other circumstances
- have their health monitored and the results reported
- attend training or advice sessions on how to reduce the risk of infecting or contaminating others
- be subject to restrictions on where they go or who they have contact with
- abstain from working or trading.

Reporting Injuries, Diseases or Dangerous Occurrences Regulations (RIDDOR) 2013

RIDDOR requires serious work-related accidents and occupational diseases to be reported. The infection must have been definitely acquired at work. Reportable diseases at work include any disease attributed to the exposure of a biological agent at work, e.g. where a worker is exposed to legionella bacteria while conducting routine maintenance on a hot-water service system. Infections that could easily be contracted in the community are not reportable.

Local policy and procedure

All health and social care organisations must have their own policies and procedures based on the legislation related to infection control. There will be common elements across the policies for different organisations and for different parts of the country, but some elements may differ slightly depending on the characteristics of the organisation, e.g. size, purpose.

> ### KNOW IT 💡
>
> 1 Define infection control.
> 2 Explain what is meant by:
>   **a)** pathogenic bacteria
>   **c)** virus
>   **d)** standard precautions.
> 3 Discuss why infection control is particularly important in hospitals.
> 4 Explain the risks associated with poor infection control.
> 5 Choose a piece of legislation and evaluate its effectiveness in supporting infection control in health and social care.

L01 Assessment activities

Below are suggested assessment activities that have been directly linked to the pass and merit criteria in L01 to help with assignment preparation they include Top Tips on how to achieve best results.

Activity 1 – pass criteria *P1 P2*

You are working as a manager in a care home and you have decided to update your policy on infection control. Produce an infection control policy that will inform staff about their responsibilities. Ensure you include:

a) a definition of infection control
b) the meanings of common words that staff might hear in relation to infection control
c) risks associated with poor infection control and how they might differ in your setting to that of other types of health and social care environments that your staff may have worked in.

> #### TOP TIPS
>
> ✔ Ensure you describe what infection control is and why it is important.
> ✔ Remember to compare different approaches to infection control.

Activity 2 – merit criteria *M1*

Write a report to circulate to your staff outlining legislation relevant to infection control in your setting.

> #### TOP TIPS
>
> ✔ Analyse the effectiveness of legislation by separating the information into components and identifying their characteristics. Discuss the pros and cons of the legislation and comment on their implications for practice.
> ✔ Use the internet or other sources to find out more about the legislation.

LO2 Know the chain of infection *P3 P4*

GETTING STARTED

(15 minutes)

Chloe is 18 and started work in a nursery ten months ago. Since starting work she has had one infection after another. She has had several colds, sore throats and tummy bugs. What advice could you give Chloe to stop her picking up bugs?

2.1 Chain of infection

Microscopic living things (germs) are all around us. Some of these germs can cause disease in people.

It is useful to refer to Unit 4, Anatomy and physiology for health and social care, to help you understand how the human body works.

Sources

Bacteria

Bacteria are found almost everywhere, including in and on the human body and lining the digestive system. Most bacteria live in close contact with us and our environment without causing any harm. However, some bacteria can cause disease. Examples of bacterial diseases include streptococcal sore throat, pertussis (whooping cough) and meningococcal disease.

Bacteria are reproduced by binary fission – the single-cell bacterium divides into two identical cells. When conditions are favourable, such as the right temperature and nutrients are available, some bacteria can divide every 20 minutes. This means that in just 7 hours one bacterium can generate 2,097,152 bacteria. After 1 more hour the number of bacteria will have risen to 16,777,216. That is why people can quickly become ill when pathogenic microbes invade their bodies.

Viruses

Viruses are tiny organisms that may cause infectious illnesses, ranging from a cold to life-threatening conditions like HIV/AIDS. The virus particles are 100 times smaller than a single bacteria cell. The bacterial cell alone is more than 10 times smaller than a human cell and a human cell is 10 times smaller than the diameter of a human hair. Viruses by themselves are not alive. They cannot grow or multiply on their own and need to enter a human cell or bacterial cell, attack it and take over its machinery to multiply and grow. An infected cell will produce viral particles instead of its usual products.

Fungi

Fungi can be single-celled or complex multi-cellular organisms and can be found anywhere. A small number of fungi cause diseases in humans including athletes' foot, ringworm and thrush.

Yeasts

Yeasts are also part of the fungi group. They are small, single cells that multiply by budding a cell off from the original parent cell. Yeasts are widely used organisms in genetic studies, for example in cancer research. Other species of yeast such as *Candida* are opportunistic pathogens and cause infections such as a vaginal yeast infection – *Candida albicans* (also called vaginal thrush) – in females who do not have a healthy immune system.

Reservoirs

The reservoir of infection is any human, animal or environmental source where an infectious agent normally lives and multiplies. The reservoir typically harbours the infectious agent and is a source from which other individuals can be infected. The infectious agent primarily depends on the reservoir for its survival. It is from the reservoir that the infectious substance is transmitted to a human or another susceptible host. In humans, micro-organisms can grow vigorously in reservoirs such as blood, skin crevices (folds), throat and nasal passages as well as open wounds.

People

Many common infectious diseases have human reservoirs. Diseases that are transmitted directly from person to person include sexually transmitted diseases, measles, mumps, streptococcal infection and many respiratory pathogens.

Human reservoirs may or may not show the effects of illness. A healthy **carrier** is a person with no signs of infection who is nevertheless capable of transmitting the pathogen to others. Healthy carriers

KEY TERM

Carrier – a person without obvious signs or symptoms of disease who harbours the bacteria or virus, and acts as a vehicle transmitting the pathogen to others.

never experience symptoms despite being infected. Carriers commonly transmit disease because they do not realise they are infected, and consequently take no special precautions to prevent transmission. Symptomatic persons who are aware of their illness, on the other hand, may be less likely to transmit infection because they are either too sick to be out and about, take precautions to reduce transmission, or receive treatment that limits the disease.

Animal

Humans are also subject to diseases that have animal reservoirs. Many of these diseases are transmitted from animal to animal, with humans as incidental hosts, e.g. brucellosis (cows and pigs), anthrax (sheep), plague (rodents) and rabies (bats, dogs, and other mammals). Many newly recognised infectious diseases in humans, including HIV/AIDS, ebola, SARS and avian flu are thought to have emerged from animal hosts.

Environment

Plants, soil and water in the environment are also reservoirs for some infectious agents. Many fungal agents, such as those that cause histoplasmosis, live and multiply in the soil. Outbreaks of Legionnaire's disease are often traced to water supplies in cooling towers, evaporative condensers and air conditioning. For soil pathogens to cause disease, the skin must be broken to allow the pathogen entry into the body.

Food

Foodborne illness (food poisoning) is common yet preventable. Many different disease-causing microbes, or pathogens, can contaminate foods, so there are many different foodborne infections. In addition, poisonous chemicals or other harmful substances can cause foodborne diseases if they are present in food.

There is no single foodborne illness. However, the microbe or toxin enters the body through the gastrointestinal tract, and often causes the first symptoms there, so nausea, vomiting, abdominal cramps and diarrhoea are common symptoms in many foodborne diseases.

> 🔑 **KEY TERM**
>
> **Foodborne illness** – (food poisoning) any illness resulting from contaminated food containing pathogenic bacteria, viruses or parasites, or from chemical or natural toxins such as poisonous mushrooms.

Infection can be reduced by promoting good food hygiene practice in the kitchen.

Water

Water is a non-living reservoir and is the source of infections in countries with poor sanitation and low levels of personal hygiene. As people cannot live without water, some regions with poor sanitation practices can have high levels of faecal contamination in the water. This causes infection to spread via the faecal–oral route of infection. However, there have been instances of infection from contaminated water in the UK.

Way out of body (portals of exit)

To enter another host, pathogens have to find a portal of exit from their current host.

Table 5.2 Common infectious pathogens and their portals of exit

Reservoir	Example of infectious pathogens	Portals of exit
Respiratory tract	Influenza Tuberculosis	Nose or mouth through coughing, sneezing, breathing, laughing, talking, mucous, sputum, phlegm exhaled air
Blood	Human Immunodeficiency virus (HIV) Hepatitis B	Open wounds, needle punctures, non-intact skin, mucous membrane surfaces
Gastro-intestinal tract	Salmonella, *E. coli*, hepatitis A, *Clostridium difficile*	Faeces, vomit, saliva

Methods of transmission

A mode of transmission is necessary to bridge the gap between the portal of exit from the reservoir and the portal of entry into the host. The two basic modes are direct and indirect. Direct transmission is the most common form of transmitting diseases and viruses.

Direct transmission

Direct transmission occurs when disease-causing micro-organisms pass from the infected person to the healthy person via direct physical contact, e.g. by touching, skin to skin contact, kissing, sexual contact, contact with oral secretions, blood or other bodily fluids, or contact with body lesions. This is known as horizontal transmission. Vertical transmission happens when micro-organisms pass from a mother to her unborn baby through the placenta. German measles and HIV can be passed this way.

Table 5.3 Examples of infectious diseases spread by horizontal transmission

Type of contact	Bacterial disease	Viral disease
Kissing	Bacterial meningitis	Herpes (cold sores) Glandular fever
Touching	Bacterial gastro-enteritis	Chickenpox
Sexual intercourse	Syphilis, gonorrhoea	HIV Hepatitis B

Indirect transmission

Indirect transmission occurs when there is no direct human-to-human contact. An infectious agent is deposited onto an object or surface (fomite) and survives long enough to transfer to another person who touches the object, e.g. telephones, computer keyboards and mice, door knobs and handles, tables, beds, cups, dishes, taps and sinks can spread infection, as can soiled towels, bedding and clothing from the infected person. This is known as vehicle-borne transmission as it involves an object carrying the disease-causing micro-organism.

Vectors (agents that act as a vehicle for spreading the infection), such as mosquitoes, flies, mites, fleas, ticks, rodents or dogs, can also spread infection.

Table 5.4 Examples of vehicle-borne infections

Vehicle	Bacterial disease	Viral disease
Droplets in air	Tuberculosis (TB)	Colds, flu
Food	Salmonella food poisoning	Hepatitis A
Water	Cholera	Polio
Sharp objects (e.g. needles)	Tetanus	HIV

Airborne

Indirect contact infections spread when an infected person sneezes or coughs, sending infectious droplets into the air. If healthy people inhale the infectious droplets, or if the contaminated droplets land directly in their eyes, nose or mouth, they risk becoming ill. Droplets generally travel between 3 and 6 feet and land on surfaces or objects including tables, door knobs and telephones. Healthy people touch the contaminated objects with their hands, and then touch their eyes, nose or mouth.

Ingestion

Micro-organisms enter the body through eating or drinking contaminated food and water. Inside the digestive system (usually within the intestines) these micro-organisms multiply and are shed from the body in faeces. If proper hygienic and sanitation practices are not in place, the micro-organisms in the faeces may contaminate the water supply. Fish and shellfish that swim in contaminated water may be caught for food.

If the infected individual is a food handler, then inadequate handwashing may result in food being contaminated with micro-organisms.

Injection

The diseases most frequently transmitted through unsafe injection practice are hepatitis B, hepatitis C and HIV/AIDS. In addition, unsafe injections can cause abscesses and lead to septicaemia. Less frequently, haemorrhagic fevers and malaria can also be transmitted.

Inoculation

Live inoculations should not be given if the person has a weakened immune system. This is because live vaccines contain a weakened form of the virus they are supposed to protect against. There is a danger of infection from any live vaccination as some of the virus is excreted from the body in bodily fluids, so thorough handwashing is needed.

Person at risk

Some people are more at risk of picking up infections than others, either because of where they work or their physical condition.

People in contact with infection

Health care workers in the NHS are at risk of infection. While clinical staff are probably most at risk, as they have direct contact with the patients through nursing, there are potential risks to other staff who come into contact with patients or soiled or infected material.

People with underlying illnesses

The immune system protects the body from harmful bacteria and other organisms. Cancer and its treatment can weaken the immune system, putting people with cancer at a higher risk of infection in a number of ways.

- Some cancers, especially lymphomas and leukaemia, may stop the bone marrow from producing enough healthy white blood cells, which work to fight off infections.
- Chemotherapy and radiotherapy can reduce the number of white blood cells the bone marrow produces.
- Surgery creates a break in the skin, which can make the person more prone to infection.

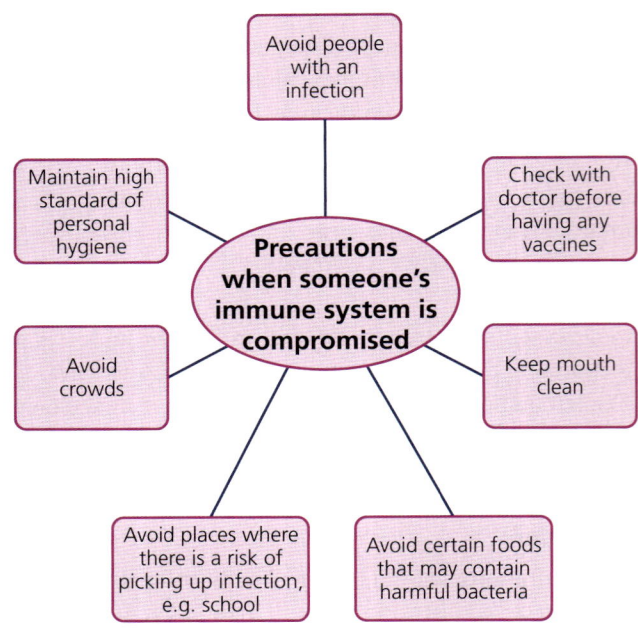

▲ **Figure 5.1** Avoiding infection when the immune system is compromised

Diabetes

Having diabetes increases the risk of infection and diabetics tend to have more serious infections than people without diabetes. Diabetes type I is an autoimmune disease where the cells of the immune system attack the cells in the pancreas. This means that the immune system is less able to cope with additional infections. In addition, the high concentration of sugar in the cells of the body and bloodstream increases the growth of bacteria in the body (as the bacteria will have more access to sugar that they use to grow). Urinary tract infections (UTIs) and infections in the feet are particularly common in diabetics.

Very young and very old

Babies and young children get infections such as colds because they have no immunity to the hundreds of different viruses as they have never had them before. Gradually they build up immunity and get fewer infections.

Advanced age can also weaken the immune system, which is why infections such as influenza can cause death in the very old.

People on certain medications

Steroids can increase the risk of infections and are often used alongside chemotherapy to treat cancer.

Way into the body (portals of entry)

A portal of entry is the site through which micro-organisms enter the susceptible host and cause disease/infection.

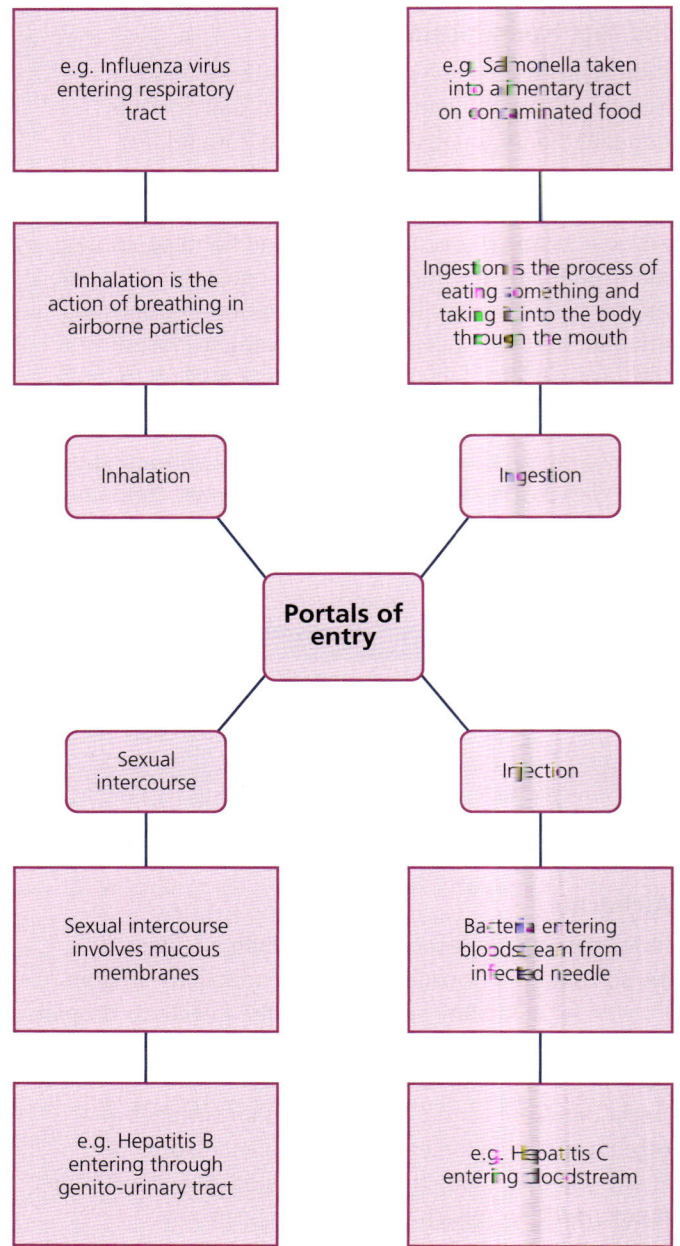

▲ **Figure 5.2** Portals of entry into the body

LO2 Assessment activity *P3 P4*

Below is a suggested assessment activity that has been directly linked to the pass criteria in LO2 to help with assignment preparation; it includes Top Tips on how to achieve best results.

Prepare a presentation for a group of care workers which will:

a) describe sources of infection
b) outline the ways in which infections can be transmitted from one body to another.

TOP TIPS

✔ Ensure you provide detailed information and present it in a way that care workers can easily understand and apply.
✔ Make sure you check your work for typos and grammatical errors.

LO3 Be able to control the spread of infection *P5 P6 P7 M2 M3 D1*

GETTING STARTED

Read:

http://tinyurl.com/m5qbmco

Explain how personal protective equipment (PPE) helped to bring the ebola virus under control.

3.1 Eradicate the source of infection

In the UK, persistent application of hygiene, sanitation, **environmental control**, vector control and vaccines has led to the eradication (removal) of infectious diseases such as cholera, typhoid, polio and dysentery. It is difficult to eradicate all sources of infection, but it is possible to control the spread of infection by following simple hygiene practices such as thorough handwashing.

The chain of infection refers to the way germs are spread (see Figure 5.3). All steps in the chain need to occur for germs to spread from one person to another. By breaking the chain, infections can be controlled and prevented.

The germ spreads from the source
There are three main ways germs can be spread: by infected droplets in air; by germs in bodily fluids; or by tiny airborne particles

The germ has a source
A person picks up germs directly from an infected person or from the environment

The germ infects another person
If a germ comes in contact with another person, it may enter the body though the nose, ears, eyes, genitals or a patch of broken skin

▲ **Figure 5.3** The chain of infection

Breaking the chain of infection by targeting one or more links can stop its spread. This usually involves:

1 eradicating the source of infection through appropriate antimicrobial treatment (using substances that kill or inhibit the growth of pathogenic micro-organisms)
2 preventing the spread through handwashing, hygiene, disposal of waste, decontamination of equipment etc.
3 protecting the individual at risk by immunisation
4 preventing microbes from entering the body by wearing protective clothing, using an aseptic technique when handling invasive devices, covering wounds and insertion sites with sterile dressings etc.

3.2 Preventing the method of spread

Most doctors would recommend that good practice in preventing the spread of infections includes the ill person staying at home.

Handwashing

Handwashing regularly and thoroughly is the most important method of preventing infection and cross-infection.

The purpose of handwashing is to remove or destroy any bacteria picked up on the hands. Bacteria and viruses can easily be spread by touch and picked up from contaminated surfaces, objects or people, then passed on to others. Effective hand decontamination – either by washing with soap and water or with an alcohol-based hand-rub – is recognised as crucial in reducing avoidable infection.

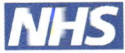

▶ **Figure 5.4**
Handwashing technique with soap and water (Source: NHS)

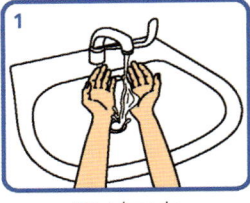
Wet hands with water

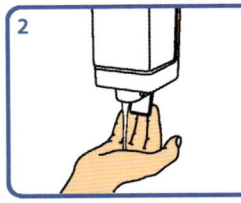
Apply enough soap to cover all hand surfaces

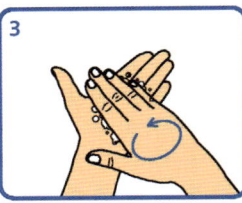
Rub hands palm to palm

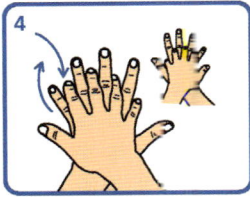
Rub back of each hand with palm of other hand with fingers interlaced

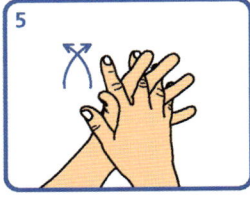
Rub palm to palm with fingers interlaced

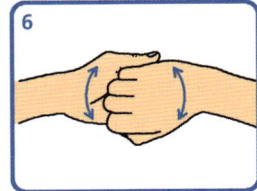
Rub with back of fingers to opposing palms with fingers interlocked

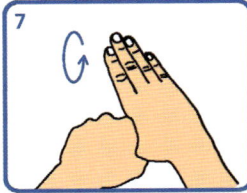
Rub each thumb clasped in opposite hand using a rotational movement

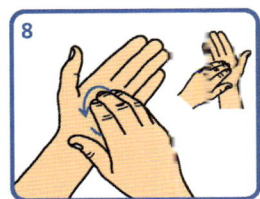
Rub tips of fingers in opposite palm in a circular motion

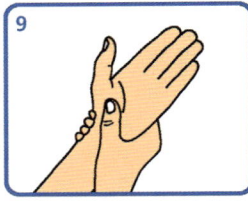
Rub each wrist with opposite hand

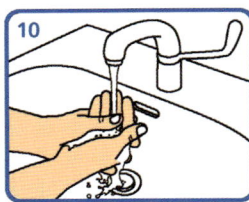
Rinse hands with water

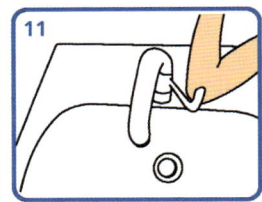
Use elbow to turn off tap

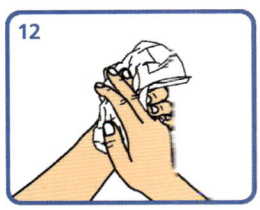
Dry thoroughly with a single-use towel

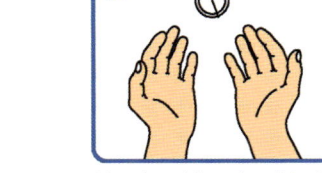
Handwashing should take 15–30 seconds

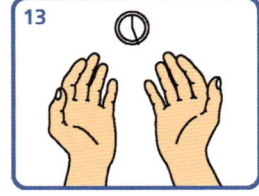

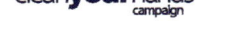
cleanyourhands campaign

NHS
National Patient Safety Agency

Adapted from World Health Organization *Guidelines on Hand Hygiene in Health Care*

(20 minutes)

Examine Figure 5.4. Do you use the correct method of washing?

Wash your hands the way you would normally. Then use a hand inspection cabinet to see if your hands are really clean. You may be surprised to find your hands are not as clean as you thought. Now wash your hands again following the steps in Figure 5.4 and retest in the cabinet. Is there a lesson to be learned here?

Now visit:

http://tinyurl.com/grdh4og

How could this information be used to encourage people to wash their hands?

Personal hygiene

Keeping clean is essential for good health. Poor hygiene can cause skin complaints and infections, and be a source of discomfort and low self-esteem.

Washing uniform

Uniforms must be clean. The Royal College of Nursing advises that there must be sufficient uniforms provided to enable freshly laundered clothing to be worn for each shift or work session, with access to spare clothing if clothing becomes contaminated (for example, splashed with blood and/or body fluids). They also suggest that uniform fabrics must withstand water temperatures of at least 60°C and tumble drying.

Tying up long hair

Loose hair can spread bacteria, which could cause infection. Cross-infection could occur if hair is allowed to trail into body fluids when a carer is cleaning up a patient. Besides this, loose long hair would get in the way of many tasks; for example, giving out food on the ward – patients could find a hair in their lunch.

Disposal of waste

The management of health care waste is essential to ensure that health and social care procedures do not pose a risk of infection. Clinical waste is defined as waste produced from health care that poses a risk of infection or that may prove hazardous.

Using correct colour waste bags/sharps bins

Clinical waste has to be separated into different containers for disposal that indicate how hazardous or infectious it might be. A colour coding system (see Table 5.5) indicates what is in each container and how it needs to be disposed of to prevent the spread of infection either to the people handling the waste or to the environment. For example, if highly infectious waste were to be sent to a landfill site instead of to an incinerator the material could leak into the water table, polluting rivers and sewers and causing disease.

Table 5.5 Colour coding of waste containers/plastic bags

Colour	Type of waste	Disposal method
Sharps bin with purple lid	Sharps used to administer cytotoxic or cytostatic (used in the treatment of cancers) and medicinal products	Incineration
Red clinical waste bin	Body parts, organs, blood bags, blood preserves	Incineration
Sharps bin with yellow lid	Sharps and syringe bodies with residue medicinal product	Incineration
Yellow waste bags	Highly infectious waste plus anatomical waste from theatres and diagnostic specimens	Incineration
Blue clinical waste bin	Waste medicines, out of date medicines, liquids in bottles, blister packs of pills	Incineration
Orange plastic bags	General infectious waste, soiled dressings and autoclaved laboratory waste	Autoclave (to treat with high temperature steam)
Sharps bin with orange lid	Sharps not contaminated with medicinal products, typically phlebotomy sharps	Either incineration or autoclave
Tiger/yellow and black striped bags	Offensive/hygiene waste, which is not infectious, e.g. nappies or incontinence pads	Recycled, incinerated or landfilled in suitably permitted/licensed facilities
Black plastic bags	General waste such as packaging, plastic containers, tissues, flowers, sandwich wrappings	Landfill or other local general waste disposal method

For the safety of everybody who will handle the waste after it has left the clinical area, the person disposing of the waste must put it in the correct container. Also, as clinical waste is expensive to dispose of, it is essential that no other type of waste is put in with the clinical waste.

Decontamination of equipment

Decontamination describes a range of processes, including cleaning, disinfection and sterilisation, which remove or destroy contamination and therefore prevent infectious agents from reaching a susceptible site in sufficient quantities to cause an infection.

Sterilisation and disinfection

It is important that a distinction between cleaning, disinfection and sterilisation is made and that the correct process is chosen.

- Cleaning is physically removing dirt along with most pathogens using detergents, water and friction. This is necessary for successful disinfection and sterilisation, which will generally be ineffective on surfaces that have not already been physically cleaned.
- Disinfection is a chemical or physical process that kills pathogens and reduces them to a level that does not pose a risk to human health. When applied to the skin this is often referred to as antisepsis. This process does not guarantee the removal of all bacterial spores.
- Sterilisation is a chemical or physical process that removes or kills all pathogens. It usually involves steam, oxygen super radicals or irradiation.

Use of correct equipment

Using the correct colour chopping boards in the kitchen will prevent cross-infection from bacteria spreading from one food to another and help keep track of which food is cut on which board. It is essential to keep raw and cooked foods apart in the kitchen, e.g. raw meat cannot be cut on the same board as cooked meat and vegetables cannot be cut on the same board as raw poultry.

Table 5.6 Colours of chopping boards

Colour of chopping board	Use
Red	Raw meat
Blue	Raw fish
Yellow	Cooked meat
Green	Salad and fruit
Brown	Vegetables
White	Bakery and dairy products

3.3 Protection by immunisation

Any vaccine-preventable disease that is transmissible from person to person poses a risk to both health care professionals and their patients. Health care workers have a duty of care towards their patients, which includes taking reasonable precautions to protect them from communicable diseases.

Vaccination

Immunisation or vaccination has cut deaths from infectious diseases. Vaccines work by stimulating the immune system to produce antibodies (substances produced by the body to fight disease), as though the body has been infected with a disease. This is called 'active immunity'. If the vaccinated person then comes into contact with the disease, their immune system will recognise it and produce the antibodies they need to fight it.

MMR, polio and tetanus

All staff should be up to date with their routine immunisations, e.g. tetanus, diphtheria, polio and MMR. The MMR vaccine is especially important to reduce the ability of staff to transmit measles or rubella infections to vulnerable groups. While health care workers may need the MMR vaccination for their own benefit, they should also be immune to measles and rubella to assist in protecting patients. The Department of Health also recommends the influenza vaccination for carers working with older service users.

INDEPENDENT RESEARCH ACTIVITY

Go to:

http://tinyurl.com/pvbvqxz

Watch the Vaccinations animations part 1 and part 2 on the right-hand side of the page.

Explain what is meant by herd immunity.

3.4 Protective clothing

Personal protective equipment (PPE) is used to protect health care workers while performing tasks that might involve them coming into contact with infectious materials.

Gloves

Disposable gloves are worn when performing or assisting in procedures that involve a risk of contact with body fluids, broken skin, dirty instruments and harmful substances such as chemicals and disinfectants. This includes procedures that involve:

- a risk of being splashed by body fluids (e.g. blood, saliva, sputum, vomit, urine or faeces)
- contact with the patient's eyes, nose, ears, lips, mouth or genital area, or any instruments that have been in contact with these
- contact with an open wound or cut
- handling potentially harmful substances, such as disinfectants.

Aprons

Aprons are not usually needed to carry out day-to-day care, but they will be needed for:

- performing or assisting in a procedure that might involve splashing of body fluids
- performing or helping the patient with personal hygiene tasks
- carrying out cleaning and tidying tasks in the patient's living space, such as bed-making.

Face masks

Face masks are effective barriers for retaining large droplets that can be released from the wearer through talking, coughing or sneezing. They may reduce wound site contamination during surgical or dental procedures. But face masks do not protect the wearer from inhaling small particles, which can remain airborne for long periods of time.

Isolation rooms

Isolation rooms are used to help stop the spread of infection, e.g. viral gastroenteritis, from one person to another. These precautions protect patients, families, visitors and health care workers from the spread of infections. When a patient is placed in an isolation room, a sign on the door reminds visitors and health care workers which isolation precautions are needed. There are two types of isolation.

1 *Source isolation* aims to confine the infectious agent and prevent its spread.
2 *Protective isolation* aims to protect an immunocompromised patient who is at special risk from environmental organisms or those carried by attending staff and visitors.

3.5 Use of aseptic technique and sterile dressings

Aseptic technique is designed to prevent contamination from pathogenic micro-organisms that cause disease. It involves applying the strictest rules and using what is known about infection prevention to minimise the risks of causing an infection. Common settings where the aseptic technique is used include surgeries, clinics and outpatient care.

Sterile materials are those that have not touched a contaminated surface. They are specially packaged and cleaned items that are put on in a way that minimises exposure to germs. It is recommended that wounds with a high risk of infection should be dressed with sterile materials.

3.6 Importance of maintaining standard precautions at all times

Standard infection prevention and control precautions (**standard precautions**) are the minimum infection prevention practices that apply to all patient care, whether or not the patient is known to have an infection, in any setting where health care is delivered. Since examination and medical history alone cannot reliably identify all patients with infections, standard precautions represent a standard of care to be used routinely for all patients.

> ### 🔑 KEY TERM
>
> **Standard precautions** – the minimum infection prevention practices that apply to all patient care, regardless of suspected or confirmed infection status of the patient, in any setting where health care is delivered.

Standard infection control precautions include:

- effective hand hygiene practices
- minimising contact dermatitis following handwashing by using hand cream
- protection of open wounds/skin lesions
- use of appropriate personal protective clothing
- avoidance of sharps injury through safe use and disposal of sharps
- appropriate decontamination of instruments and equipment, including safe management of blood spillage
- maintaining a clean hospital environment
- safe disposal of waste
- safe handling and laundering of used linen.

3.7 Last offices and care of the deceased

'Last offices, sometimes referred to as "laying out", is the term for the nursing care given to the deceased patient which demonstrates continued respect for the patient as an individual.'

(Source: Dougherty and Lister, 2008)

Last offices refers to the care rituals immediately following a person's death that are usually performed prior to viewing of the deceased by relatives. These rituals are often carried out by the nurses that attended the person during their illness and include washing the body, shaving, replacing dentures, tidying the hair, closing the mouth and eyes and dressing the body.

Clear communication regarding the possibility of an infection risk must be maintained between health care staff, mortuary attendants and funeral directors to enable effective infection control measures to be maintained. Standard precautions that would have been taken when the patient was alive should be continued to protect all who handle deceased persons against infections.

Examples of infectious conditions and pathogens in the recently deceased that present particular risks include: tuberculosis, group A streptococcal infection, gastrointestinal organisms, the agents that cause transmissible spongiform encephalopathies (TSEs), such as Creutzfeldt-Jakob disease, hepatitis B and C viruses and HIV.

KNOW IT

1 Explain how handwashing can prevent the spread of bacteria.
2 Explain why it is essential to wash care workers' uniforms at 60°C.
3 Discuss the importance of using the correct colour waste bags or bins.
4 Explain the difference between sterilisation and disinfection.
5 Discuss the advantages of having six different coloured chopping boards for food preparation.
6 Choose two pieces of personal protective equipment and explain how they can protect the care worker.
7 Explain the meaning of aseptic.
8 Discuss the importance of standard precautions.

LO3 Assessment activity

Below is a suggested assessment activity that has been directly linked to the pass, merit and distinction criteria in LO3 to help with assignment preparation; it includes Top Tips on how to achieve best results.

Activity 1

Elziz is a student nurse who is on work placement at a teaching hospital. He is shocked by some of the practices he has noticed over his ten weeks at the hospital. Some staff do not wash their hands properly and do not seem to know about standard precautions. He has observed one member of staff using the same gloves for several patients as well as for a patient in an isolation room. He overheard one of the nurses saying her immunisations were not up to date as she had not had time to go for her booster injections. Elziz has mentioned his worries to his mentor, the staff nurse on the ward, who is keen to improve the practices of the staff. She has asked Elziz to produce a booklet where he:

a) demonstrates methods used to prevent the spread of infection **P5**
b) describes why standard precautions for infection control should be maintained at all times **P6**
c) explains why not just one but a number of different methods of preventing the spread of infection are needed on the ward **M2**
d) explains the purpose of protective clothing in controlling the spread of infection **P7**
e) explains different methods of caring for the deceased and why infection control remains important **M3**
f) analyses the effectiveness of immunisation in controlling infection. **D1**

Write Elziz's booklet, covering these points.

TOP TIPS

✔ Remember that explaining something is to give an account of the purposes and reasons for it. Consider what Elziz would need to say to convince his colleagues to change their behaviour.
✔ Ensure you provide detailed evidence for how to reduce the spread of infection.

LO4 Understand the role of the health and social care worker in controlling infection *P8 P9 P10 M4 D2*

GETTING STARTED

(10 minutes)

Go to:

http://tinyurl.com/lb3un6g

What are the benefits of the staff having their portrait on the front of their PPE?

4.1 Role of worker in maintaining high standards of cleanliness in HSC setting

Following policy and procedures

All staff working in health and social care must have access to a written infection control policy and receive training in infection prevention and control.

The Health and Social Care Act 2008: Code of Practice on the prevention and control of infections and related guidance sets out a number of criteria that should be taken into account when health and social care settings are formulating infection control policies and procedures. In particular, these policies should ensure that:

- procedures are in place for the prevention and control of infections and staff are aware of their role, such as effective hand decontamination procedures, policies on wearing of sterile gloves, use of PPE, dress code, safe use and disposal of sharps
- a person is identified as the infection control lead for the centre, and management systems are in place to ensure infection control issues are dealt with.

All care workers must be aware of their local infection prevention and control arrangements and whom they can contact for advice or guidance in the event of an incident. Many infection prevention and control problems can be resolved quickly if immediate action is taken and advice is received from specialists. All staff have a duty to be aware of, and comply with, their organisation's requirements. All organisations have policies and procedures on cleaning to control infection.

Food hygiene

Level 2 Food Hygiene training is mandatory for anyone preparing and serving meals in any organisation because all foods are potentially hazardous if they are not handled correctly. Good food handling practices minimise the risk of food poisoning. This is especially important in residential care settings where food is being prepared and served to large numbers, and where service users are at particular risk from foodborne illnesses. Food poisoning can cause serious illness and even death, particularly in the elderly. Everyone involved in preparing and serving food must be aware of how to reduce the risk of food poisoning.

Working with individuals who require care and support

Prevention and management of infection is the responsibility of all staff working in health and social care, so it is their duty to ensure that vulnerable people are protected from infection.

Promoting best practice

All health care organisations in the UK must comply with national statutory or regulatory standards for infection prevention and control. All staff need to be aware of their regulatory or statutory requirements to support their employers in meeting and improving the expected standards.

Standard infection control precautions underpin routine safe practice. By applying standard precautions at all times and to all patients, best practice becomes second nature and the risks of infection are minimised.

Explaining procedures

It is useful if the care worker begins by explaining to the patient that they have a written infection control plan, which describes the specific measures the care team has to follow to ensure the safety of both patients and staff.

It is helpful to show patients the PPE that is used during the patient care. For example, gloves are changed for each patient and, in some instances, more than once with the same patient.

Monitoring practice

It is essential to monitor practice in controlling infection to check if the policies and procedures are successful in bringing down the rate of infection in the organisation.

It is good practice for the manager of a care home to produce an annual report on the systems in place for the prevention and control of infection and how these are monitored. The report should contain information on incidents and outbreaks of infection, risk assessment, training and education of staff, and infection control audit and the actions that have been taken to rectify any problems.

Managers should also periodically undertake an assessment of the infection risks in their workplace and ensure that everything is in place to manage those risks. An effective monitoring programme with regular feedback of results to staff is crucial to the development of action plans to reduce HCAIs.

Choice and control

Patients who do not comply with treatment for infectious diseases are likely to fall into one of the following three categories.

- Patients who have capacity to consent to treatment (as defined by the Mental Health Capacity Act section 3) but who refuse to comply with treatment may need to have compulsory admission and detention to hospital to ensure that they are closely monitored under sections 37 and 38 of the Public Health Act. Compulsory medical examination can also be required under section 35 of that Act. Compulsory treatment is not allowed under the Public Health Act.
- Patients who do not have capacity to consent to treatment as defined by the Mental Capacity Act section 3 can usually be treated, if necessary by admission to hospital if it is in their best interests that treatment should be given. Any treatment must conform to the principles of the Mental Health Capacity Act.
- Patients who refuse treatment for infectious disease due to mental disorder may in some cases be detained under the Mental Health Act 1983. The Mental Health Act does not provide a power for compulsory treatment of a physical condition. If the patient is incapable of consent to treatment for the infectious disease due to their mental disorder, treatment can be provided.

By law they do not have a choice about going to hospital but they can refuse treatment. However, the care worker could give them all the facts about the treatment so they could make an informed decision. While they are in hospital it is up to the care workers to ensure that the infected patient is put in an isolation room so that they will not infect other patients.

Waste disposal

The safe disposal of clinical waste, particularly when it might be contaminated with blood, other potentially infectious body fluids, secretions or excretions, is part of the standard infection control precautions (see LO3.2, page 102). Any waste that is not clinical waste is classed as household domestic waste. This is usually stored in a black landfill bin, which should only be used for household rubbish that cannot be reused, recycled or composted. Examples of items that go into the domestic waste bin include nappies, black bags, polystyrene and tissue paper.

Any special non-clinical waste cannot go to non-hazardous landfill sites. Examples include garden chemicals that include pesticides, oil-based paints, household cleaning products, lawn treatments and car

anti-freeze. Disposal of hazardous household waste requires specialist help and advice.

Cleaning practices

The environment (e.g. door handles, flush handles, taps) plays an important role in cross-infection. Therefore, special attention must be paid to these fittings during outbreaks. In addition, accumulations of dust, dirt and liquid residues will increase infection risks and must be reduced to the minimum by regular cleaning and by using good design features in buildings, fittings and fixtures.

The role of the health and social care worker in cleaning

A written cleaning schedule should be devised, based on Control of Substances Hazardous to Health (COSHH), to include the regular removal of dust by damp dusting both high and low horizontal surfaces. All health and social care settings should have a decontamination policy and cleaning schedule stating how and when to clean the environment, fixtures, fittings and specialist equipment (for example a hoist); what products and equipment to use when cleaning; what to do and what products to use if there is a spillage of blood or body fluids; and what training staff need to implement the policy, and describe individual responsibilities for cleaning.

The function of a detergent

Detergents and soaps are used for cleaning because pure water cannot remove oily, organic soiling. Soap cleans by acting as an emulsifier as it allows oil and water to mix so that oily grime can be removed during rinsing. Thorough cleaning with a neutral detergent and/or biological cleaning solution and warm water (at body temperature) will remove large numbers of micro-organisms from a surface, especially if the item can be rinsed. Micro-organisms reduce further as the surface dries. Devices cannot be effectively disinfected or sterilised without having first been thoroughly cleaned and dried.

The function of disinfectant

Disinfectant reduces the number of micro-organisms to a level that is considered safe, but it may not destroy some viruses or bacterial spores. Disinfection is usually acceptable for items that pose a medium risk of infection if these items cannot be effectively sterilised. Chemical disinfection is not as effective as heat disinfection. Heat disinfectants, such as dishwashers, washing machines and washer-disinfectors clean the item and then expose it to hot water for the required time to achieve thermal disinfection: 65°C for 10 minutes, 71°C for 3 minutes, 80°C for 1 minute and

90°C for 1 second. While most chemical disinfectants inactivate bacteria and some viruses, many are not so effective against the hepatitis viruses, cysts and bacterial spores.

The function of sanitiser

Hand sanitisers are an alternative to handwashing when soap and water are not available. Alcohol rub sanitisers kill most bacteria and fungi and stop some viruses.

Hand sanitisers are common at the entrance to wards in hospitals so that staff and visitors do not bring infections in to or out of the ward.

INDEPENDENT ACTIVITY

(10 minutes)

Read http://tinyurl.com/qyp8zp3

Do you use hand gels? After reading the article would you still use them?

The function of sterilising agents

Sterilisation is used for food, medicine and surgical instruments. To sterilise means to kill all microbes and their spores – whether harmful or not – present on a surface or object. This can be done by using machines called autoclaves that use steam heated to 121–134°C. Another method is to use heat, including incineration, boiling in water and dry heat, which deactivates and kills micro-organisms in glass and metals. Items that can be damaged by heat are subjected to chemical sterilisation, e.g. biological materials, fibre optics, electronics, and plastics. Irradiation, high pressure and filtration are other agents used in the sterilising process.

Cleaning facilities for different rooms

Kitchens

Risks can be avoided by keeping all equipment and work surfaces hygienic and clean, using the correct cleaning solutions and water temperatures. Kitchen surfaces must be cleaned after each use and floors swept and washed regularly. All utensils, equipment and crockery should be washed after use with a strong detergent, and hot, clean water, especially when changing to different food types, and then dried, preferably by air rather than using towels, and stored away in a clean space. Taps and sinks should be cleaned after every use; and cloths and sponges should be reserved for separate tasks and washed thoroughly after use.

Bathrooms

Bathrooms can cross-infect people who are using them if they are not kept scrupulously clean. This involves cleaning, with disinfectant, all toilets, baths and washbasins twice daily plus another check to make sure everything is clean and not soiled. It is also important to replenish soap and hand towels twice daily with an extra check for cleanliness, as dirty towels do not remove bacteria from people's hands. All ledges and surfaces should be damp dusted, mirrors cleaned and floors should be mopped daily with another check during the day.

All NHS organisations should adopt the national colour coding scheme for hospital cleaning materials and equipment. All cleaning items, for example cloths (reusable and disposable), mops, buckets, aprons and gloves, should be colour coded. This also includes those items used to clean catering departments.

Table 5.7 National colour coding scheme for hospital cleaning materials and equipment

Colour	Application
Red	Bathrooms, washrooms, showers, toilets, basins and bathroom floors
Blue	General areas including wards, departments, offices
Green	Catering department, ward kitchen areas and patient food service at ward level
Yellow	Isolation areas

CLASSROOM DISCUSSION

(20 minutes)

Discuss the ways that organisations can prevent infections from spreading.

Monitoring and recording procedures

Rotas

A cleaning rota will have a clear allocation of responsibilities for cleaning all areas within the home/hospital (resident/patient rooms, communal areas, toilets, bathrooms etc). It must clearly identify who has responsibility for cleaning these areas and regularly used residential equipment items such as wheelchair, commodes hoists, shower chairs etc.

The cleaning rota must state the areas and frequency of cleaning activities, for example daily, weekly, monthly, annually. It must include clear cleaning instructions following a patient's discharge, isolation or death, and deep cleaning activities. Cleaning rotas must respond to the changing needs of a particular area or ward.

Records

The person in charge should identify and record what requires cleaning, disinfection and sterilisation and how it is to be achieved. For example, high-touch surfaces such as toilets, commode chairs, computer keyboards, chairs, bedrails, call bells and telephones must be cleaned and then disinfected regularly. Routine and managerial cleaning audits must take place and a timeframe to put cleaning problems right should be included. They must ensure that staff are competent by providing instruction, information and training as appropriate.

Reporting outbreaks of infectious and communicable diseases

RIDDOR (see LO1.5, page 96) requires employers to report infectious diseases to the director of public health for the local authority so that service users, carers and the wider community can be protected. This is particularly important in any care setting with vulnerable people as it is essential to monitor and manage outbreaks of infectious diseases.

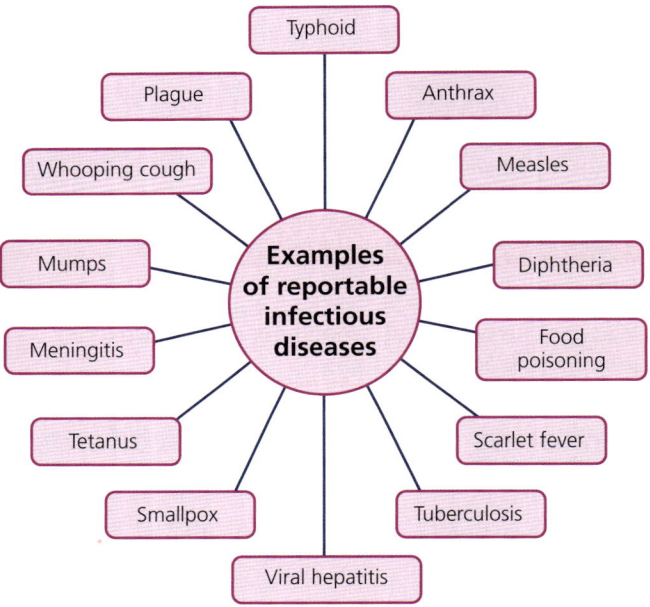

▲ **Figure 5.5** Reportable infectious diseases

Managing self

You have a responsibility to prevent the spread of infections by having appropriate vaccinations (e.g. the flu jab) and maintaining good standards of personal hygiene. Pay attention to areas where disease-causing germs and parasites can grow and multiply, e.g. the skin and in and around the openings to the body. Good personal hygiene habits include:

- washing the body often, e.g. having a shower or a bath every day; when this is not possible, a wash all over the body with a wet sponge or cloth will do
- cleaning teeth at least once a day
- washing hair with soap or shampoo at least once a week
- washing hands with soap after going to the toilet
- washing hands with soap before preparing and/or eating food
- changing into clean clothes.

All staff working in care homes or hospitals must inform their management if they have:

- diarrhoea or vomiting (during working hours or their line manager at the beginning of the next working day, and not return to work until they have been symptom-free for 48 hours)
- throat infections
- skin rashes
- boils or any other skin lesion.

Managers monitoring sickness must inform the person responsible for infection prevention and control if they have more than one member of their staff off duty at one time with a gastrointestinal illness.

KNOW IT

1 Explain why staff need to follow policies and procedures in health and social care settings.
2 Explain how staff in health and social care settings can promote good practice.
3 Describe the function of a detergent.
4 Describe the function of disinfectant.
5 Explain how to clean a kitchen to ensure there is no risk of food poisoning.
6 Discuss the importance of maintaining a good standard of personal hygiene particularly when working in health and social care settings.

LO4 Assessment activity

Below is a suggested assessment activity that has been directly linked to the pass, merit and distinction criteria in LO4 to help with assignment preparation; it includes Top Tips on how to achieve best results.

Activity 1

Farxiya has been promoted to Nurse Manager of a large nursing home called The Willows. The recent CQC report for The Willows highlighted concerns, including inadequate cleaning in some areas of the home. Some staff were criticised for having dirty uniforms and for ignoring policies and procedures for infection control. A number of residents at The Willows have dementia and inspectors were keen to find out how the staff would cope if the residents with an infection refused to comply with the home's policy on infection control. Farxiya wants to ensure these concerns are addressed.

a) Describe how she can ensure that there is adequate cleaning in the home. **P8**

b) Describe she can make sure the staff manage themselves to prevent the spread of infection. **P9**

c) How can Farxiya explain to staff the importance of following the home's policies and procedures for effective infection control? **M4**

d) Suggest how the staff at The Willows could deal with residents who refused to comply with the home's infection control measures. Analyse how effective these proposals would be. **D2**

TOP TIPS

✔ Consider how best to present your response, e.g. in an assignment or as a presentation to the rest of the group.
✔ When analysing, separate the information into components and identify the steps that might be taken and why. This could be in the form of a policy or procedure.

Read about it

Dougherty, L. and Lister, S. (2008) *The Royal Marsden Hospital Manual of Clinical Nursing Procedures* (Student Edition), Wiley-Blackwell.

Koutoukidis, G. et al. (2013) *Tabbner's Nursing Care: Theory and Practice*, Churchill Livingstone

Useful websites

Infection control in health and social care environments:

www.rcn.org.uk

www.kch.nhs.uk

www.gov.uk/government/organisations/Public-health-england

www.hse.uk

The safe use of PPE in care settings:

http://tinyurl.com/zxjkp8r

What are standard precautions and why are they necessary?

www.rcht.nhs.uk

Last offices and care of the deceased:

www.mhsc.nhs.uk

Promoting best practice:

www.rcn.org.uk

Importance of thorough cleaning in hospitals:

http://tinyurl.com/gpgvavk

http://tinyurl.com/zox66dz

The importance of the correct disposal of health care waste:

www.hse.gcv.uk/healthservices/healthcare-waste

Unit 06

Personalisation and a person-centred approach to care

ABOUT THIS UNIT

Personalisation had its origins in the 1990s as a result of campaigning by disability rights groups, but it took until 2008 for the government to fully embrace the concept. It has changed individuals' lives, as they are allowed choice and control over the support they need to live life to the full.

In this unit you will learn about what is meant by personalisation and how the health and social care sector can achieve this by adopting a person-centred approach. You must develop a positive, professional approach to caring that will empower and support individuals who need services to help them in their daily lives.

You will explore how attitudes towards caring have changed and how government policies have resulted in health and social care professionals adopting a person-centred approach to care. You will be introduced to the practical tools and approaches that are used by professionals in their work.

LEARNING OUTCOMES

The topics, activities and suggested reading in this unit will help you to:

1 Understand personalisation in health and social care
2 Understand what is meant by a person-centred approach to care
3 Understand methods used to implement a person-centred approach
4 Know how to plan and conduct review meetings using a person-centred approach

How will I be assessed?

You will be assessed through an external assessment set and marked by OCR.

LO1 Understand personalisation in health and social care

1.1 Definition of personalisation

Personalisation is defined by the Department of Health as follows: 'every person who receives support, whether by **statutory services** or funded by themselves, will have choice and control over the shape of that support in all care settings'. However, this definition is limited as it does not imply that the individual receiving the support will be at the centre of the process. Personalisation means recognising that the person has individual strengths, preferences, wishes and aspirations. It means putting them at the centre of the process by identifying their needs and supporting them to make choices about the services they want so they can live the way they want to.

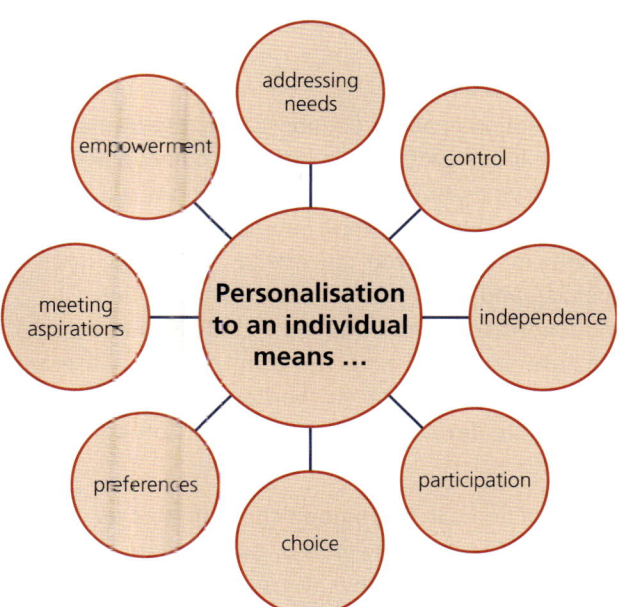

▲ **Figure 6.1** What personalisation means to individuals

Personalisation means that individuals will have to decide which outcomes they wish to achieve, and how their needs and **aspirations** may be met. It is a **proactive** approach for the individual rather than the traditional approach which determined what services they would receive and where and how these services would be provided. They are involved in all aspects of their care needs and must take part in all the aspects of decision making.

1.2 Key features of personalisation

🔑 KEY TERMS

Statutory service – a service provided by local authority as laid down by legislation/law.

Aspiration – a strong desire to achieve something.

Proactive – when a person creates or controls a situation by causing something to happen rather than responding to it after it has happened.

Personal budget – the amount of money an individual is awarded by the local authority to spend on the help they need to achieve what is important to them.

Support plan – the document where day-to-day requirements and preferences for care and support are detailed to enable an individual to live with dignity and respect in the community. It may be known by other names e.g. care plan, or an individual plan.

Social care outcomes – the results of receiving social care that is desired by the individual, e.g. living independently, finding employment.

Means-tested payments – payments based on an individual's financial circumstances to determine whether an individual is eligible or has the right to claim assistance.

Personal budgets

A **personal budget** is an agreed amount of money that is used to carry out or deliver certain aspects of provision set out in an individual's **support plan**. In December 2007 the government stated:

> 'all people who are eligible for social care and support should have access to a personal budget with the intention that they could use it to exercise choice and control in meeting their agreed **social care outcomes**. It is a **means-tested cash payment** made in the place of regular social service.'

There are two ways that a personal budget may be taken by an individual.

Direct payments

These are a direct (cash) payment, held by the person or, where they lack the **mental capacity** to look after themselves, by an 'authorised or nominated person', usually a carer, family member or friend, or an independent advocate identified by the **local authority**. This method of payment underpins personalisation as individuals are given responsibility for making decisions; and can spend the money as they please as long as it relates to their support plan.

Individuals who are **eligible** for a community care service, such as home care, respite or day services, can choose to receive an agreed amount of money from social care instead of having care provided for them, so they can arrange their own help. They are responsible for making sure their personal budget is spent appropriately and they need to keep accurate records to demonstrate this. The money can be used to arrange services (including equipment) that adult social care services have agreed they need. For example, the individual may choose to employ their own personal assistant, or pay for support provided by a care agency or self-employed person. They are not allowed to employ their partner or a close relative living with them, unless there is no alternative and this has been agreed. Direct payments cannot be used to pay for long-term permanent residential care or for services provided by social services.

Managed accounts

This account is managed by the local authority in line with the person's wishes. This may include paying for community care services provided or commissioned by the local authority. Local authorities sometimes provide services directly but they increasingly commission non-government providers, such as private companies or charities, to provide services on their behalf.

As with direct payments, anyone who opts for a managed personal account must know what sum of money is available and they also have choice and control over the support provided. It is, however, unlikely that a managed arrangement will offer the same level of user choice and control as a direct payment.

Co-production

Co-production is about collaboration or working together. It is a partnership between citizens and public services, such as Neighbourhood Watch or Healthy Schools, to achieve valuable outcomes. The idea is to **empower** citizens to contribute time, expertise and effort to their local communities. Co-production recognises that individuals who use social care have skills and expertise that they can share with others. For example, social workers, service users and carers could develop new, local support organisations together.

Co-production can strengthen communities as everyone involved can feel empowered by contributing. Although it is a straightforward idea, it is not so easy to put into practice as it may be a new idea for those who use services.

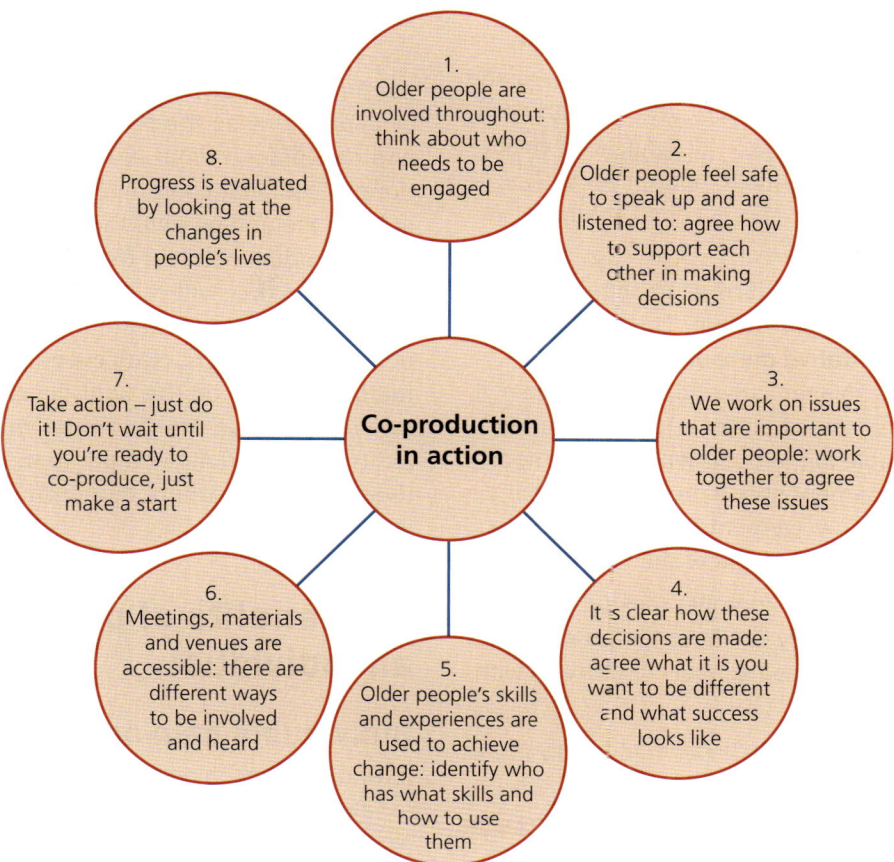

▲ **Figure 6.2** Co-production in action with older people (Source: *Personalisation: Don't just do it, coproduce it and live it!*)

🔑 **KEY TERM**

Empower – to give someone the authority or control to do something; the way a health, social care or early years worker encourages an individual to make decisions and to take control of their own life.

Choice and control

Personalisation is a commitment to giving individuals more choice and control, supporting and enabling them to make their own decisions about where and how care is provided and the support they need to live a full and independent life. Individuals may decide, for example, that they need to have better:

- housing options
- person-centred support plans
- personal budgets
- support in the form of a personal assistant.

These would give them choice and therefore control over what happens to them. This is liberating. For example,

before personalisation someone who needed assistance to get ready for bed would have to fit into their personal assistant's (PA) time schedule. Now many direct budget holders employ their own personal assistant to come at the time convenient to them and not the personal assistant. There is also the reassurance that the PA is a single person who they know. PAs increase **autonomy**, enabling and sustaining the rights of individuals to make choices about how they live their lives.

🔑 **KEY TERM**

Autonomy – self-rule, independence or freedom to do as an individual wishes.

Self-assessment of needs

Self-assessment is led as far as possible by the person who uses the services, or in partnership with a professional, and focuses on the outcomes they want to achieve. The professional will talk to the individual about the support they need in different areas of their life.

Self-assessment involves the individual working with professionals to look at the circumstances, situation and needs of the individual, carers, family members and others who provide informal support. The local authority will decide if the person is eligible for long-term social care support and, if so, how much money they will need to pay for this support. This is called an indicative personal budget.

The assessment will collect information about how the individual's care needs might be met. This could include identifying how **preventative measures** like simple aids (such as devices to open jars and tins more easily), **home adaptations** (such as handrails) or information about support available in the community might meet their need. The assessment should be carried out in a way that ensures their involvement and that takes the right amount of time to capture all of their needs.

If they have a friend or family member looking after them as an unpaid carer they can have their own carer's assessment to see if they need support to carry on with their role.

The local authority must give the individual a copy of their **needs assessment** or carer's assessment.

> ## 🔑 KEY TERMS
>
> **Preventative measures** – using methods to stop or prevent something, e.g. providing a jar-opening device for an individual to allow them to open jars safely and prevent injury.
>
> **Home adaptations** – changes to the home to make it safer for the individual to live independently, e.g. a stair-lift to enable an individual to go upstairs in their home, making it accessible.
>
> **Needs assessment** – the overall process for identifying and recording the health and social care risks and needs of an individual and evaluating their impact on daily living and quality of life so that appropriate action can be planned.
>
> **Universal services** – services that are available to everyone, such as transport and housing.
>
> **Service led** – a service-led provision is where an individual has to fit into existing traditional services such as day centres.
>
> **Centre for Independent Living** – centres that promote the principles of independent living and provide services for individuals who use direct payments.
>
> **Self-esteem** – the value an individual gives themselves.

Changing role of professionals

The control has moved from the professional to the person. Obviously, everyone has their own dreams or aspirations so the professional must be sensitive and non-judgemental. By listening to the individual, the professional can empower them to take control of their life and be able to make their own decisions. The individual will feel that their judgements are valued and they will respond to the professional in a positive way. It is about letting an individual make decisions for themselves even if the professional feels it may not be the right decision. Part of their role is to provide the individual with all the relevant information and allow them to make their choice and their decision, without compromising safeguarding issues.

1.3 Benefits of personalistion to an individual

Individuals gain and maintain control

Individuals can gain and control a budget if they opt for direct payments. If they have employed a personal assistant, they also control everyday aspects of their lives that other people take for granted, such as getting up and going to bed when they want to. They do not have to fit into other people's timetables.

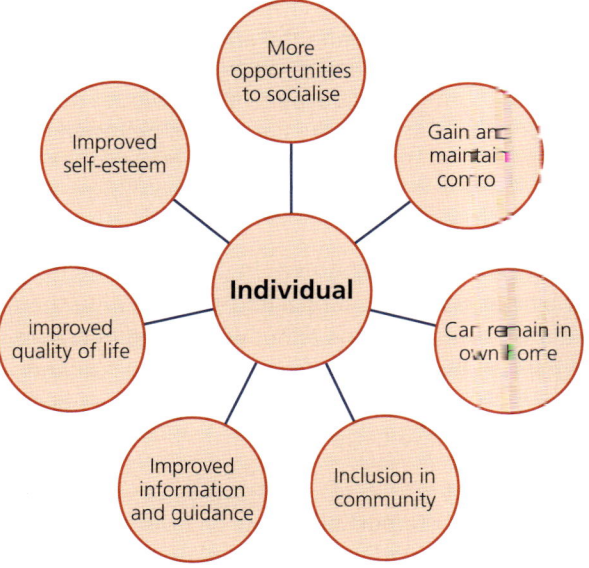

▲ **Figure 6.3** Benefits of personalisation for the individual

Individuals can remain in their own home when receiving care

Remaining in their own home is important for most individuals as they may feel they will leave their memories and possessions behind if they have to go into residential care. They may think they will become dependent on others if they move into care. Remaining in their own home, with support, will mean the individual can choose to do what they want, when they want to do it.

Inclusion in community

Inclusion means that individuals are involved in the same activities as the rest of the community. They feel valued, are treated with respect and feel part of the community. An individual could use previous experience from job roles or skills. This involvement provides access to social networks so the individual can widen their social group.

Improved information and guidance

To make good decisions about the support they need, everyone must have access to the right advice, guidance, information and advocacy. Individuals must have as much information as possible to give them the widest choice in how their needs can be met by **universal services** such as housing, health, education, transport and leisure. It also widens the opportunity of employment, regardless of age or disability. Local authorities should ensure that information, advice and support are available through a single point of access, which should not be online. It is the government's policy to have at least one **service-led** disabled persons' organisation, such as a **Centre for Independent Living**, for each local authority area to provide advice.

> **CLASSROOM DISCUSSION**
>
> **(10 minutes)**
>
> *Which?* is a consumer magazine offering advice on household items, services, etc. Why do people use it? Draw parallels with the need for access to advice and guidance, before deciding which services to buy, for individuals who have a direct budget.

Improved quality of life, self-esteem and socialisation

These are all interrelated. If an individual has more control over their everyday life then their quality of life improves as they have choices. This in turn improves **self-esteem**, and if people feel good about themselves they are more willing to meet new people and socialise. It can be difficult to build and maintain social relationships without confidence. It also works the other way round – if someone's social life improves, so too will their self-esteem and confidence and they will be more likely to try new things.

> **KEY TERM**
>
> **Degenerative condition** – medical problems that worsen over time.

> **? THINK ABOUT IT**
>
> ### Case study: Mo's experience of personalisation
>
> Mo is 46 years old. She has multiple sclerosis, a long-term **degenerative condition**. Until her mother died seven years ago, Mo lived in the family home and was looked after by her mother, who was very protective.
>
> After her mother's death, Mo felt she could not continue to live alone without support. She was assessed by her local authority, was offered a suitable house and opted for direct payments. She employed a personal assistant and other health and social care professionals.
>
> Mo enjoyed the opportunity to start a new life and take part in activities that in the past would have been difficult. She enjoyed the freedom of being able to do what she wanted when she wanted, as she could arrange her support around her lifestyle.
>
> Feeling confident for the first time in her life, Mo decided to go to university. She had a fantastic experience meeting new people from a variety of backgrounds. During summer vacations she was invited to visit some of them in Europe and Asia. She went clubbing and partying until the early hours with her new friends.
>
> Mo felt life was worth living as she looked forward to each day. After she finished her degree she applied for a part-time job as an advisor working for the local authority. She now assists and offers advice to families with children who have needs. She loves her job and the feeling of self-worth it has given her.
>
> 1 Discuss how a personalised budget has changed Mo's life.
> 2 Explain how three professionals from the health and social care sectors might work in partnership to support Mo. State the advantages of this approach.

117

1.4 Impacts of personalisation

There are many impacts of personalisation: some positive and some that provide challenges.

Positive impacts of personalisation

1 Direct payment for care allows rapid access to services and means the individual can have support as and when they need it. There is no need for the individual to have to wait for the local authority to organise or approve payment of care. They have the money to be able to pay for it immediately.

2 Inclusion within communities means individuals do not have to go into a residential home where they are separate from everyday life. They can be supported to live, work and socialise in the community in the same way that those who do not require care and support are able to.

3 Remaining in own home where there is familiarity and a sense of belonging adds to quality of life. The individual feels comfortable and safe. They know their home and the surrounding area. They have all their belongings and memories around them. They know their neighbours and use the local shops.

4 Access to information and guidance allows for better choices. Individuals feel more confident about making a choice if they feel they have all the facts. It is the local authority's duty to ensure individuals have all the information they need.

5 New opportunities, such as employment, further and higher education, are open to individuals who need services as they can pay for the necessary support they need to access these opportunities. Support is available and given at the time when they want it.

Challenges of personalisation

There are some challenges related to personalisation. The main ones are described below.

1 Care is limited to the prescribed budget. The individual is given a set sum of money. When the money is spent it is likely that no more will be available until the next financial year. Individuals need to know their plans for the coming year so that when they are assessed they can apply for the relevant support; otherwise they could miss out on funding, particularly with government cuts. If individuals don't stay within budget they may be short of funds towards the end of the month. This could be an added worry.

2 Availability and access to some services may be restricted, particularly if the individual lives in a rural area and travel is difficult because of poor public transport. High-demand services may be provided only for individuals with the greatest needs, so some people will miss out. There could also be a lack of trained carers.

3 Worry about spending the budget as all the money has to be accounted for. If an individual has opted for direct payments, the local authority will ask them for copies of bank statements, invoices and receipts to justify how their budget has been spent

1.5 Legislation underpinning personalisation

> ### 🔍 INDEPENDENT RESEARCH ACTIVITY
>
> **(30 minutes)**
>
> Go to independentliving.org/docs6/evans2003.html
>
> Read the document on the Independent Living Movement.
>
> Discuss the progress of the Independent Living Movement since its origins in 1996 to the current situation today.

Health and Social Care Act 2012

Improving the quality of care was at the heart of the Health and Social Care Act 2012. Although predominantly related to health, the Act reinforced personalisation in social care and empowers patients to make choices. It enables patients to choose services that best meet their needs, including from charity or independent sector providers, as long as they meet NHS costs. Patients can choose to have their treatment in a hospital of their choice. The Act also established new Healthwatch patient organisations to give patients a voice. **Monitor** was established as a specialist regulator to protect patients' interests.

The key legislative changes were as follows.

- The Act strengthened the collective voice of patients. Service providers and commissioners should welcome feedback as a means of assessing the quality of their services.
- The Act provided the basis for better collaboration, partnership working and integration across local government and the NHS.
- The NHS Commissioning Board, **Clinical Commissioning Groups**, Monitor and Health and Wellbeing boards all have duties to involve patients,

carers and the public. Commissioning groups have to consult the public on their annual commissioning plans and involve them in any changes that affect patient services.

- The Act provided for the establishment of **Healthwatch England** as a statutory committee of the **Care Quality Commission**. Healthwatch England is a national body representing the views of users of health and social care services, other members of the public and local Healthwatch organisations. It advises and provides information to the Secretary of State, the NHS Commissioning Board, Monitor, English local authorities and the Care Quality Commission on the views and experiences of users of health and social care services.

💬 CLASSROOM DISCUSSION

(30 minutes)

Discuss the effect the Health and Social Care Act 2012 has had or will have on the health and social care services.

🔑 KEY TERMS

Monitor – the sector regulator for health services in England. Monitor's job is to make the health sector work better for patients.

Clinical Commissioning Groups (CCGs) – most of the NHS commissioning budget is now managed by 209 CCGs. These are groups of general practices that come together in each area to commission the best services for their patients and population.

Healthwatch England – the national consumer champion in health and care, with statutory powers to ensure the voice of the consumer is heard by those who commission, deliver and regulate health and care services.

Care Quality Commission (CQC) – an independent regulator of health and social care in England. They monitor, inspect and regulate services to make sure they meet fundamental standards of quality and safety.

Local Authority Circular (DH) 2008 – Personalisation Guidance

'Everyone who receives social care support, regardless of their level of need, in any setting... will have choice and control over how that support is delivered. It will mean that people are able to live their own lives as they wish, confident that services are of high quality, are

safe and promote their own individual requirements for independence, wellbeing and dignity.'

(Source: Social Care. Local Authority Circular LAC (DH) (2008)1, 17 January 2008)

The statement reinforces the commitment to personalisation. It seeks to reassure individuals that, whatever their circumstances, they will have a voice and a choice in their care, enabling them and their supporters to maintain or improve their wellbeing and independence rather than relying on intervention at the point of an emergency or crisis. This is about prevention rather than waiting for something to go wrong.

The Care Act 2014

The Care Act 2014 puts people and their carers in control of their care and support. The Act combined existing pieces of legislation but aimed to give greater control to those in need of support. It sets out what local authorities have to do to provide support. The most significant developments relating to personalisation are:

- people in need of support are encouraged to think about what outcomes they want, for a better sense of physical or emotional wellbeing
- if a carer has needs and is eligible for support, they have a legal right to assessment and to receive support
- local authorities will encourage and help people to lead healthy lives, reducing the chances of them needing more support in the future
- local authorities should provide clear guidance to help individuals make informed choices and enable them to stay in control of their lives
- a greater emphasis on the use of advocates
- greater regulation for those who provide professional care and support, and tougher penalties for those who do not provide care and support of a high enough standard
- greater emphasis on safeguarding vulnerable individuals from neglect and abuse
- greater emphasis on personalised budgets and payments
- people may appeal against council decisions on eligibility and funding for care and support.

The Care Act reinforces personalisation in the guidelines for health and social care professionals working with individuals. These guidelines are:

- the individual knows themselves and their needs best
- the individual's views, wishes, feelings and beliefs should always be considered

- professionals' focus should be on the individual's wellbeing, reducing their need for care and support, and reducing their need for care and support in the future
- any decisions should take into account all relevant circumstances
- any decisions should be made with the individual's involvement
- an individual's wellbeing should be balanced with that of involved family and friends
- professionals must protect the individual from abuse and neglect
- professionals should ensure that any actions taken to support the individual affect their rights and freedom as little as possible.

? THINK ABOUT IT

Case study: James

James is 55 and has learning difficulties. He is in hospital recovering from a severe stroke. His social worker has told him that his only choice, when he is discharged from hospital, is to go into a residential home. James is very unhappy about this as he would like to stay in his own home.

1 Explain how the Care Act 2014 would help James.
2 Explain how the social worker has not followed the guidelines for professionals working with individuals.

Children and Families Act 2014

The Children and Families Act 2014 focuses on putting children and young people at the heart of planning and decision making through co-production and person-centred practice. It emphasises the importance of engaging young people and their families in all processes.

In terms of personalisation, the Children and Families Act 2014 focuses on:

- the importance of involving young people and their parents/carers in all decisions
- choice and control for the children, young people and families involved in decision making
- the duty of the local authority to integrate services across health, care and education
- a single, co-ordinated assessment
- a single Education, Health and Care Plan (EHCP)
- empowering young people so they are engaged and supported to plan for their future
- the duty of the local authority to carry out a Child's Needs Assessment (CNA) for young people who may need support to make informed choices for their future
- the duty of the local authority to provide information, advice and support (IAS) on health, social care and education.

1.6 Role of local authority

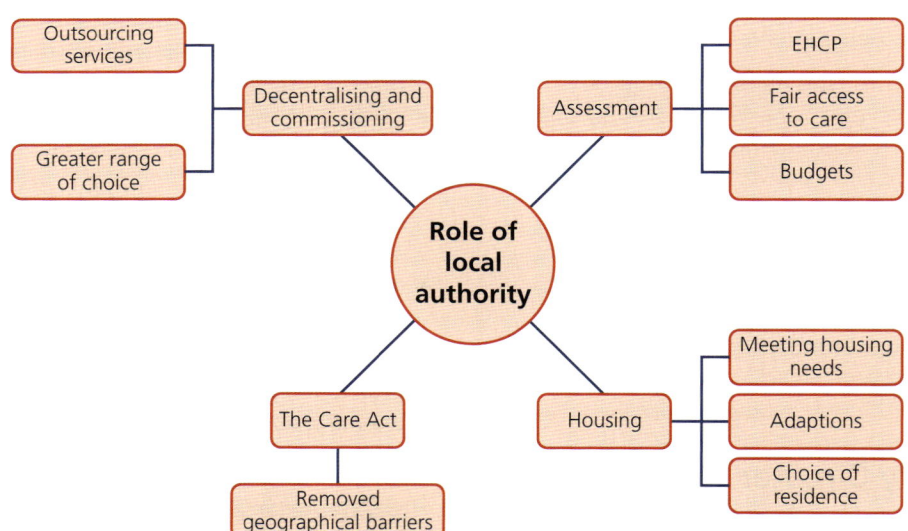

▲ **Figure 6.4** The role of the local authority in promoting personalisation

Assessment

Education, Health and Care Plan (EHCP)

It is the role of the local authority to carry out an assessment for an Education, Health and Care Plan (EHCP).

An EHCP is a legal document which sets out a description of a child's or young person's needs. It documents what they can and cannot do and what has to be done to meet those needs by education, health and social care. Few children are issued with an EHCP, usually those with complex and severe needs which require high levels of support.

CLASSROOM DISCUSSION

(20 minutes)

Visit enfield.gov.uk/downloads/file/9922/ehcp_example to view an example of an EHCP. Decide if the child in the example would be issued with an EHCP. Explain your answer.

Fair Access to Care

Fair Access to Care Services (FACS) guidelines were introduced by the government in 2003 to provide local authorities with a common framework for determining individuals' eligibility for social care services and to address inconsistencies in outcomes across the country.

The framework is based on individual needs and associated risks to independence, and includes four eligibility bands – critical, substantial, moderate and low. When placing people in these bands it should not only be immediate needs that are addressed, but also needs that would worsen with a lack of timely help.

Individual budgets

If the goal is independent living, then the individual will need to be assessed by the local authority for an individual budget. This is the money that individuals use to buy the support and services they need to meet the outcomes they have identified in their support plans.

How much money people are entitled to is determined by completion of the Self Assessment Process (SAP). This process aims to assess people's care needs thoroughly and accurately, without procedures being needlessly duplicated by other agencies.

People don't have to hold or manage the individual budget themselves. If they wish, someone appointed as an agent, a trust or an organisation can act on their behalf to hold and manage their individual budget.

See also direct payments on page 114.

Housing

The local authority must meet the individual's needs and so should consider the following.

Choice of residence

For local authorities, personalisation means offering individuals choice over where and how they live. Local authorities must ensure that homes are accessible, flexible and designed with individuals' needs in mind. There should be a core service for specialist housing with a range of additional options as required to meet individuals' needs.

Housing adaptations

These could be to the individual's own home or be in an already adapted house. They are assessed by the local authority's social services to enable an individual to live independently. For example, if a kitchen needs to be suitable for using in a wheelchair, units, the cooker or sink could be lowered so everything is within reach. Another adaptation could be a hoist in the bedroom or bathroom making it easy for individuals to go to bed or have a bath.

INDEPENDENT RESEARCH ACTIVITY

(10 minutes)

Visit livingmadeeasy.org.uk to check out the range of adaptations available to help individuals live independently.

Meeting housing needs

If the individual wants to stay in their own home, social services will do their best to help them stay there by using special equipment and adaptations. If it is not possible to adapt the house then the options would be:

- purpose-built or adapted accommodation that is accessible and meets the individual's needs; for example, a ramp might already be in place to the front door or it may have wider doors to accommodate a wheelchair
- sheltered accommodation that gives an individual the independence of having their own bungalow or flat

with the security of an alarm system and a warden to check on residents and help in an emergency; they would not provide care or carry out household tasks; most sheltered accommodation has a common room for social activities

- a residential home that would be suitable for an individual who finds it difficult to look after themselves and cannot receive the care needed in their own home. Residential care would ensure all the individual's physical needs were met. Care assistants would be available to help day or night.

? THINK ABOUT IT

Case study: Molly

Molly is 82 and lives alone in her three-bedroom house. Recently she tripped over her cat and fell down the stairs. She broke her arm and was badly shaken. She is otherwise in good health.

Outline the housing options that are available to Molly and the advantages and disadvantages of each.

The Care Act's removal of geographical barriers

The Care Act 2014 removed geographical barriers as it wanted continuity of care so that, when an adult who is receiving care and support in one area of England moves home, they will continue to receive care in the new area. There should be no gap in care and support when people choose to move.

The Act describes the process to be followed so that local authorities know when someone wants to move areas, and what must happen to make sure that their needs are met when they arrive in the new area.

Decentralisation and commissioning

Decentralisation is the process of redistributing or shifting functions from a central authority or location. In its simplest form commissioning is the process of planning, agreeing and monitoring services. Key to commissioning is working in equal partnership with individuals who use services, their families, communities and organisations.

Outsourcing services

When applied to personalisation, outsourcing means that the services will not necessarily come from the local authority but may be bought from other organisations. This could give more value for money and a better choice of services. For example, individuals can choose which hospital they would prefer to carry out their operation. The local authority commissioner must demonstrate that services reflect comments from consultation with individuals who use them. Individuals must be engaged from the start of the process through implementation, monitoring and evaluation.

Promoting greater range of choice

Before personalisation, the services on offer to an individual would come from inside the local authority. If the service was not available then the individual had no choice. Now services can be sourced from many different organisations, so the individual can choose the service that best meets their needs.

KNOW IT

1. Explain what is meant by personalisation.
2. Identify two positive impacts of personalisation.
3. Name two Acts that underpin personalisation.
4. Explain what is meant by an Education Health and Care Plan (EHCP).
5. Explain what is meant by an individual budget.

LO2 Understand what is meant by a person-centred approach to care

GETTING STARTED

(15 minutes)

Research asylums and workhouses. What were conditions like for individuals who lived there? Compare and contrast these institutions with the way health and social care is organised today.

2.1 Person-centred approach

A person-centred approach is to see the person as an individual, focusing on their personal needs, wants, goals and aspirations. The individual becomes central to the health and social care process. The support the individual needs must be designed in partnership with the individual, their family and/or carers.

Key concepts of a person-centred approach are:

- knowing the person as an individual
- empowerment and power
- respecting the individual's values and preferences
- choice and autonomy
- respect and dignity
- empathy and compassion.

Balance between what is important to and what is important for a person

Individuals receiving support are entitled to take risks if they want to. As part of person-centred care, carers need to see risk taking as positive rather than negative. It is now recognised that risk taking can have positive benefits for an individual, allowing them to do things just like other people. Risks are part of everyday life.

Enhancing voice, choice and control

A balance has to be achieved between levels of protection and levels of choice and control. The wishes of the individual and the duty of care must also be carefully balanced. There may be some level of compromise on behalf of the individual, their family, carer or a professional. Empowerment should mean allowing an individual to make their own decisions that carers may disagree with.

Clarification of roles and responsibilities

It is the role and responsibility of the carer/personal assistant to provide support for the individual to enable them to live the life they want. Professionals are no longer in charge of making decisions about an individual's life. It is the duty of the individual to make their wishes clear to the carer.

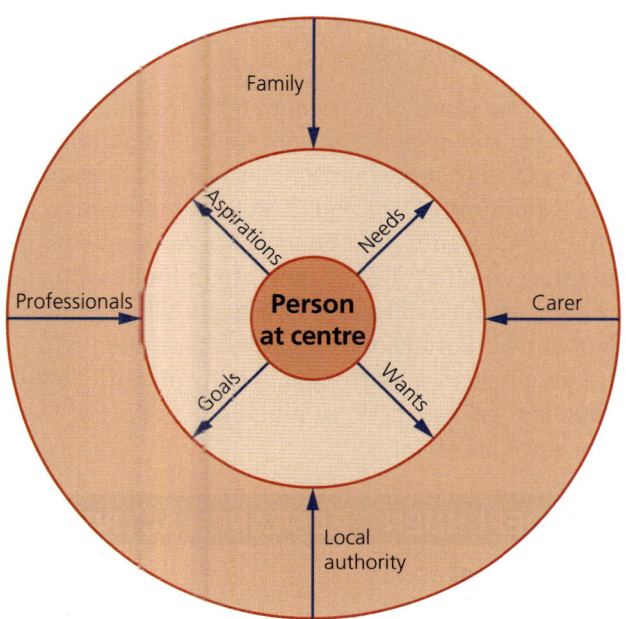

▲ **Figure 6.5** Putting the individual at the centre of a person-centred process

Professionals of all disciplines, including GPs, housing specialists, financial advisors and social workers, are there to give advice so that the individual can make an informed decision. Professionals need to respect preferences and treat the individual as a partner in setting goals, planning care and making decisions about care, treatment or outcomes. In sharing power and responsibility, it is essential to acknowledge the different expertise and experience of individuals both using and providing the support.

2.2 Principles of a person-centred approach and how they support person-centred care

Independence and rights

These can include:

- to live the way they want to (see LO1.3, page 116)
- to be employed – the Equality Act 2010 ensures an individual with a disability is not discriminated against; a carer can help an individual to produce a CV which identifies academic qualifications, strengths, interests, competences and resources; volunteering, in the short term, may also help an individual find employment
- to form meaningful relationships – if an individual is able to spend more time in the community there is more chance of them meeting new people and making friends.

Co-production, choice and control

Such as to:

- be treated as an equal partner in decision making about their care
- be able to make decisions about their life/care
- have more of what is important to them.

These are all interrelated. Further information can be found in LO1.2 (page 113).

Inclusive and competent communities

Individuals should have the opportunity to participate in community activities, to volunteer in their community and, ultimately, to feel they belong.

For an individual to have a part in a community it helps if they:

- feel valued as a neighbour, friend, tenant, employee or volunteer

- have friends, social contacts, ways of contributing, reasons to go out each day, a real home, meaningful work, hobbies, freedom to make decisions
- can use community resources such as sports clubs, libraries, interest groups and leisure centres.

See LO1.3 (page 117) for further information about community involvement.

2.3 Current context of the person-centred approach

The policy landscape

All of the Acts, summarised in LO1.5 (page 119), confirm the government's commitment to personalisation. Personal budgets featured earlier in the Health and Social Care Act 2001.

Role of a person-centred approach in achieving good practice in the delivery of care services

An individual who is involved in their own treatment is more likely to continue with the treatment and be happy with the outcome. When involved in the decision-making process they are more knowledgeable and less anxious as they understand the risks and benefits. They have been able to ask any questions to clarify concerns as well as to feel that their opinion counts. They also have a better relationship with the professional as they will feel valued and treated with respect for what they could bring to the partnership.

2.4 Historic overview

Institutional history of public services

In the nineteenth century, a rapid expansion of new institutions meant many individuals with disabilities were moved from their homes and communities into asylums and workhouses. These were long-stay institutions with most people confined there until they died. Institutions often regarded their disabled residents as second-class citizens and showed them little respect. Staff often made little attempt to empathise with disabled people's experiences, denying them autonomy, choice and dignity.

These institutions lasted into the twentieth century. In the 1940s and 1950s, Leonard Cheshire, RNIB and the Spastics Society established residential homes for people with disabilities. Prior to this the only option for people with some disabilities was to be forcibly put into mental institutions. However, the movement for equal rights for people with disabilities was gaining momentum.

The 1990s saw the introduction of direct payments and the growing influence of the People First movement (see below).

The 2000s saw the closure of the last remaining institutions, signalling the end of **segregated** institutional living.

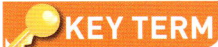

KEY TERM

Segregated – to be set apart from others.

Disability Rights Movement and links to person-centred approach

The person-centred approach originated from individuals with disabilities who wanted independent living, participation, choice, control and empowerment. These concepts have their origins in the social model of disability and the Disability Rights Movement which led to the Independent Living Movement.

In 1995, protests by disabled people lead to the landmark introduction of the Disability Discrimination Act. This makes it illegal to discriminate against disabled people in connection with employment, the provision of goods, facilities and services or the disposal or management of premises. Service providers must make reasonable adjustments to enable disabled people to access their services.

In 1996, after years of campaigning by people with disabilities, the government produced legislation allowing for direct payments. This was enshrined in the Community Care and Direct Payments Act 1996. In 2001 Health and Social Care Act made it mandatory to offer direct payments to those with an assessed need. The Valuing People White Paper (2001) aimed to make direct payments available to more people with a learning disability and officially introduced 'person-centred planning' as part of social work practice.

INDEPENDENT RESEARCH ACTIVITY

(30 minutes)

Research the Disability Rights Movement further, then compare and contrast the life of an individual who needs support today with the life of an individual in the 1980s.

2.5 Challenges to adopting a person-centred approach

Resistance to change

Resistance to change is an emotional reaction based on fear of loss. Some individuals may not want to lose the safety net of someone else making decisions for them. Professionals may feel loss of power as they are no longer in control.

Institutional history of public services

Traditionally, it was common practice for individuals to accept professionals' decisions as they 'knew best'. This culture will not be changed overnight.

Institutions promoting a medical model of health

The medical model of health sees disability as a problem belonging to the individual; therefore, they are limited by their condition and cannot participate in society. Institutions such as the NHS focus on curing or fixing the individual as they can deal with disabilities using medical advances such as surgery or medication.

Lack of staff training

As person-centred care is a relatively new concept, if it is to be successful, staff, at all levels, should be re-trained as they will need a different set of skills.

Communication barriers

Good communication is the basis of a person-centred approach as it helps to establish trusting relationships and ensures that information is passed on and understood. Barriers can lead to resentment, frustration, misunderstanding and demoralisation for both individuals and professionals.

Respecting choice when alternatives may promote better health or wellbeing

Sometimes it can be difficult for professionals to accept an individual's choice, particularly if their choice could potentially affect their health; for example, when an individual decides they will not go for **screening**.

> 🔑 **KEY TERM**
>
> **Screening** – process of identifying healthy people who may be at risk of disease; for example, the breast screening programme.

Focusing on deficits rather than capacities

In the past, professionals assessed individuals in terms of what they could not do; that is, deficits. They then set the individual goals to overcome the deficits instead of focusing on the individual's strengths, as the person-centred approach does.

Lack of clarity over roles and responsibilities

In a person-centred approach everyone is an equal partner, so roles and responsibilities are shared between the individual, the family, carers and professionals.

2.6 Methods for overcoming challenges

Values-based recruitment

Staff values have a major impact on the quality of care. The values-based recruitment model is designed to help and support employers in recruiting staff with social care values. Part of this process involves asking questions at job interviews that enable candidates to give examples of behaviours in their previous roles that demonstrate their values in action. It focuses on how and why candidates made certain choices in their work and explores the attitudes and reasons underpinning their behaviour, giving the employer a good insight into the applicant's values.

Staff training

Staff training can reduce job stress and reduce staff turnover as well as adding job satisfaction. Staff must have the confidence for delivering person-centred care through skills and knowledge gained in education and training.

Regular review of support provided

Regular reviews are essential as they are as important as the support/care plan. Reviews should be conducted in a person-centred way when the individual, their family and the professionals feel it is necessary. The reviews should be included in the support plan.

Recognising when provision is not person-centred and taking action to rectify this

This could happen if the professional working with the individual fails to constantly check that the individual is aware of what is happening and that they are in control of the process. If the individual does not feel in control then this is easily rectified by the professional. Another factor could be if the individual takes a passive role.

Modelling behaviour

Modelling behaviour is observing good practice, of how other professionals carry out person-centred care, and then imitating or copying it. This can be a good starting point for professionals who need to gain confidence, as they are able to watch and then follow the example they have observed.

> **KNOW IT**
>
> 1 Explain what is meant by a person-centred approach.
> 2 Discuss three key concepts of a person-centred approach.
> 3 Analyse the effects of the Disability Rights Movement in the person-centred approach.
> 4 Describe challenges to adopting a person-centred approach.
> 5 Explain how the challenges described in question 4 may be overcome.

LO3 Understand methods used to implement a person-centred approach

GETTING STARTED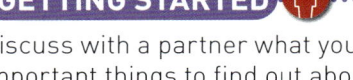

Discuss with a partner what you think are the most important things to find out about an individual, other than any relevant medical details. How would you find out this information?

3.1 Tools to find out what is important for a person

Good days/bad days

This tool encourages an individual to describe a typical good day so the carer/professional can learn what makes a good day and what support is needed to achieve it. Factors for bad days can also be identified and avoided. It enables an individual to make changes in their own life to help them have more good days. The information can be used to inform assessment, care plans and support plans. It can also be used in reviews to better understand how to support individuals in the future.

Routines

Getting an individual to talk through their daily routines will provide an idea of what is and what isn't working for them. For example, if they tell you that it typically takes two hours to get out of bed and dressed, they may need further support in their morning routine.

Top tips

The purpose of 'top tips' or the 'two minute drill' is to learn what is most important to, and for, the individual and the critical aspects of support they need. It is useful when the carer has only a few moments of someone's time. They have two minutes to find out what they should know and what they need to do to create a meaningful, safe and enjoyable day for the individual.

Relationship circles

Also known as relationship maps, relationship circles help to identify who an individual knows, how they know them, who else in the circle knows them and how these networks can help support an individual to live the life they want. It identifies who is closest to the individual and who is further away. There are many different types of relationship maps or circles.

One-page profiles

This is a summary of what matters to a person produced on a single page of A4 paper.

> **? THINK ABOUT IT**
>
> **Case study: Andy**
>
> Andy has learning difficulties and a hearing impairment. He has been admitted to hospital seriously ill with pneumonia. Staff are struggling to communicate with Andy and this has had an impact on how he is responding to treatment.
>
> Discuss how a one-page profile would help Andy and the hospital staff.

3.2 Tools that enhance voice, choice and control

Communication charts

Communication charts are an essential tool when individuals do not use words to communicate. They describe the ways an individual chooses to communicate so that other people can understand them. They can reduce the frustration of not being understood, protect dignity and can create a more inclusive environment. A communication chart has four headings, like the example in Table 6.2.

Table 6.1 Elements of a one-page profile

A one-page profile must have	What this section is	What this section is not
1 What people like and admire about the individual.	List of positive, strong statements about the individual and their talents and strengths.	A list of things the individual has done.
2 What is important to the individual.	What really matters to the individual. Information from all aspects of their life, including hobbies, routines and people, so someone who does not know them can understand who they are and who and what is important to them.	A list of likes and dislikes.
3 How to support the individual.	Creating best situations and outcomes for the individual. Includes what others need to know so they can help in a positive way.	A list of general hints; it must be specific information.

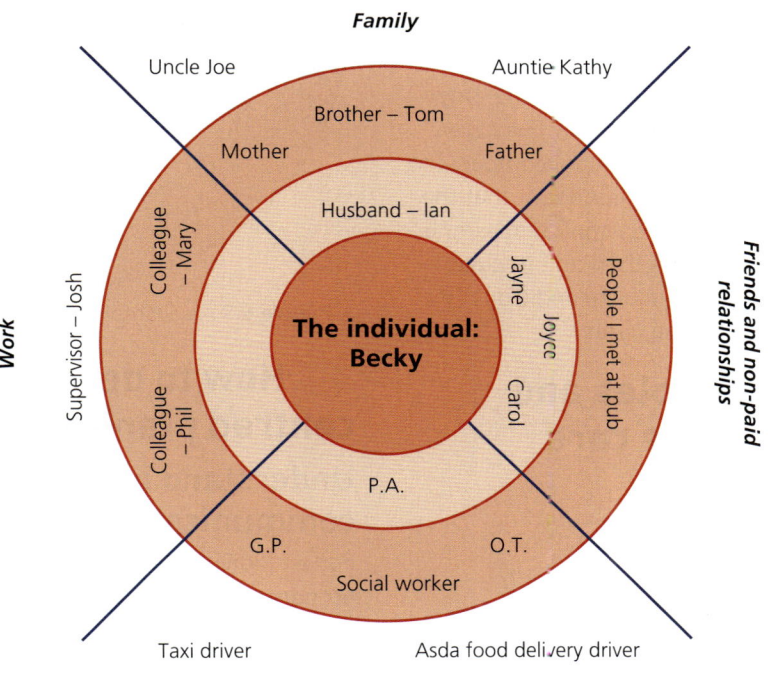

▲ **Figure 6.6** Example of a relationship circle

Table 6.2 An example of a communication chart

What is happening – describes circumstances	What the person does – clearly describes individual's behaviour	What this is thought to mean – best guess at meaning	What should staff do – how should staff respond
For example, staff go to help Lucy out of bed in the morning.	Lucy hides under the bed covers.	She does not want to get out of bed.	Go back to Lucy later.

Decision-making charts

Also known as the decision-making agreement, this helps a carer/professional support an individual to make decisions by breaking them down into three easy sections as follows:

1 Important decisions in my life.
2 How must I be involved?
3 Who makes the final decision?

This process helps the carer/professional think about how much choice and control an individual has in their life. It can lead to thinking about ways to increase choice and control for the individual.

Building effective relationships with individuals who require care or support

Learning to talk to and listen to individuals is the only way to get to know them and build up trust. The carer should always treat individuals with dignity, compassion and respect. Once an individual feels confident that the carer is honest, trustworthy, can keep confidences and is committed to their best interests then an effective relationship is more likely to be built. The individual will know they can trust and rely on the carer.

3.3 Tools to clarify roles and responsibilities in the care relationship

Doughnut (donut) chart

This tool was developed by Charles Handy in *The Empty Raincoat* (1994). It helps different professionals and agencies, supporting individuals and their families, to clarify their roles and responsibilities. The tool is useful if a carer is unsure about their responsibilities.

This tool helps the carers to see:

- what they must do (core responsibility). These are the things carers are expected to do correctly; for example, to encourage an individual to eat healthily and stay safe
- where they can use their own creativity and judgement (middle ring of doughnut); for example, support an individual to make new friends and go out more. They are learning what works and what does not work

- what is not their responsibility (on the outside of the doughnut), for example, parts of an individual's life where a carer would not get involved – things that go beyond what should be asked of a paid carer.

The chart can inform a family support plan.

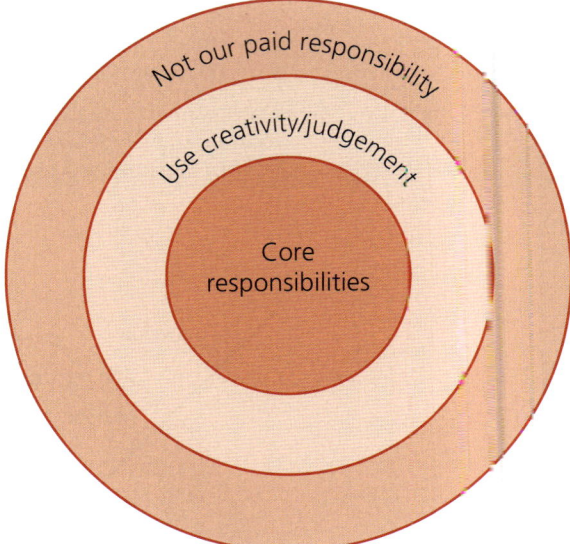

▲ **Figure 6.7** An example of a doughnut chart

3.4 How to develop person-centred plans and records

Understand how the individual communicates their wishes and needs

For an individual who does not communicate verbally, prepare support for their preferred method before the planning session. This could be through photographs, DVD clips or objects of reference. An advocate may speak on behalf of the individual.

Focus on the individual's capabilities and how they can best be supported to make decisions

This is focusing on what an individual is good at and what other people think are their strengths. Personal strengths could form the basis of the types of employment, career paths, educational courses and social activities they may wish to pursue. An individual will need to identify the key areas in which they need support and decide how they can get that support.

Finding out what is important to a person to have a good quality of life

Services used to focus on what was important *for* an individual, for example keeping them safe, but now the emphasis is on what is important *to* an individual. Person-centred planning sees the individual first, not just what is the matter with them. A balance must be found that is satisfactory to the individual.

Finding out who is important in a person's life

See LO2.1 (page 123) and 3.1 (page 126) for further information on clarity of roles and responsibilities.

See LO2.1 (page 123) and 3.1 (page 126)

KNOW IT

1 Discuss three tools to find out what is important to a person.
2 Explain what is meant by a one-page profile.
3 Explain what must be in the one-page profile.
4 List the tools that enhance voice, choice and control.
5 Describe two of the tools you have named in question 4.
6 Explain how to develop person-centred plans and records.

LO4 Know how to plan and conduct review meetings using a person-centred approach

GETTING STARTED

Planning a review meeting (10 minutes)

Write down five ways of putting the individual at the centre of their review meeting. Share your ideas with a partner.

4.1 Review meetings

Review meetings check that the individual's support and care plan is still right for them and change it, if necessary

The importance of reviews in health and social care

Putting the individual at the centre of the meeting

An individual can meet with their local authority at any time, at least once a year, to discuss whether their support plan is working. It is their opportunity to discuss whether the goals have been achieved or if the goals have changed so the plan may need to be altered. Just as the individual is at the centre of the planning process, it is essential for them to play a major role in the review process as only they know what does and does not work for them.

Builds and shares information collaboratively

Everyone involved in the individual's care – the individual, carers, family and professionals – should share information regarding what is working and what is not. This will provide as full a picture as possible. This collaborative approach means there is an open forum for opinions, experiences, information and suggestions to meet the outcomes set.

Generates actions

If some areas are found not to be working then something must be done to rectify the issue. This should be in the form of an updated support plan documenting the next steps toward achieving the revised or new goals.

The purpose of review meetings

A review meeting could be arranged to:

- meet charging needs
- review the budget
- ensure care relationships are effective
- review the person-centred description.

These are interrelated; if the needs of the individual change, then the budget will need reviewing and care relationships that were effective may suddenly become ineffective.

For example, Shiva's needs have changed as her degenerative illness has worsened and she now needs a lot more help in her personal care and also in her home. This means that she will also need a larger budget to pay for the extra help. Shiva's person-centred description would also have to be updated as her circumstances have changed.

4.2 Planning and preparing for review meetings

Understanding the role of the facilitator

The trained facilitator supports the person whose review it is and considers them to be at the centre of the meeting. They make sure that those at the meeting focus on the individual and their strengths by asking questions such as:

- What are these person's strengths and capabilities?
- What can we do to help this individual achieve their objectives?
- What is important now for this person?
- What is important for this person in the future?
- What is working/not working from this person's perspective?

The facilitator:

- invites contribution from the people at the meeting
- helps the group compare and explore their different perspectives, enabling them to see the individual, and their relationship with them, in a different way
- assists the group in agreeing a common direction, based on what they learn from their focus on the individual
- checks with the individual that they are happy with the way the review is going.

How the individual can be made to feel as comfortable as possible during the meeting

Ways of ensuring the individual is comfortable include giving them a choice over the people present at the meeting. They can invite whoever they wish so that the meeting brings together the people who give most care to the individual. This includes family, friends, carers and professionals who work with the individual.

Both the timing and the location should be the choice of the individual whose review is taking place. It should be at a convenient, accessible place for all those who have been invited. The timing also should suit everyone.

4.3 Conducting review meetings
Person-centred tools during the meeting

MAPS (making action plans)

MAPS is a planning tool that builds on a shared commitment to support the individual to move towards a more positive future. MAPS has several stages and is drawn from the different areas of an individual's life:

- What is their history?
- What are their dreams?
- What are their nightmares?

- What are their strengths, talents and capacities?
- What are their needs?

It should result in an action plan to set out who will do what and when, in order to meet their wishes and needs.

PATH (planning alternative tomorrows with hope)

PATH aims to identify the individual's hopes/dreams/goals and what it would entail to move nearer to these. There are several stages to this tool:

- Create a picture of where they would like to be.
- Identify the goals – focus on the year ahead.
- First steps to meeting these goals.
- Identify the people who will enrol to help reach dreams/goals.
- Recognise ways of building strength.
- Action plan for interim goals, for example three months ahead.
- Longer term plan, for example six months ahead.

Essential Lifestyle Planning

Essential Lifestyle Planning uses detailed planning to focus on an individual's life now and how it could be changed to provide a more enhanced lifestyle. It recognises what is important to the individual and what support would be needed to achieve this. This approach uses seven tools.

- Doughnut chart: see LO3.3 (page 128)
- Relationship circle: see LO3.1 (page 127).
- Communication chart: LO3.2 (page 127).
- Sorting importance to/for an individual. The user needs to separate what is important *to* and what is important *for* the individual and find a balance between the two.
- Matching staff. If an individual is advertising for staff to support them, a job description and a personal profile helps the applicant know what is required in the role and if they match criteria for the role.
- Learning log. This tool requires thinking through activities and events to find their strong/weak points and what worked/did not work, and learning from them so the individual can benefit more from the activities.
- What's working/what's not. If used regularly, this tool can prevent problems from escalating into a crisis. It is an effective way, for professionals, of evaluating and improving practice and support.

Personal Futures Planning

This is a detailed plan developed for an individual with complex support needs. It starts with their current situation and focuses on changes for the future. It is an effective way of mapping how an individual may be included into a community, highlighting changes that may need to be made within the community to facilitate this inclusion.

Asking appropriate questions

To find out if the support plan is working it is very important that the individual is asked the following questions:

- What is important to you now?
- What will be important to you in your future?
- What do you need to stay healthy, safe and well supported?
- What is working and not working from different perspectives?

Answering these questions will allow issues and concerns to be addressed early in the process so there is less chance of an escalation.

Review budget

A review of the budget is necessary to keep an individual's support needs under scrutiny in order to ensure that these needs are successfully being met by the agreed budget.

Generate actions

Any issues picked up at the review meeting will have an action plan with specific deadlines. For example, if an individual is concerned about their lack of inclusion in the community then this will be targeted.

KNOW IT

1 Explain the purpose of review meetings in health and social care.
2 Discuss the importance of review meetings in health and social care.
3 Explain the role of facilitator in health and social care.
4 Describe how the individual can feel comfortable during their review meeting.
5 Compare and contrast two of the person-centred tools that can be used during a review meeting.

Read about it

Fisher, A. et al. (2012) Applied AS Health & Social Care for OCR, revised edition, Oxford University Press.

Moonie, N. et al. (2007) Core Themes – Health and Social Care, Heinemann.

Morris, C., Ferreiro Peteiro, M. and Collier, F. (2015) Level 3 Health and Social Care Diploma, Hodder Education.

National Development Team for Inclusion/Helen Sanderson Associates et al. (2010). Personalisation: Don't just do it, co-produce it and live it! www.ndti.org.uk.

Unit 6: Assessment practice

Below are practice questions for you to try.

1   Alice is 89 years old and lived alone without any help until she had a stroke which left her with vascular dementia and problems with mobility. Now she needs help from social services as she wishes to stay in her own home. She has been assessed by her local authority and her personal budget has been agreed. Her son has offered to act as her authorised person.

   a) Identify two ways that Alice may receive her personal budget. (2)

   b) Identify two challenges Alice may face with regard to her personal budget. (2)

   c) Identify two adaptations Alice may need so that she can live in her home. (2)

   d) Explain how a personal assistant could help Alice to have choice and control over the care she receives. (5)

   e) Evaluate the advantages for Alice of remaining in her own home. (4)

2   a) Identify one piece of legislation (other than the Care Act 2014) that underpins personalisation. (1)

   b) Evaluate how your chosen piece of legislation helps professionals to reinforce personalisation. (6)

3   Shula is a 47-year-old primary school teacher. Two years ago a serious car accident left her quadriplegic. She is depressed about her continuing ill-health and that she can no longer teach. She is unable to carry out any personal care. She is in rehabilitation but wishes to go home as she always played a big role in her local community and wishes to do so again. She has no family who could support her.

   a) Shula will be assessed by her local authority using Fair Access to Care Services (FACS). Describe what FACS is. (1)

   b) Identify the four bands of the FACS eligibility framework. (4)

   c) Explain how Shula could participate in her local community. (5)

4   a) List three key concepts of a person-centred approach. (3)

   b) Explain why it is important to clarify roles and responsibilities in the person-centred approach. (4)

   c) Which piece of legislation ensures that an individual with a disability is not discriminated against when applying for employment? (1)

   d) There are many challenges in adopting a person-centred approach to care. Evaluate the methods for overcoming these challenges. (6)

5   Monty is 44 and has severe learning difficulties and limited communication skills. He lives in a residential home with seven other residents with similar learning difficulties. He has lived there for five months since his elderly parents were no longer able to look after him. Recently his parents have noticed that he seems depressed and has little enthusiasm for life. They are very concerned and ask for a meeting with the care manager. The manager suggests using the good day/bad day tool.

   a) Describe what is meant by the good day/bad day tool. (1)

   b) Describe how this tool can help a person-centred approach. (2)

   c) Explain how the care home should develop a person-centred plan for Monty. (5)

   d) Analyse the importance of review meetings in the person-centred approach. (6)

Total marks: 60

Unit 07
Safeguarding

ABOUT THIS UNIT

Safeguarding involves promoting the human rights, needs and interests of adults, children and young people as well as protecting them from potential and actual harm and abuse. It is fundamental to the provision of high-quality, safe and professional health and social care.

In this unit you will learn about the different types and signs of abuse as well the factors that may lead to abusive situations occurring. You will also learn more about the legislation and guidance in place to safeguard adults, children and young people Finding out how to respond to **suspicions** and **disclosures** of abuse as well as the procedures to follow for reporting abuse will help you to understand your safeguarding responsibilities. Knowing how to reduce the likelihood of abuse occurring will be crucial to the effective safeguarding and protection of adults, young people and children.

LEARNING OUTCOMES

The topics, activities and suggested reading in this unit will help you to:

1 Understand types and signs of abuse
2 Understand factors which may lead to abusive situations
3 Understand legislation, regulatory requirements and guidance that govern the safeguarding of adults, young people and children
4 Understand how to deal with suspected abuse and disclosures of abuse
5 Understand working strategies and procedures for the safeguarding and protection of adults, young people and children
6 Understand how workers within health, social care and child care environments can minimise the risk of abuse

KEY TERMS

Suspicions of abuse – when you suspect an individual is likely to be at risk of being harmed or abused, or when you suspect harm or abuse has occurred.

Disclosures – when an individual or another person tells you either directly, or indirectly through their behaviour, that they have been, or are being, abused.

How will I be assessed?

You will be assessed through an external assessment set and marked by OCR.

LO1 Understand types and signs of abuse

GETTING STARTED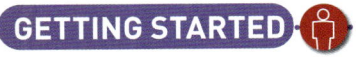

Abuse (10 minutes)
What do you understand by the term abuse? Discuss with a partner.

1.1 Types of abuse

What is abuse?
The UK government's guidance Working Together to Safeguard Children (2015) defines abuse of a child as:

'A form of maltreatment of a child. Somebody may abuse or neglect a child by inflicting harm, or by failing to act to prevent harm. Children may be abused in a family or in an institutional or community setting by those known to them or, more rarely, by others (e.g. via the internet). They may be abused by an adult or adults, or another child or children.'

Action on Elder Abuse (AEA), a national charity, defines abuse in relation to older adults as:

'a single or repeated act or lack of appropriate action, occurring within any relationship where there is an expectation of trust, which causes harm or distress to an older person'.

Abuse can occur anywhere, may happen once only or may be repeated over and over again; more than one type of abuse may also occur at the same time or at different times. Table 7.1 provides you with additional information about the current meanings of the different types of abuse.

Table 7.1 Types of abuse

Type of abuse	Definition
Physical	'A form of abuse which may involve hitting, shaking, throwing, poisoning, burning or scalding, drowning, suffocating or otherwise causing physical harm to a child. Physical harm may also be caused when a parent or carer fabricates the symptoms of, or deliberately induces, illness in a child.'* Physical abuse of adults includes 'hitting, slapping, pushing, misuse of medication, restraint or inappropriate physical sanctions'.**
Sexual	'Involves forcing or enticing a child or young person to take part in sexual activities, not necessarily involving a high level of violence, whether or not the child is aware of what is happening. The activities may involve physical contact, including assault by penetration (for example, rape or oral sex) or non-penetrative acts such as masturbation, kissing, rubbing and touching outside of clothing. They may also include non-contact activities, such as involving children in looking at, or in the production of, sexual images, watching sexual activities, encouraging children to behave in sexually inappropriate ways, or grooming a child in preparation for abuse (including via the internet).'* Sexual abuse of adults includes 'rape and sexual assault or sexual acts to which the adult has not consented or was pressured into consenting'.**
Emotional/psychological	'The persistent emotional maltreatment of a child such as to cause severe and persistent adverse effects on the child's emotional development. It may involve conveying to a child that they are worthless or unloved, inadequate, or valued only in so far as they meet the needs of another person. It may include not giving the child opportunities to express their views, deliberately silencing them or "making fun" of what they say or how they communicate. It may feature age or developmentally inappropriate expectations being imposed on children.'* Emotional/psychological abuse of adults includes 'threats of harm or abandonment, deprivation of contact, humiliation, blaming, controlling, intimidation, coercion, harassment, verbal abuse, isolation or unreasonable and unjustified withdrawal of services or supportive networks'.**
Neglect	'The persistent failure to meet a child's basic physical and/or psychological needs, likely to result in the serious impairment of the child's health or development.' It may involve a failure to 'provide adequate food, clothing and shelter (including exclusion from home or abandonment), protect a child from physical and emotional harm or danger, ensure adequate supervision (including the use of inadequate caregivers) or ensure access to appropriate medical care or treatment.'* Neglect of adults includes 'ignoring medical or physical care needs, failure to provide access to appropriate health, care and support or educational services, the withholding of the necessities of life, such as medication, adequate nutrition and heating'.**

Financial	A form of abuse that includes 'theft, fraud, exploitation, coercion in relation to an adult's financial affairs or arrangements, including in connection with wills, property, inheritance or financial transactions, or the misuse or misappropriation of property, possessions or benefits'.**
Institutional	A form of abuse that can include 'neglect and poor care practice within an institution or specific care setting like a hospital or care home, for example. This may range from isolated incidents to continuing ill-treatment.'**
Bullying	Although there is no legal definition of bullying, it is usually defined as behaviour that is repeated, intended to hurt someone and often aimed at certain groups, e.g. because of race, gender or sexual orientation. It can include physical assault, teasing, name calling, making threats and cyberbullying – bullying via mobile phone or online (e.g. email, social networks and instant messenger).
Discrimination	Something that underlies many forms of abuse and includes treating a person less favourably on, for example, 'grounds of race, gender and gender identity, disability, sexual orientation, religion, and other forms of harassment, slurs or similar treatment'.**
Exploitation/mate crime	A form of abuse that can occur 'either opportunistically or premeditated'; it involves 'unfairly manipulating someone for profit or personal gain', often when the abuser pretends to be their friend.**

*(Source: Working Together to Safeguard Children: A Guide to Inter-agency Working to Safeguard and Promote the Welfare of Children, March 2015)

**(Source: Care and Support Statutory Guidance Issued under the Care Act 2014)

GROUP ACTIVITY

Types of abuse (45 minutes)

Post up on one wall examples of different types of abuse. Post up on another wall the definitions of different types of abuse. Work in small groups to match each type of abuse to its correct definition. Record and present your findings to the rest of the groups.

1.2 Signs of different types of abuse

Recognising different types of abuse involves being aware of the signs that abuse is taking place as well as the symptoms individuals may experience as a result. Remember, all individuals are unique so signs and symptoms will also be different and may or may not be indicators of abuse.

Table 7.2 overleaf shows a list of some of the signs and symptoms of the main forms of abuse to look out for that may indicate that abuse is occurring or has occurred.

? THINK ABOUT IT

Case study: Gemma

Gemma is 10 years old and every Tuesday night, after dance class, stays overnight at her cousin's house. The following morning at school, her maths teacher notices that Gemma appears to have been crying and seems a little anxious; he also notices a bite mark on her arm. When he asks Gemma if she is alright she kicks her chair back and runs out of the class.

Analyse Gemma's behaviour. What types of abuse could this be a possible indicator of and why?

KNOW IT

1 Define emotional/psychological abuse.
2 Define institutional abuse.
3 Identify the signs of institutional abuse.
4 What are the signs of discrimination?
5 How can abuse affect an individual's behaviour?

Table 7.2 Signs of abuse

Types of abuse	Signs to recognise	Symptoms to recognise
Physical abuse	Unexplained injuries that are the shape of objects, finger marks, bruises, black eyes, fractures, breaks, cuts, scars, scratches, bite or slap marks, burns, weight loss.	Individual becoming anxious or fearful in particular in the presence of the abuser, less confident, withdrawn, deterioration in health, reluctance to undress in front of others.
Sexual abuse	Bruises, scratches, soreness, or bleeding around genital and rectal areas, incontinence, pregnancy, blood on clothing, unexplained stomach pains and cramps.	Individual becoming withdrawn, anxious, frustrated, aggressive, displaying inappropriate uninhibited sexual behaviour, reluctance to undress.
Emotional/ psychological abuse	The individual avoiding making eye contact, being fearful and anxious, incontinence, self-harming, the individual telling you that they are not worthy and not able.	Individual displaying changes in eating and sleeping, low self-esteem, becoming withdrawn from people and situations, having mood swings, anxious, fearful, frustrated, aggressive.
Neglect	Poor standards of care by others that do not meet the individual's needs, e.g. poor personal hygiene, malnourishment, dehydration, dirty surroundings, development of pressure sores, untreated medical conditions, repeated falls. Self-neglect can include unexplained injuries to arms, face and body including bruises, scratches and cuts.	Individual becoming anxious, depressed, suicidal thoughts, withdrawn. Individual becoming passive, social withdrawal, losing interest in themselves and their values in life.
Financial/ material abuse	Unexplained lack of money or wish to spend money, sudden debts and unpaid bills, possessions disappearing, sudden changing of the individual's will, enduring power of attorney obtained when individual is unable to consent.	Individual becoming anxious over money and increasingly talking about inability to make payments and buy items.
Institutional abuse	Poor working practices and low standards of care and support, inadequate staffing, withholding as well as lack of access to care, support, activities and visitors, failure to uphold individuals' rights to choice, privacy and dignity.	Individual becoming withdrawn, passive, frustrated, feeling isolated, social withdrawal, losing interest in themselves and others.
Bullying	Unexplained physical injuries, asking for or stealing money to give to a bully, self-harming that can include bruises, scratches and cuts.	Individual becoming fearful of going out and carrying out day-to-day activities, anxious, withdrawn. Low self-esteem, changes in eating and sleeping, suicidal thoughts.
Discrimination	Failure to respect an individual's needs, exclusion from activities or services, a cold or intolerant attitude towards the individual.	Individual becoming withdrawn from people and situations, anxious, withdrawn, low self-esteem, frustrated.
Exploitation/mate crime	Unexplained physical injuries, bills not being paid, losing weight.	Individual becoming withdrawn from people and situations, low self-esteem, mood swings, changes in friends.

LO2 Understand factors which may lead to abusive situations

GETTING STARTED

Why abuse? (10 minutes)

Discuss as a whole group why abuse happens. You could think about a specific example of adult or child abuse you have heard or read about.

2.1 Adults, young people and children most at risk from abuse

Some individuals may be more vulnerable to abuse than others due to their individual needs. Figure 7.1 details examples of what these needs may include and how they can increase individuals' risk of being abused.

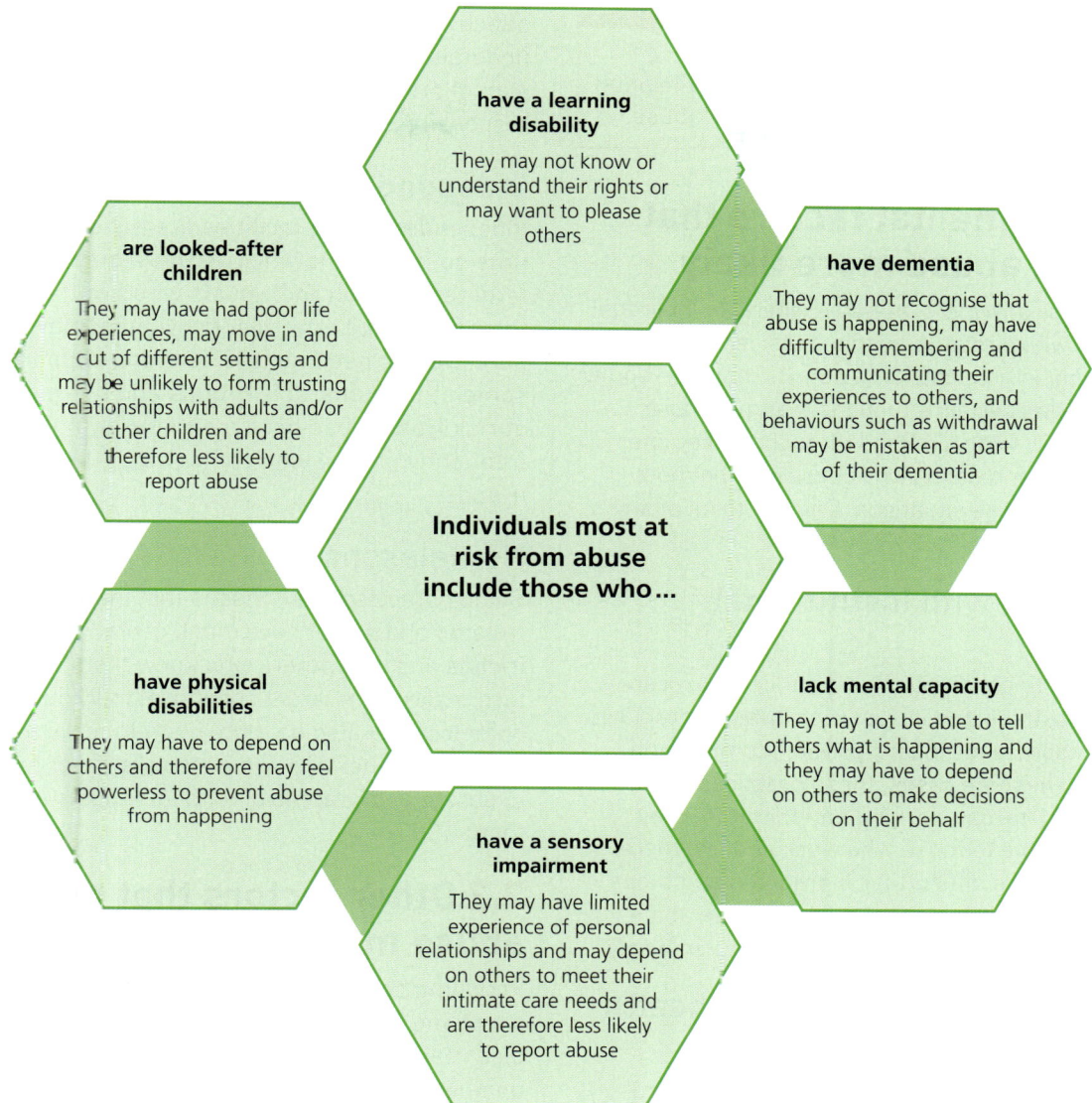

▲ **Figure 7.1** Individuals most at risk from abuse

It is important to remember that just because these needs are present it does not mean that an individual will be abused, but they may make the circumstances for abuse more likely.

One hundred and thirty-two councils submitted data on **safeguarding alerts** in 2012–13. A total of 176,000 safeguarding alerts were reported by the 132 councils. In the 172,000 alerts where the key information was known:

- 60 per cent were over the age of 65
- 40 per cent were adults aged 18–64
- almost half of the alerts (49 per cent) were about adults who have a physical disability
- 24 per cent were adults who have mental health needs
- 19 per cent were adults who have learning disabilities.

(Source: HSCIC, Abuse of Vulnerable Adults in England 2012–13, Final Report, Experimental Statistics, 6 February 2014)

2.2 Environmental factors that may make abuse more likely

Abuse can occur anywhere: at home where an individual lives alone or with a relative, within a residential or nursing setting, in hospitals or in public. There are some environments and certain situations that may make abuse more likely to occur. Read through the key ones below and note the reasons why abuse may be more likely to occur in these situations. Can you think of any other reasons?

Care services with institutional practices

Institutional settings, as you found out in LO1.2, can involve rigid routines and intrusive or invasive practices that do not respect individuals' privacy, comfort and unique needs. In some cases, these practices could form part of day-to-day working and therefore may become acceptable to those who work and live there. It then becomes more difficult for individuals and those who work in these settings to report or speak about these institutional practices if they are in the minority.

Adults and children residing in health and social care settings

Adults and children living in health and social care settings usually perceive these settings as safe and those who work there and/or live there with them as being in positions of trust and power. Adults and children may therefore be afraid to speak out about abuse that is happening as they may fear that they could lose their home or be responsible for a health and care professional losing their job or going to prison.

Health services

Health services, such as GP surgeries and physiotherapy practices, will be visited by individuals with a wide range of needs; again, practitioners are usually viewed as being in positions of trust and power. If staff are not trained well, or do not have the necessary skills to communicate and problem solve effectively, then individuals may not receive safe and effective care. In addition, these settings may also be understaffed and this may mean that staff will be under a lot of pressure and have less time to carry out their responsibilities safely.

Independent living facilities

Independent living facilities are not staffed all the time so individuals who live there may become targeted by other individuals who live there by staff, their visitors or relatives. Individuals may also be perceived as needing less care and support than some other vulnerable groups and therefore may be at risk from abuse because they may not be visited as frequently or may lose contact with their family and friends.

Homelessness

Being homeless often means that individuals become isolated and do not have much contact with family and friends and with others who know them; this can in turn make them targets of abuse. Individuals who are homeless will also be more likely to move from one place to another and could also stay from time to time in unsafe public areas or with individuals who abuse them.

2.3 Other factors that may make abuse more likely

Providing care and support to individuals can be a very satisfying and enriching experience, but it can also be a real challenge to ensure that every individual's unique needs are fully met; it is also difficult for an individual to accept that their needs have changed and that they have to depend on others. Situations where individuals are dependent on others as well as other factors may make abuse more likely to occur; see Figure 7.2.

CLASSROOM DISCUSSION

Taking stock (30 minutes)

As a class, discuss how you felt about the different types of abuse you've learned more about; were there some types of abuse that you found more difficult to talk about? Were you surprised by the factors that make some individuals more vulnerable to abuse? Did you know about the range of places where abuse can take place?

Situations where people are dependent on others	Relationships where there is an imbalance of power	Social isolation
e.g. an older individual who has dementia and depends on others for personal care and management of money. Care givers may experience high levels of stress particularly if the individual displays challenging needs such as verbal or physical aggression, and that can lead to abuse.	e.g. a child who has autism and depends on others for all aspects of their care. The caregiver may not be receiving practical or emotional support from others and may also have other family and work commitments; these factors may cause the child's needs to not be met or to be ignored.	e.g an individual who has mental health needs and is living independently with no care or support. The individual may show signs of mental illness and may become a target for abuse, particularly if the abuser knows that the individual lives alone.

Situations where there is an invasion of privacy	Staffing issues
e.g. a health or social care setting where individuals' doors and/or curtains are not kept shut whilst they are getting dressed or undressed. Individuals may become the targets of abuse as they may be feeling vulnerable and embarrassed at having to depend on others for their personal, intimate care.	e.g. lack of staff or lack of staff training may also lead to the abuse of individuals as unsafe and abusive practices may result. Staffing issues may also remain unchallenged by staff, management and/or individuals and therefore may make it even more difficult to speak out.

▲ **Figure 7.2** Other reasons why abuse may occur

 THINK ABOUT IT

Case study: Maurice

Maurice is 74 years old and lives on his own in the flat that he shared with his partner Mike for 30 years until Mike died recently from a sudden illness. Once a week his nephew visits and helps him with reading his letters as his sight has deteriorated and he finds it increasingly difficult to read small print. Last week Maurice noted that his nephew seemed different; he was a little impatient with him when he couldn't find the letter that had arrived from the hospital and kept on asking him about his finances. Maurice feels uncomfortable about his nephew visiting him again this week and so thought he would talk to his GP about the situation as she has known Maurice for a long time. However, the surgery receptionist tells him that his GP has left. As Maurice said that it's not too urgent, there are no appointments available until next week.

What factors may make Maurice more at risk from abuse?

KNOW IT

1. Define 'lacking mental capacity'.
2. How can institutional practices lead to abuse happening?
3. Describe different environments where abuse may be more likely.
4. Describe different situations that may make abuse more likely.
5. How can staffing issues lead to abuse of adults, young people and children?

LO3 Understand legislation, regulatory requirements and guidance that govern the safeguarding of adults, young people and children

GETTING STARTED

Safeguarding (10 minutes)

What do you understand by the term **safeguarding**? Share with the whole group.

3.1 Current applicable legislation

Legislation refers to the process of making laws and defines the duties organisations and practitioners must carry out by law. Guidance, by contrast, refers to the process of how legislation should be implemented and complied with by organisations and practitioners.

🔑 KEY TERM

Safeguarding – proactive measures to reduce the risks of danger, harm and abuse.

Table 7.3 Relevant legislation and guidance

Name of legislation	How it protects and safeguards individuals	Useful sources of additional information
Human Rights Act 1998	• The Act enables specific rights to be given to every person living in the UK. It promotes for example the right to life, freedom from degrading treatment and respect for private and family life.	http://tinyurl.com/2b4rax5
Health and Social Care Act 2008 (Care Quality Commission)	• The Act established the Care Quality Commission (CQC) as the regulator to provide registration and inspection of health and adult social care services together for the first time, including primary care services such as hospitals, GP practices, dental practices and care homes.	http://tinyurl.com/4yszqqe
Care Act 2014	• The Act requires local authorities to make enquiries if an individual is being abused or neglected or is at risk of abuse or neglect. • It requires local authorities to set up multi-agency safeguarding adult boards to review cases when individuals die as a result of abuse or neglect. • It introduced the Duty of Candour and Fundamental Standards on which all service providers are inspected.	http://tinyurl.com/rew4d8
Safeguarding Vulnerable Groups Act 2006	• The Act implemented the vetting and barring scheme to ensure that people considered unsuitable to work with vulnerable adults and children are not able to do so.	http://tinyurl.com/zz5nw7e
Mental Capacity Act 2005 and Deprivation of Liberty Safeguards	• The Act aims to protect and empower individuals who are unable to make choices and decisions for themselves. • The Mental Capacity Act Deprivation of Liberty Safeguards (MCA DOLS) were introduced into the Mental Capacity Act 2005 through the Mental Health Act 2007 and came into effect on 1 April 2009.	http://tinyurl.com/zbqkgus
Equality Act 2010	• The Act protects people from discrimination, harassment and victimisation due to protected characteristics including: race, gender, disability, sexual orientation, transgender, religion and age.	http://tinyurl.com/gwz7j3m
Public Interest Disclosure Act 1998 (the 'whistleblowing' act)	• The Act protects workers who disclose information about malpractice including abuse at their current or former workplace and provides the legal framework for whistleblowing.	http://tinyurl.com/2uydlcq
The Rehabilitation of Offenders Act 1974	• The Act exists to support the rehabilitation into employment of reformed offenders. • It aims to give those with convictions or cautions the opportunity to start afresh as some convictions or cautions can become spent after a specified period of time known as the rehabilitation period. • Section 139 of the Legal Aid, Sentencing and Punishment of Offenders Act 2012, which was brought into force on 10 March 2014, made two key changes to the 1974 Act. The first change was to extend the scope of the Act to cover custodial sentences of up to 48 months (previously prison sentences over 30 months never became spent), and the second was to change the length of some of the rehabilitation periods (in most cases by reducing them).	http://tinyurl.com/jx5f34m

Name of legislation	How it protects and safeguards individuals	Useful sources of additional information
Children Act 2004 – Every Child Matters	• The Children Act 2004 established for England many reforms that underpin children's services including: a Children's Commissioner to champion the views and interests of children and young people, a duty on local authorities to make arrangements to promote co-operation between agencies and other appropriate bodies including setting up local safeguarding children boards. • The Act gave legal force to the five outcomes included in Every Child Matters and are key to wellbeing in childhood and later life – 1) being healthy 2) staying safe 3) enjoying and achieving 4) making a positive contribution and 5) achieving economic wellbeing.	http://tinyurl.com/hfrrcjg
Data Protection Act	• The Data Protection Act 1998 regulates the way in which personal data needs to be handled and therefore protects people's data from being placed in the wrong hands which might make them more vulnerable to abuse.	http://tinyurl.com/nzdksfd
Disclosure and Barring Scheme, 'No Secrets' (Department of Health 2000)	• The 'No Secrets' (England) and 'In Safe Hands' (Wales) 2000 guidance documents set out how different agencies must work together to respond to, investigate and prevent abuse of vulnerable adults wherever possible.	http://tinyurl.com/mfg2h6z
Working Together to Safeguard Children (2006)	• Working Together 2006 sets out how organisations and individuals should work together to safeguard and promote the welfare of children and young people in accordance with the Children Act 1989 and the Children Act 2004. • This guidance was updated in 2013 and 2015.	http://tinyurl.com/ppcndw3 http://tinyurl.com/pxdtntn
Safeguarding Adults (2005)	• This guidance document provides a national framework of 11 sets of good practice standards to ensure the implementation of high-quality and consistent work in protecting vulnerable adults from abuse.	http://tinyurl.com/zjg5bmq
Mental Capacity Act Code of Practice 2014	• This code of practice gives guidance to people who work with and care for individuals who can't make decisions for themselves.	http://tinyurl.com/mfyf3hh

INDEPENDENT RESEARCH ACTIVITY

What the law says (60 minutes)

Conduct some independent research around two pieces of legislation and two guidance documents described in Table 7.3.

Note down in your own words the main points of each, in relation to protecting and safeguarding individuals. You can use the internet and books as sources of information.

THINK ABOUT IT

Case study: Nana

Nana has recently returned from maternity leave and is feeling anxious and not very confident about resuming her duties as a care worker as she is unsure if her knowledge and practices are still up to date in relation to protecting and safeguarding adults.

Imagine you are Nana's supervisor, explain how you could support her.

LO4 Understand how to deal with suspected abuse and disclosures of abuse

4.1 People who might suspect or be told about abuse

As you read in LO1, abuse can happen anywhere, can show itself in different ways and can have a number of different signs and symptoms. A wide range of people might suspect or be told about abuse in relation to adults, young people and children.

Peers

An individual may find it easier to tell one of their peers or friends about being abused. This could be because the individual might feel guilty about the abuse and therefore will want to share this with a friend who will be likely to believe them and listen to them. The individual may also find it easier to speak to one of their friends about being abused because they can use their own language and terminology and not worry about how it will sound.

Family

Family members may be another source of emotional support for an individual being abused. An individual may turn to a family member they trust and feel comfortable with. Family members who know the individual well may be more likely to notice that the individual's behaviour has changed and might suspect that abuse is happening.

Siblings

An individual may also be likely to tell a sibling about being abused; particularly if the individual has an older brother or sister who they see as a role model who they look up to and can confide in. Some siblings can also notice, due to their close bond with the individual, when something is wrong and might suspect that abuse is happening.

Teachers

Teachers' roles involve close monitoring of children and young people's learning and development, so they may notice when an individual's behaviour changes or when they behave in an unusual way and suspect abuse is happening. A student may have a good relationship with one particular teacher and may choose to confide in them. They may also be found by a teacher when they are upset or anxious and speak to them about being abused.

Social workers

Social workers are professionals who are qualified and trained to identify evidence to suggest that an individual is being abused. They may also receive suspicions of abuse from other professionals such as teachers, GPs and school nurses. For some young people, social workers are their only main contact and so may be the first person they approach about being abused; in addition, a social worker who has worked with a young person for a long time may also identify when something is wrong.

Other professionals

Professionals such as doctors, nurses and health visitors may suspect abuse while carrying out their roles. Like social workers, they are trained to identify signs and symptoms and if they have come into contact with the individual on a number of occasions they may have noticed a deterioration in their physical or emotional health. In addition, a private appointment may provide the environment where an individual may be more likely to disclose that they are being abused.

Other members of the public

Other members of the public, such as neighbours, may notice changes in an individual's behaviour or the individual behaving in an unusual way. They may, for example, notice that they haven't seen the individual for a long time or that the individual becomes withdrawn when they are spoken to or in the presence of a particular person.

4.2 How to deal with disclosures of abuse and suspected abuse

Whether abuse is disclosed directly or suspected there are certain principles that must be upheld.

Duty to report

It is important to not ignore the signs that an individual may be at risk of abuse or is being abused; doing nothing is not an option as it may result in the individual not being safe because the abuse continues. It is therefore your duty to not delay reporting any suspicions or disclosures of abuse, to ensure the individual is protected from any further risk of abuse.

Report appropriately

Each organisation will have its own reporting procedures for both disclosures of abuse and suspected abuse. It is important that you familiarise yourself with these so that when you report your concerns, you are doing so in line with your workplace procedures. This may involve reporting your or others' suspicions to the named person in your workplace, such as a line manager, or making a referral to an external agency such as the NSPCC, CQC, social services or the police. Not reporting abuse appropriately may lead to you failing to carry out your role and responsibilities effectively; this may in turn result in an individual and others being in danger.

Reporting procedures

Reporting procedures will also include more information about the actions your organisation expects you to take; for example, how to ensure that any evidence is preserved and how to record accurately the details of what you have noticed, others have witnessed or you have been told. Figures 7.3 and 7.4 include more information about the reporting procedures that must be followed when dealing with suspected abuse and disclosures or allegations of abuse.

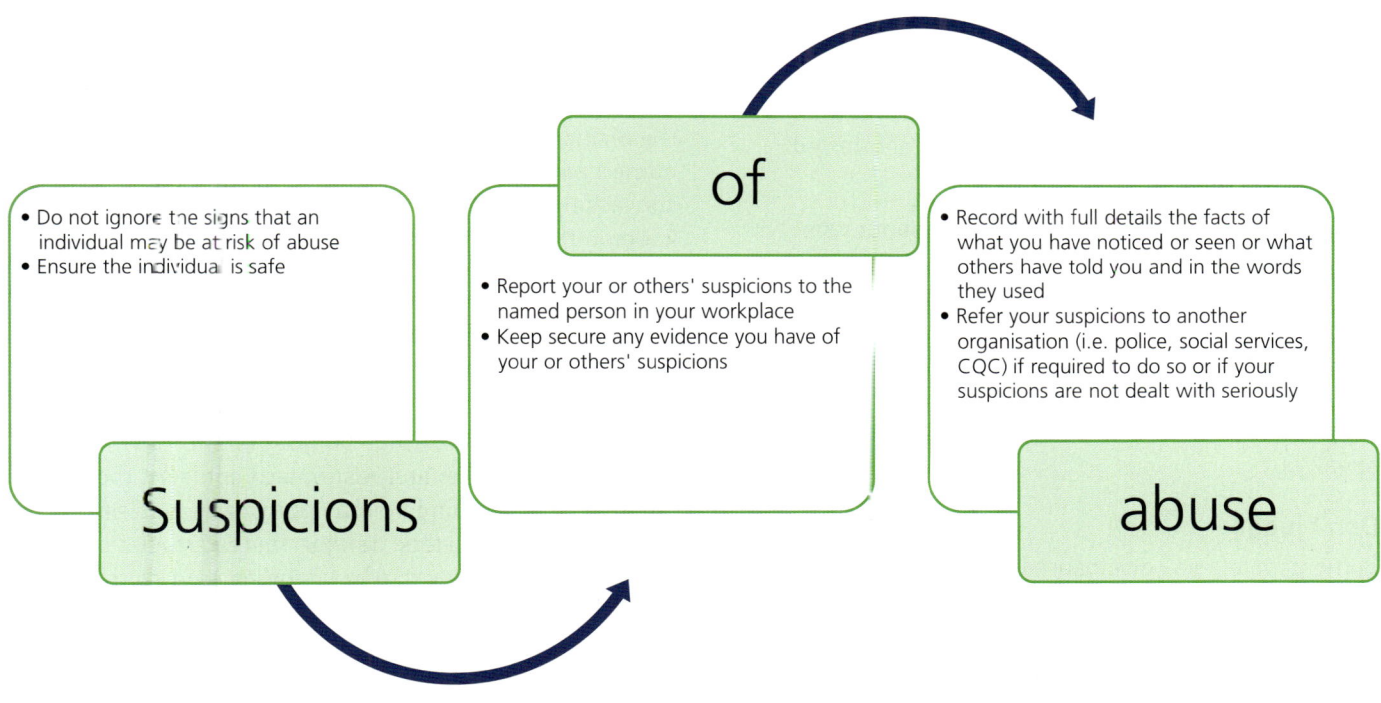

▲ **Figure 7.3** Actions to take when there are suspicions of abuse

Suspicions

- Do not ignore the signs that an individual may be at risk of abuse
- Ensure the individual is safe

of

- Report your or others' suspicions to the named person in your workplace
- Keep secure any evidence you have of your or others' suspicions

abuse

- Record with full details the facts of what you have noticed or seen or what others have told you and in the words they used
- Refer your suspicions to another organisation (i.e. police, social services, CQC) if required to do so or if your suspicions are not dealt with seriously

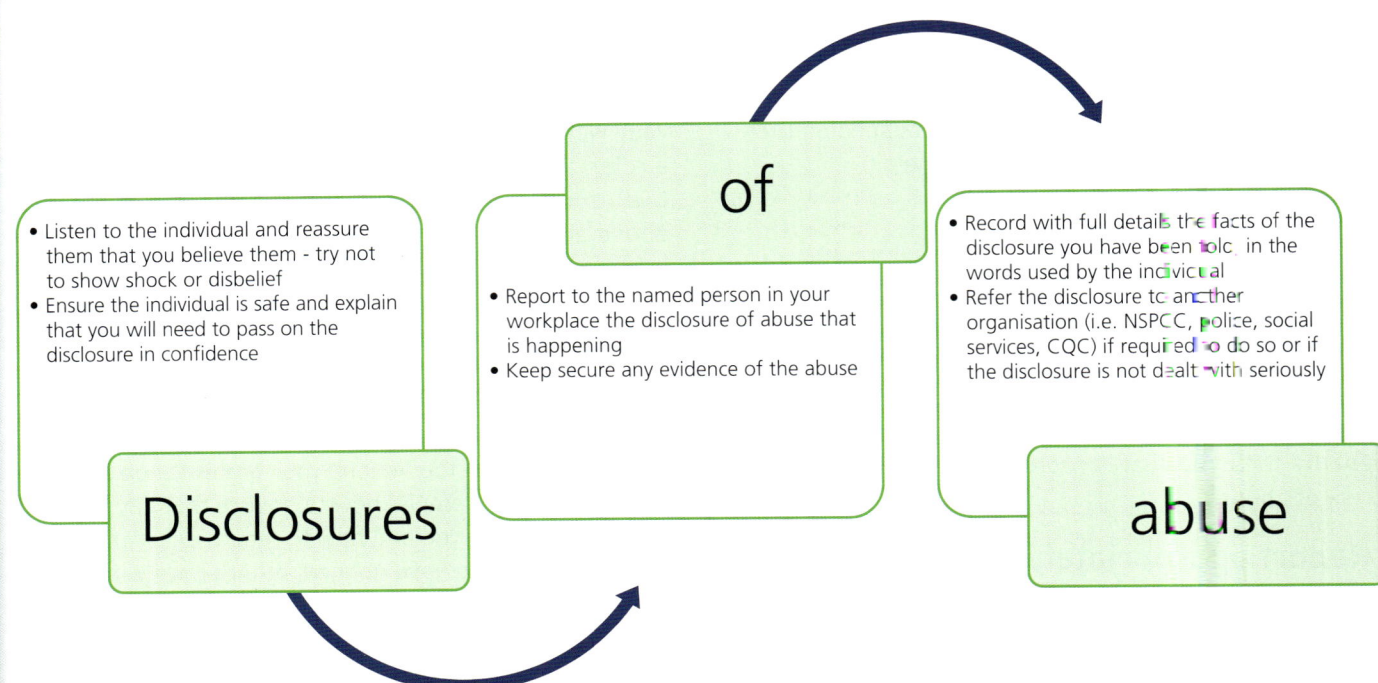

Listen to the individual and reassure them that you believe them - try not to show shock or disbelief
Ensure the individual is safe and explain that you will need to pass on the disclosure in confidence

Report to the named person in your workplace the disclosure of abuse that is happening
Keep secure any evidence of the abuse

of

Record with full details the facts of the disclosure you have been told, in the words used by the individual
Refer the disclosure to another organisation (i.e. NSPCC, police, social services, CQC) if required to do so or if the disclosure is not dealt with seriously

Disclosures

abuse

▲ **Figure 7.4** Actions to take when there are disclosures of abuse

Support and comfort

Disclosures and suspicions of an individual being abused can make individuals feel distressed, anxious and/or angry. Recognising this is important as the individual will need to be supported and comforted through this difficult time.

An individual may also have concerns about what will happen to them or to their abuser; it is important that you reassure the individual by explaining what will happen next with the disclosure or suspected abuse and the support that is available to them. Remain calm, do not look shocked, take the individual seriously and reassure them that they were right to speak out.

Don't judge

Some people delay disclosures of abuse for many years because they fear that they will not be believed or will be judged. It is for this reason that you must not make any judgements about the truth of what the individual is telling you or express any doubts; you may also want to tell the individual that they are not to blame for anything that has happened.

Maintain confidentiality

Maintaining confidentiality is crucial when dealing with disclosures of abuse and suspected abuse. This must not be confused with promising an individual that what they have told you will be kept secret; you must report the disclosure to stop the abuse. Maintaining confidentiality will involve reporting the disclosure in the strictest of confidence to the named person in your organisation, recording the conversation in private as soon as possible and keeping the record in a secure place.

Protect self

While it is important to acknowledge to an individual how difficult it is to make a disclosure or suspicion of abuse, it is also important to maintain one's own safety and wellbeing. Do not question the individual, ask leading questions or confront the alleged abuser; doing so may put you as well as the individual in further danger. Instead, focus on and listen attentively to what is being said so that the information that is recorded and reported is accurate.

Listening to disclosures and suspicions of abuse can be upsetting and stressful; if you are a survivor of abuse yourself then doing so may evoke other feelings and thoughts. It is important that you know about all the different sources of information and advice that are available to you if you require additional support or guidance at any time.

LO5 Understand working strategies and procedures for the safeguarding and protection of adults, young people and children

5.1 The policies and procedures that health and social care settings should have in place to safeguard vulnerable adults from abuse

Health and social care settings have a range of policies and procedures in place that influence how they keep vulnerable adults safe from danger, harm and abuse. Policies contain a set of principles that outline how an organisation plans to deliver its services. Procedures describe how each policy will be put into practice by, for example, detailing specific roles and responsibilities, the steps that will be taken as well as the documentation that must be used. Policies and procedures will vary between settings and organisations to reflect the organisation's specific values and the work approaches that best meet individuals' needs.

Staff training, recruitment procedures

Clear and effective recruitment procedures minimise the risk of unsuitable people working with vulnerable adults. This involves having, for example, job descriptions and codes of practice that indicate the skills, qualifications, behaviours and qualities needed to work or volunteer in the setting, and a recruitment process that provides information about the setting, its aims and the tasks involved in the work or volunteer roles available.

Health and social care settings have a duty to ensure that they recruit people who are of good character and have integrity. Information in relation to past work roles, previous convictions and investigations is essential and must be requested and reviewed through an application form, during the interview process, by requesting and following up all references and carrying out checks on whether a person is registered with a health and social care professional regulatory body.

Staff should undertake safeguarding vulnerable adult training courses that provide up-to-date information to ensure knowledge and skills remain current and effective. Government guidance states that safeguarding training must be undertaken by staff at least every three years and at least every two years if for designated officers. It must be appropriate to job roles and include an understanding of the possible signs and symptoms of vulnerable adult abuse, how to respond when abuse is disclosed or suspected and the latest safeguarding legislation, national and local policies and procedures.

A clear induction process for all new staff and volunteers prepares them for the work they will be carrying out. The Care Certificate is an important aspect of this process; it is a set of standards that have been specifically designed for those who work across both the health and social care sectors. It forms part of the induction process as it can help new staff to learn and understand more about their roles and the standards of care that will be expected from them.

A probationary period is part of all work and voluntary roles. It is the 'trial period' during which a manager or supervisor decides whether the staff member or volunteer has met the standards and expectations of the job, as set out in their induction or job description, and whether they are suitable to carry out the role on a permanent basis.

A combination of formal and informal systems of support must also be provided by organisations so that staff knowledge and skills remain current.

Appraisals are part of a formal process to ensure that staff achieve agreed goals and usually take place once a year. As part of this process employees agree with their manager or supervisor a series of personal goals that are designed for them to achieve over the year ahead. A **personal development plan** is usually the outcome of this process.

Formal supervision is the process by which an employee's manager monitors the staff member's progress towards the goals agreed in the appraisal. It happens more regularly than appraisals and can take place monthly, bi-monthly or at three-monthly intervals. Supervision can also take place with experienced colleagues (peer supervision) and/or as a team (group supervision).

Formal and informal supervision from others can be useful for staff to review what has been learned and/or achieved, identifying any gaps in knowledge and skills that exist as well as planning how to address them.

Linked to formal and informal supervision is the technique of mentoring that is used by employers. Mentoring, when used as a source of support, can be effective in providing encouragement, support, guidance and feedback around staff's personal development needs. The mentor is usually an experienced staff member who has a good understanding of both the organisation's goals and the staff member's learning and training needs, and can therefore transfer their knowledge and skills when necessary.

> ## 🔑 KEY TERM
>
> **Personal development plan** – a way of staff recording their past achievements and future learning objectives.

Disclosure and Barring Service

The Disclosure and Barring Service (DBS) works closely with the police and helps to safeguard vulnerable groups, including adults and children, from harm and abuse by preventing unsuitable people from working with them, by:

- processing requests for criminal records checks by searching police records and barred list information
- deciding whether it is appropriate for a person to be placed on or removed from a barred list
- placing people on the DBS adults' or children's barred list for England, Wales and Northern Ireland
- requiring people on the DBS adults' or children's barred list not to obtain paid or volunteering work with vulnerable adults
- requiring employers not to offer paid or volunteering work with vulnerable adults or children to people on the DBS adults' or children's barred list
- requiring employers and agencies to refer people to the DBS who have harmed or put at risk a vulnerable adult or child.

Multi-agency approach

Safeguarding children, young people and adults from abuse and promoting their welfare is everyone's responsibility. Agencies such as schools, social services, health services, youth organisations, charities and the police can work alongside one another to protect children, young people and vulnerable adults from abuse and prevent further harm and abuse. A multi-agency approach can help to:

- ensure all concerns are identified early and reported
- ensure professionals and agencies that may have different insights and experiences of individuals and their families come together and share the information they have
- provide a better insight into the needs and views of children, young people and adults
- ensure professionals and agencies work in consistent ways that focus on building trust, mutual respect and providing support to children, young people and adults.

In order for a multi-agency approach to be effective, all agencies involved must understand the role they have to play as well as the role others have in safeguarding. All professionals must be committed to working alongside other professionals who may work in different agencies and have different roles.

Risk assessments

Safeguarding individuals from abuse involves thinking about any risks that may cause them potential harm as well as the actions that may be taken to prevent that harm from occurring. This is known as risk assessment and is required by law. Risk assessments involve identifying, managing, recording and reviewing any risks that have the potential to cause harm. In this way, abuse can be prevented, its likelihood of occurring reduced and employers and employees can respond effectively when it occurs. Risk assessments also promote vulnerable adults' rights to take risks and are a way of enabling them to identify and manage potential and actual risks to themselves and others.

Accessible complaints procedures

Accessible complaints procedures enable individuals and others who work in and visit health and social care settings to openly raise and discuss any concerns and complaints. This will in turn promote an environment of mutual trust and respect, where individuals take an active role in making their own decisions. Responding promptly to complaints and concerns and ensuring complaints procedures are available in formats that are understood and reinforced will mean that individuals and others will be more likely to raise any concerns in relation to safeguarding vulnerable adults.

Designated protection officer

Health and social care organisations are required to have in place a designated protection officer; more than one may be nominated in larger organisations. This person provides information and support to staff and volunteers in relation to disclosures and suspicions of abuse.

GROUP ACTIVITY

New staff (45 minutes)

Work in small groups to agree on the five most important qualities and the five most important skills for workers of health, social care and child care settings to have to be able to safeguard adults and children from abuse. For example, you may think that being patient and approachable are important qualities, as well as excellent communication skills and the ability to stay calm under pressure. Share your findings with the other groups.

5.2 The policies and procedures that health, social care and child care settings should have in place to safeguard children from abuse

Safeguarding children is also vital to health, social care and child care settings and part of the legal requirements. It is important therefore that you are also aware of the range of measures in place to safeguard children from abuse.

? THINK ABOUT IT

Case study: Mariana

Mariana is a new volunteer at Abby Crèche and has never worked with children and their families before. During her induction training she meets with the manager and asks to see the main policies and procedures that the crèche has that are specifically related to safeguarding children from abuse.

Imagine you are the Manager of Abby Crèche and explain what policies and procedures you think are the most important for safeguarding children from abuse and that Mariana should be aware of.

KNOW IT

1 What is the role of the Disclosure and Barring Service?
2 What is meant by the term a 'multi-agency approach' when safeguarding vulnerable adults?
3 What is your understanding of an accessible complaints procedure?
4 What is the role of a designated protection officer?
5 What measures should be taken when recruiting and training staff in relation to safeguarding children and vulnerable adults?

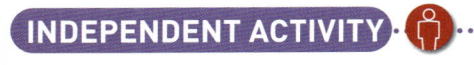

(10 minutes)

Read through the following extracts from a range of policies and procedures developed by Little Daisies

Children's Centre and think about how these compare to the policies and procedures that adult settings have in place to safeguard adults from abuse.

LITTLE DAISIES CHILDREN'S CENTRE – POLICIES & PROCEDURES

Safeguarding policy

Our safeguarding policy aims to protect all the children in our care by providing a safe and secure environment.

It is aimed at all staff including senior management and volunteers. It reflects our commitment to ensure through training and supervision, that all staff and volunteers know how to identify and report disclosures and suspicions of abuse of a child.

Confidentiality policy

Little Daisies Children's Centre makes all its staff, volunteers and visitors aware of the importance of keeping the information it receives confidential. It is committed to ensuring that information about each child is only shared with staff, volunteers and other professionals on a 'need to know basis'.

Children's parents or carers can ask to see the information held about their child at any time; parents or carers will not have access to information held about other children who attend the Children's Centre. Information held about staff and volunteers who work at the Centre will not be given out without the person's permission.

Risk assessment

Little Daisies Children's Centre aims to ensure at all times the health, safety and welfare of all its children, staff, volunteers and visitors.

As part of our health and safety management regular risk assessments are undertaken and reviewed. We undertake regular risk assessments of the following:
- all rooms in the Children's Centre's premises
- all activities provided at the Children's Centre, such as classroom activities
- all activities away from the Children's Centre, such as educational outings
- fire safety
- lone working
- manual handling.

Staff recruitment/training

The Children's Centre Manager, Deputy Manager and Senior Management have undertaken safer recruitment and selection training and this is implemented across the appointment of all staff and volunteers, including senior management.

All staff and volunteers that work in the Children's Centre must complete the structured induction programme and safeguarding training. All persons working with the children and their families are required to undertake an enhanced check as well as a check of the DBS barred lists.

Disclosure and Barring Service (DBS)

Our service complies with the Disclosure and Barring Service's checks in relation to all staff and volunteers working on our premises.

All persons working with the children and their families that attend the Centre are required to undertake an enhanced check as well as a check of the DBS barred lists.

The Children's Centre will take the necessary actions to suspend or dismiss staff and volunteers from employment and undertaking their roles if the person concerned acquires a criminal record, has withheld information about a criminal record, or appears on a list of individuals held by the DBS that are unsuitable for working with children.

Designated Child Protection Officer

The Centre Manager has overall responsibility for safeguarding the children in our care and is the Designated Safeguarding Child Protection Officer.

In the absence of the Centre Manager, the Deputy Manager will act as the Designated Safeguarding Child Protection Officer. The Designated Safeguarding Officers are responsible for receiving all concerns from staff and volunteers and acting on these to protect the child at risk.

▲ **Figure 7.5** An example of policies and procedures in a child care setting

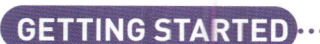

LO6 Understand how workers within health, social care and child care environments can minimise the risk of abuse

Empowering individuals (10 minutes)

Discuss as a class what empowering an individual involves. How can doing so minimise the risk of abuse?

6.1 Minimising the risk of abuse

Person-centred planning

Person-centred planning is a good way to minimise the risk of abuse to vulnerable adults and children because it enables individuals to be in control of their own safety. It ensures workers within health, social care and child care environments:

- place individuals at the centre of their care and support
- value individuality
- promote individuals' privacy and dignity
- promote individuals' rights to independence and to make their own informed choices and decisions
- promote mutual trust and respect
- work together in partnership.

See Unit 6 (page 112) for a detailed look at person-centred approaches.

INDEPENDENT RESEARCH ACTIVITY

Person-centred planning (30 minutes)

Conduct some independent research on why effective record keeping is important and how it can reduce the likelihood of abuse. You could interview professionals such as those who work in your GP surgery about what effective record keeping involves. You could also use your books and the internet as sources of additional information.

Duty of care

All workers and organisations that provide care and support services within health, social care and child care environments have a professional **duty of care** to safeguard vulnerable adults and children by minimising the risk of danger, harm and abuse by ensuring:

- decisions made are led by the individual's needs, wishes and preferences
- risks are identified and reduced while respecting individuals' rights to make their own choices and decisions
- individuals are supported and protected from the risk of danger, harm and abuse
- individuals are not placed in situations that may cause danger, harm and abuse.

KEY TERMS

Duty of care – the legal obligation professionals have to safeguard individuals who they care for and support from danger, harm and abuse.

Need to know basis – when information is given to people only if and when it is needed.

Effective record keeping

Effective record keeping that includes accurate, complete and up-to-date information as well as secure storage and handling practices can minimise the risk of abuse by:

- clearly identifying potential risks of danger, harm and abuse
- providing guidance on the actions to take when risks are identified
- providing consistent information that is accessible by all workers who access it on a **need to know** basis
- providing accurate information that can be shared between professionals and agencies who access it on a need to know basis.

Following policies and procedures

As you will have read in the previous section, following policies and procedures designed to protect and safeguard vulnerable adults and children can minimise the risk of abuse by:

- upholding individuals' rights to live safely and free from danger, harm and abuse
- focusing on preventing danger, harm and abuse
- managing risks and concerns of danger, harm and abuse
- providing a set of standards that workers can work to and comply with.

Building a trusting professional relationship

Vulnerable adults and children who have been or are being abused are often left feeling unsafe, fearful and suspicious of others. By building a trusting and professional relationship with individuals, workers can minimise the risk of abuse by:

- enabling individuals to confide in them when abuse is happening to them and/or others
- building mutual respect so that the individual feels in control of their life
- encouraging open discussions and therefore minimising the risk of abusive relationships.

Effective communication channels

Effective verbal, non-verbal and written communication (topics you learned about in Unit 1) between workers, individuals, their families, professionals and agencies can minimise the risk of abuse by:

- creating an open environment where it is encouraged to be open about and discuss any concerns or risks of abuse happening
- ensuring all concerns are responded to and acted on quickly to lessen the risk and extent of abuse happening
- diffusing situations that have the potential to cause distress and frustration and that could potentially lead to abuse occurring.

Continuing professional development

Continuing professional development provides workers within health, social care and child care environments with opportunities to maintain and develop their knowledge and skills in minimising the risk of abuse by:

- equipping them with current knowledge and up-to-date practices in safeguarding and protecting individuals to be able to practise safely and legally

- enabling them to identify when individuals may be at risk of being abused or abusing others
- knowing about how to reduce the opportunities for abuse to occur
- developing ways of working that reduce the likelihood of abuse happening, i.e. person-centred approaches.

> 🔑 **KEY TERM**
>
> **Continuing professional development** – opportunities for professionals to maintain and develop their knowledge and skills, not just through training but also through experience, self study and sharing best practice.

6.2 Developing the confidence and resilience of individuals who receive care and support

Workers within health, social care and child care environments can minimise the risk of abuse by developing an individual's belief in their own abilities and their trust in others (i.e. confidence) as well as their ability to recover from difficulties they've experienced and adapt to changes (i.e. resilience).

Table 7.4 provides you with some additional information about a range of strategies used by workers to develop the confidence and resilience of individuals who receive care and support. Can you think of any other ways that these strategies can help?

Table 7.4 Strategies for developing confidence and resilience

Strategies	How the confidence of individuals who receive care and support is developed	How the resilience of individuals who receive care and support is developed
Supporting positive risk taking	Empowering individuals to take responsibility for their own choices and decisions will lead to individuals becoming less dependent on others and thus minimise the scope for abuse to take place.	Creating a safe environment where individuals can take risks, make mistakes and learn from them will make individuals less vulnerable to abuse.
Promoting active participation	Promoting the rights of individuals, including their independence, will result in increasing their wellbeing and self-esteem and thus create more of a partnership with others, reducing the risk of abuse.	Providing opportunities for individuals to participate in day-to-day tasks increases the individual's awareness of their abilities and what they can achieve for themselves and thus makes them less vulnerable to abuse.
Promoting choice	Enabling individuals to think through what options are available, the advantages and disadvantages of each and then make their own choices will lead to them being in control of their lives and less likely to be abused.	Supporting individuals in developing their problem-solving skills when making choices and knowing how to make positive choices in their lives will make them less vulnerable to abuse.
Teaching personal safety	Equipping individuals with the knowledge and skills related to personal safety will give individuals a sense of ownership and involvement in what this involves and they will be more likely to be able to protect themselves from abusive situations.	Equipping individuals with the understanding and awareness of how risks and difficult situations can be managed safely will reduce the opportunity for abuse to take place.

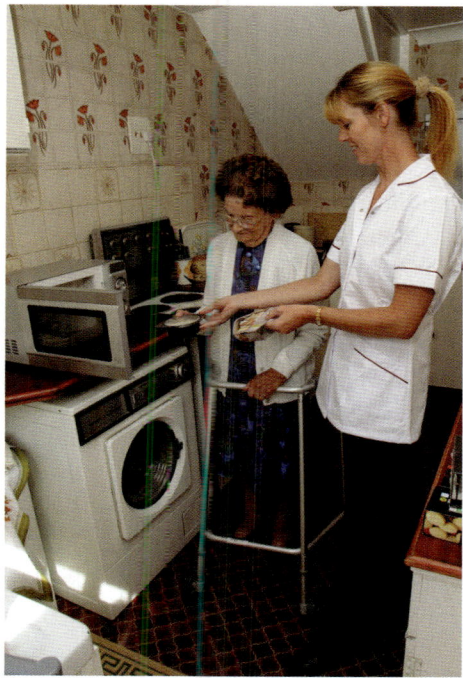

▲ Figure 7.6 Promoting active participation in the home

Read about it

Heller, T., Reynolds, J., Gomm, R., Muston, R. and Pattison, S. (1996) *Mental Health Matters*, Macmillan Press Ltd.

Morris, C., Ferreiro Peteiro, M. and Collier, F. (2015) *Level 3 Health and Social Care Diploma*, Hodder Education.

Read, J., and Reynolds, J. (1996) *Speaking Our Minds: An Anthology*, Macmillan Press Ltd.

Useful websites

Abuse Survivors: abuse-survivors.org.uk

Action on Elder Abuse: elderabuse.org.uk

Care Quality Commission: cqc.org.uk

NSPCC: nspcc.org.uk

Public Concern at Work: pcaw.co.uk

? THINK ABOUT IT

Case study: Sam

Sam is 22 years old and, having been made homeless due to living in an abusive family situation, is now living in a short-term housing scheme aimed at young people at risk. The housing scheme aims to provide individuals like Sam with support for a maximum of two years to enable them move on and live independently.

Imagine you are one of the workers at the housing scheme where Sam lives. Describe the strategies that you could use with Sam to enable him to develop confidence and resilience.

Case study: Ceri

Ceri, who is 48, lives with her younger sister at home. Two years ago, Ceri was diagnosed with Parkinson's and has recently also developed memory problems and depression. Her sister is finding it difficult to care for and support her sister and is getting frustrated with the current situation at home.

1 Why could this situation become abusive?
2 How could the risk of Ceri being abused be minimised?
3 What would you advise Ceri's younger sister to do in this situation and why?
4 How can developing Ceri's confidence and resilience minimise the risk of abuse?

Unit 7: Assessment practice

Below are practice questions for you to try.

1 **a)** Define the following four types of abuse:
   i) physical abuse (1)
   ii) neglect (1)
   iii) institutional (1)
   iv) bullying. (1)
   b) Describe two signs for each of the following types of abuse:
   i) sexual (2)
   ii) emotional/psychological (2)
   iii) financial (2)
   iv) discrimination. (2)
   c) Ana is 14 years old and lives with a foster family. Ana left her family home because she had been physically and emotionally abused by her brother. Explain the effects of both types of abuse on Ana. (4)

2 Gillian has a learning disability and lives independently. She tells her best friend Marion that she no longer wants to go to college. Last week Marion noticed that Gillian appeared to be fearful around certain people in her Tuesday college class.
   Analyse five factors that may make abuse more likely in Gillian's situation (10)

3 **a)** Describe two environmental factors that may lead to abuse happening in a children's residential home. (4)

   b) Describe two other factors that may make abuse more likely in a children's residential home. (4)

4 Explain how the following pieces of legislation help to safeguard and protect vulnerable adults from abuse:
   a) Safeguarding Vulnerable Groups Act 2006 (2)
   b) Mental Capacity Act 2005 and Deprivation of Liberty Safeguards. (2)

5 Identify two types of people who might suspect that abuse is happening to a child. (2)

6 Abraham works on a project for young homeless people. One lunchtime he notices that one of the young men who visits the project is sitting on his own in the café and is being laughed at by a group of four other young people.
   Explain the actions that Abraham must take as part of his duty to report abuse. (6)

7 Shelly has been newly recruited as a home manager in a residential care home for individuals with dementia. She has been asked to review all of the home's policies and procedures that relate to safeguarding individuals from abuse.
   a) Identify two policies or procedures that Shelly may need to review. (2)
   b) For each policy or procedure that Shelly may need to review, describe the main points included in each. (6)
   c) Explain three ways in which Shelly can support the staff in the residential care home to minimise the risk of abuse. (6)

Total marks: 60

Unit 08

Creativity and activity for children and young people

ABOUT THIS UNIT

Children and young people need opportunities to be creative and this, in turn, will enable them to develop a wide range of skills. Creativity allows us to express our emotions, solve problems and explore and experiment. Creativity is key to stimulating and developing imagination, confidence and self-esteem.

In this unit you will learn the importance of creativity for children and young people and how this will support them in later life. You will learn how creativity develops as the child or young person grows and you will explain the adult's role in this process. This unit will also give you the skills needed to design, plan, deliver and evaluate an activity for a group of children or young people in a relevant setting.

LEARNING OUTCOMES

The topics, activities and suggested reading in this unit will help you to:

1 Understand the importance of creativity for children and young people
2 Understand how creativity develops in children and young people
3 Understand the role of adults in promoting creativity for children and young people
4 Be able to design and plan an activity/creative activity for use with a group of children or young people
5 Be able to deliver and evaluate an activity/creative activity to a group of children or young people

How will I be assessed?

You will be assessed through a series of assignments and tasks set and marked by your tutor.

How will I be graded?

You will be graded using the following criteria.

Learning outcome	Pass assessment criteria	Merit assessment criteria	Distinction assessment criteria
You will:	To achieve a **pass** you must demonstrate that you have met all the pass assessment criteria	To achieve a **merit** you must demonstrate that you have met all the pass and merit assessment criteria	To achieve a **distinction** you must demonstrate that you have met all the pass, merit and distinction assessment criteria
1 Understand the importance of creativity for children and young people	**P1** Understand the importance of creativity for children and young people	**M1** Analyse the importance of using developmental stages and the link between creativity and learning	**D1** Evaluate how theory of play underpins the promotion and importance of creativity
	P2 Describe examples of when a child is being creative		
2 Understand how creativity develops in children and young people	**P3** Explain what children need to be creative		
3 Understand the role of adults in promoting creativity for children and young people	**P4** Explain the role that adults take when promoting creativity in children or young people	**M2** Assess the role adults should take in the cycle of planning, implementing, observing, recording and assessing creativity	
4 Be able to design and plan an activity/creative activity for use with a group of children or young people	**P5** Plan an activity/creative activity that is appropriate for a group of children or young people in health and social care settings		
	P6 Explain health and safety considerations for a chosen activity/ creative activity *Synoptic link to Unit 3 Health, safety and security in health and social care*		
5 Be able to deliver and evaluate an activity/ creative activity to a group of children or young people	**P7** Deliver a planned activity that is appropriate for a group of children or young people in health and social care settings	**M3** Evaluate the effectiveness of the activity and identify areas of weakness and suggest improvements	

L01 Understand the importance of creativity for children and young people *F1 M1 D1*

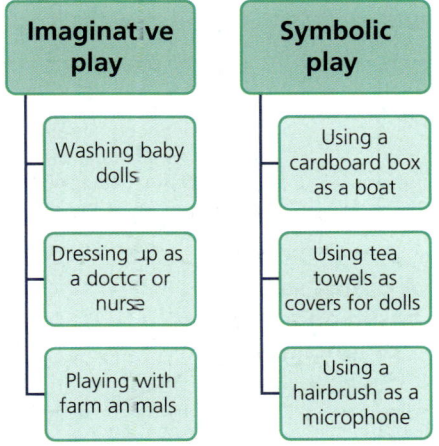

GETTING STARTED

How far will it fly? (10 minutes)

Take one sheet of paper and make a paper aeroplane. When you are told to, see how far it will fly. Once all of the paper aeroplanes have been picked up, consider the following.

- Did you enjoy making the paper aeroplane?
- Do you like trying to create things from scratch?
- Did this activity annoy you?
- Why?

1.1 Definition of creativity

KEY TERMS

'Little c' creativity – an everyday process whereby children and young people are able to be resourceful and problem solve.

'Big C' creativity – a process linked to new ideas, sudden understandings and creative excellence.

'Little c' and 'big C' creativity

Children and young people need the time, opportunity and space to be creative and to use their problem-solving skills. Their **'little c' creativity** skills are used on a daily basis to help them create and problem solve. A child trying to make a model out of junk boxes needs to work out how to make them stick and stay together; this experience will also develop their resourcefulness. Working out that they need to put a larger box at the bottom is part of 'little c' creativity.

Children need to have confidence and self-esteem in order for them to make the most of **'big C' creativity** opportunities. A child who is confident in their environment could make suggestions that could affect several people, for example suggesting a different way

of organising a group activity would mean that they have used initiative and have the conviction to discuss their ideas with other people.

1.2 Ways children express creativity

KEY TERMS

Imaginative play – involves children pretending to be, or making up stories about, something or someone else, e.g. pretending to be a cat.

Symbolic play – involves children using one thing to represent something else, e.g. using a banana as a phone.

Expressing creativity through imaginative play and symbolic representation

Early years settings will provide opportunities for children to express their creativity through **imaginative** and **symbolic play**. Most settings will have a home corner where children can pretend to be someone or something else. This area often has a theme and you may change the resources so that the area becomes a hospital, vets or shop. While you will provide the resources, the children will use their imagination to create elaborate stories and scenarios.

Imaginative play	Symbolic play
Washing baby dolls	Using a cardboard box as a boat
Dressing up as a doctor or nurse	Using tea towels as covers for dolls
Playing with farm animals	Using a hairbrush as a microphone

▲ **Figure 8.1** Examples of imaginative and symbolic play

1.3 The importance of creativity for individuals

🔑 KEY TERMS

Fine motor skills – actions that require small movements, e.g. writing, threading and playing with dough.

Gross motor skills – actions that require large movements, e.g. running, jumping and skipping.

Perceptual skills – the ability to become aware of things around us, mainly through our senses.

Creative experiences allow people to develop physical and perceptual skills

Developing potential

While being creative, children explore, experiment and push themselves to try new things. Creative experiences therefore enable children and young people to discover their talents, develop new skills and gain confidence in themselves.

Improving capacity for thought, action and communication

Children can develop their creative skills through drama and role play. For young people this can be a way of exploring other people's views and perspectives on life. An improvised drama session can encourage them to be someone they are not, leading to discussion and a reflection on thoughts, actions and consequences. By doing this through a creative activity they can feel safe to explore feelings and express their own views.

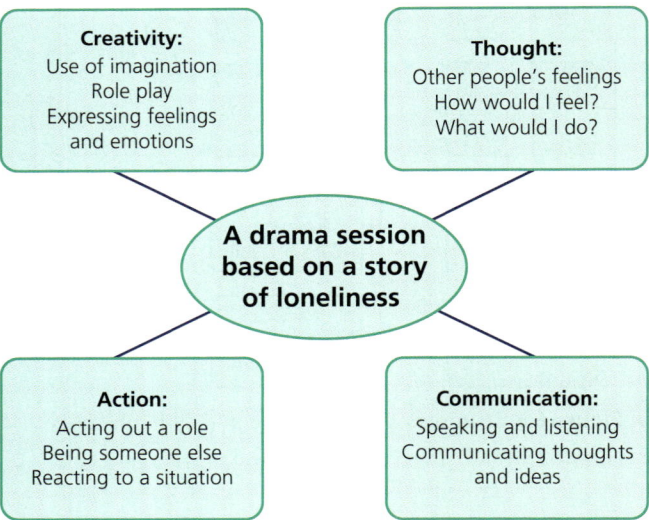

▲ **Figure 8.2** An example of how a creative drama session can develop a young person's thoughts, actions and communication skills

Nurturing their feelings and sensibilities

Creative activities will enable children to express and sometimes deal with their emotions. Table 8.1 shows how you can help a child deal with their feelings in a frustrating situation.

Table 8.1 An example of how to nurture feelings and sensibilities through a creative activity

A two year old is trying to put a basic train track together and because she cannot do it she throws a piece of track across the room and starts stamping and screaming	
The correct response to nurture her feelings and sensibilities	**The incorrect response that may affect her feelings and sensibilities**
Go down to her level and talk with a calm voice	Shout at her from across the room
Give her a little time to be angry	Tell her to stop immediately
Talk to her about how she might be feeling	Tell her to stop being silly
Offer to help her with the piece of track	Tell her to go and play with something else
Sit with her until she calms down	Walk away from her
Play with her and talk to her about how well she is doing now that she is calm	Ignore her for the rest of the session

The first column shows how the child was supported to calm down and work through her anger. This gave her the opportunity to learn through this experience and perhaps deal with her feelings differently in the future. The examples in the second column would have left this child feeling confused, angry, upset and embarrassed. She would probably react in the same way if this were to happen again.

Extend physical and perceptual skills

Creative activities can develop **fine** and **gross motor skills**. Running around outside and playing pirates requires gross motor and **perceptual skills** While children are running to catch someone, they are judging the space around them to make sure they do not bump into or trip over anything. A child sitting at a table making an intricate collage is developing their fine motor and perceptual skills by manipulating the glue stick and collage pieces.

Explore their values and understand their own and others' cultures

All settings should plan activities and experiences to reflect a range of festivals from other cultures.

(20 minutes)

Research the traditional story of why each year is represented by a different animal in the Chinese calendar. Consider the following.

- Did you already know the story of the animals?
- Why is it important for young children to know about different cultures?

Creative activities will enable children to explore and understand other people's values and cultures. They will also enable them to develop a greater understanding of their own values and culture.

Retelling key stories from a range of cultures will encourage children to understand that we are all different. This could include the stories of Christmas, Diwali, Hanukkah and Chinese New Year. While they may make a Diwali lamp at the setting, children may not celebrate that festival at home. Creative activities allow children to discuss differences and then develop their knowledge of other people's values and cultures as well as their own.

1.4 The importance of creativity for society

Creative activities can help children deal with problems and issues in the future. By problem solving through creative outlets children will develop essential skills that can be useful in society.

1.5 Creativity should be inclusive

Being creative does not mean you have to be good at art, music or drama. Creativity is within everyone and everyone's creativity should be recognised.

Creativity is not elitist

Being creative is not about being the best – it is about having a go and enjoying the activity or experience. A child may think someone else's creative work is better than theirs so they should not be made to feel inferior. All creative work should be praised and all children should be made to feel positive about the outcome.

Creativity makes the most of the talents of all children

Adults should plan creative activities for children that will develop a range of skills. All work should be valued, even if the end product is not what was expected.

For example, you have laid out a table for young children to create a card with their handprint on. One child decides to make a symmetrical pattern using just the tip of their finger; they should not be told to stop but be praised for their imagination. If a handprint is essential then you could offer a second card and ask if they can do a handprint for you, so that the child does not feel they have done something wrong.

Recognising that all children have the ability to be creative

Settings and schools have display areas for creative work and everyone should have the opportunity for

Table 8.2 How different situations can help children and young people in the future

Current situation	Future situation/s
A 2 year old is playing with a new age-appropriate puzzle. They have played at the puzzle table before but they are struggling to place the first piece. They try it in all the holes until it fits.	- Extend current knowledge to new situations - Persevering to solve a problem
A group of children are playing in the home corner, which has been set up as a shop. A 'customer' asks for carrots but there are no toy carrots in the shop. After some discussion the children hand over some beanbags and pretend they are carrots.	- Dealing with the unexpected - Problem solving - Working with others - Being flexible
A group of Year 5 children has been set the task of creating the tallest tower they can using just newspaper and sticky tape. They take time to listen to one another's ideas and decide to create a solid base before building upwards. This design wins because of its strength.	- Working as a team - Taking risks - Trying new ideas - Using previously unconnected information
Five young people are going to perform a short anti-bullying play at a Year 8 assembly. On the day, one of the group is absent and the space in which they are going to perform is smaller than anticipated. They work together to rewrite the play for four people and decide to perform all around the audience instead of in just the small space. The Year 8 children are totally engaged by the performance.	- Use previous knowledge and skills to solve current problem - Think flexibly - Take risks - Be innovative - Deal with change

their work to be displayed. This will give them a sense of pride and achievement and show that their work is valued. Praise and encouragement will boost their confidence in all areas of learning and development.

Creativity promotes access for all

Creativity should be inclusive and present no barriers to children. Those working with children and young people play a crucial role in ensuring this happens. They plan activities that can be adapted if necessary so that everyone can be included.

- Culture and ethnicity: some families may ask that their child is not included in certain activities based on festivals and you should respect this request and plan accordingly, ensuring that the child does not feel left out. For example, as not all children celebrate Christmas at home there should be choice of activities, e.g. draw a picture of Father Christmas or a snowman.
- Socio-economic status: some children and young people might have limited opportunities to engage in creative activities outside school, e.g. dance and music lessons tend to be expensive. All children should have opportunities to be creative, e.g. money isn't needed for playing cars using stones and sticks in the park, or climbing into or making models with cardboard boxes.
- Gender: stereotypes should be challenged. For example, while playing at being firefighters, a boy may tell another child that she cannot join in because she is a girl. This should be challenged by discussing why the boy feels that girls cannot join in. This may be due to stereotypical views of adult roles, e.g. that only men can be firefighters. Children must understand that the girls can be firefighters and be encouraged to join in.
- Additional needs: e.g. a hearing or visual impairment, mobility difficulties, behavioural difficulties or learning disabilities should not be a barrier to creativity. Activities can be adapted to ensure all children can participate. For example, if a child cannot stand for a long time you could make sure that they can sit down during the activity. If a child has difficulty concentrating for long periods, offer them quick creative activities or give them the chance to complete the task over a series of short sessions.

Creativity should differentiate

According to ability

All children develop at their own rate and their abilities may differ. A cutting and sticking activity should offer a range of equipment and material to suit all abilities. Some 3 year olds will be able to cut paper independently while others may have never used scissors before.

Some scissors have four finger holes, so that you can guide a child and show them what the action for cutting is, or have springy rubber between the handles so that when the child closes the scissors they spring open. You should also plan for children who cannot or will not use scissors at all, by having a variety of pre-cut pieces that can be stuck straight on to the paper.

According to stage of development

Similar creative activities can be offered to children and young people of all ages but you will have to adapt each activity according to their stage of development.

According to interest

Children often will respond positively to an activity that is based on something that connects with their interests. Get to know the children well and find out their likes and interests, even though they will be constantly changing and developing, e.g. bugs, cars, animals, space and stars, trains or dressing up.

1.6 How creativity supports children's learning and development

Creativity helps children to explore and understand their world

Helping children to understand their world involves them understanding what is immediately around them as well as the world in a wider context. Creative activities will help children to explore their world.

- Small world toys: these will encourage children to role-play real life situations through imaginative play, e.g. if they are playing with a dolls' house, placing characters and furniture in different rooms, you can talk with them about where things go e.g. 'I can see the baby is in the cot and the dog is in the garden'.
- Bug hunt: young children delight in finding bugs under rocks and stones and often give them names or characteristics. They may create stories about what the bugs are doing or where they are going. Through this experience you can develop their knowledge and understanding of habitats and where different bugs live.
- Stories: reading stories to children will give them an insight in to the world around them. Stories from different cultures and countries such as *Handa's Surprise* will encourage children to think about how different people live – they probably have never seen a child walking with a basket of fruit on their head but they will soon be re-enacting the story through role play or artwork.

```
┌─────────────────────────────────────────────────────┐
│        Creative activity using dough or clay          │
└─────────────────────────────────────────────────────┘
```

Under 2s	2–5 year olds	5–11 year olds	11+
Will explore textures and properties	They will be more curious about what they can do with the dough	Their creativity skills will develop rapidly through this age range	They now only have to be given the the modelling material and they will use their imagination and skills to develop their own ideas
They do not need anything other than the dough itself	They will copy others	They should still be given the opportunity to work with modelling materials but the final outcome or expectation will be more advanced	
They will squeeze it, poke it, tap it and taste it	They will delight in making snakes or sausages and lots of little balls		

You will have to closely monitor them to keep them safe. You should also play with the dough and narrate what you and the children are doing	You will offer a range of equipment, e.g. cutters, rollers, scissors and plates. You can also introduce other modelling materials such as clay. You will encourage children to explore and experiment and ask more advanced questions such as 'What happens if?'	You may give a group of 8 year olds a piece of clay each and then show them a design that you would like them to copy using their own interpretations	You will support them to decide on the equipment they may need to complete their creation and you may have to help them if they feel their ideas are not working. You will be more of an observer but it is still important that they are offered these types of creative activities and experiences

▲ **Figure 8.3** An activity that has been tailored to meet participants' stage of development

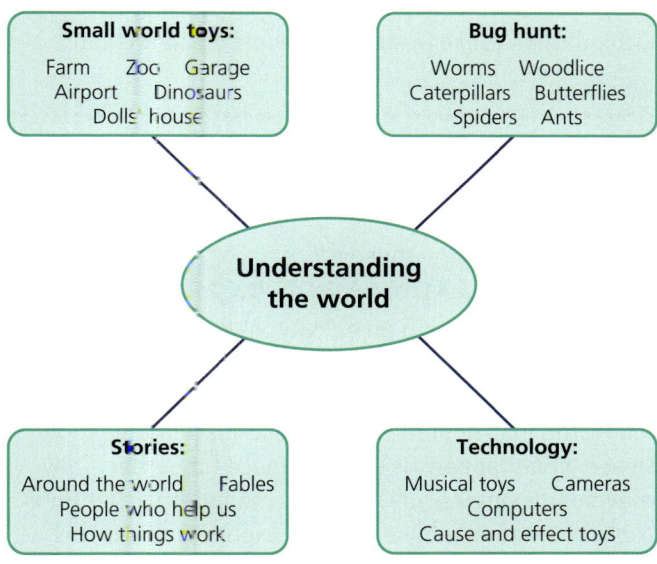

Small world toys:
Farm   Zoo   Garage
Airport   Dinosaurs
Dolls' house

Bug hunt:
Worms   Woodlice
Caterpillars   Butterflies
Spiders   Ants

Understanding the world

Stories:
Around the world   Fables
People who help us
How things work

Technology:
Musical toys   Cameras
Computers
Cause and effect toys

▲ **Figure 8.4** Examples of activities and experiences to support children's understanding of the world

● Technology: using a paint package on the computer to create a picture is not only creative but children learn that their actions cause something to happen on screen.

Creativity gives children opportunities to make new connections

Creative activities enable children to problem solve and link ideas and thoughts, to enable them to make connections to real situations.

Creativity is allowing these children to connect imaginative scenarios to real ones they may have already experienced. A child playing with a farm set will link the model of a pig to the real thing and make it move around and make pig noises. When children visit a farm for the first time they can connect the real animals to the toys.

Creativity allows children to communicate their feelings in non- or pre-verbal ways

Children show emotions and feelings during creative play, through actions, gestures, movement and dance, often without using words.

When watching a performance of their favourite story, they may be sitting silently but their expressions and body language can demonstrate how they are feeling, for example:

- leaning forward in their seat – anticipation, excitement
- hands over their mouth – worry, horror, humour
- arms folded, leaning back – bored, cross, defeated.

In a music and movement session children may be asked, for example:

- Show me an angry bear – the children stomp around the room, arms raised while taking large, slow footsteps
- Show me a happy butterfly – the children spread their arms, smile and gently move around the room
- Show me a sleepy snake – the children lie on the floor, yawn and roll and slither around.

Creativity increases self-esteem

Self-esteem is how you feel about yourself, your abilities, your talents and your skills. Opportunities to be creative will develop and **nurture** a child's self-esteem.

> 🔑 **KEY TERM**
>
> **Nurture** – to care for and protect something as it grows.

Children and young people will either be keen or reluctant to have a go at things, depending on their level of self-esteem. Creative experiences can give children a sense of pride and achievement which boosts self-esteem. Children may say, 'I can't' when invited to join in a creative activity and they will need to be encouraged to participate and praised for their efforts.

For example, children may be shy but when presented with a box of puppets they may feel more confident to play with others through a puppet. This activity may make them confident enough to begin to interact with others without puppets.

When children feel a sense of satisfaction and accomplishment from their creative work and play their self-esteem, self-worth and confidence will grow.

> 💡 **KNOW IT**
>
> 1 Define 'big C' and 'little c' creativity.
> 2 Give two examples of imaginative play and two examples of symbolic play.
> 3 Explain how your setting celebrates all children's work.

L02 Understand how creativity develops in children and young people
P2 P3 M1 D1

> **GETTING STARTED** 👤
>
> **Which comes first? (10 minutes)**
>
> Below is a list of creative stages all associated with the development of drawing and painting. Put them in order from the least to most difficult.
>
> 1 Using own imagination to create imaginary figures, creatures or worlds.
> 2 Using a pencil to make marks on the paper.
> 3 Touching the paper with a chubby crayon.
> 4 Painting and drawing recognisable scenes or objects.
> 5 Holding a short paint brush to paint.
> 6 Giving a face to a bubble figure.
> 7 Drawing figures that represent families.
> 8 Drawing a basic stick figure.
> 9 Creating pictures with more detail including sky, sun and houses.
> 10 Colouring in a picture while staying in the lines.
>
> Do you think there is a definitive 'order' to this list?
>
> Why?

2.1 When children are being creative

When they explore and experiment

Any child undertaking an activity that encourages them to experiment is developing their creative skills. A child playing with a basic construction set does not always follow the instructions, but will use their imagination to see what happens if they put pieces together. They may push seemingly random pieces together but their experimentation allows them to expand and explore their creativity.

When they use language or play to make sense of the world

Children chatting to themselves about what they are doing or talking to imaginary creatures are making sense of the world around them.

A child may be playing with a doll in a high chair, feeding it and talking to it, telling it that it is a 'good boy' or saying 'one more'. They are role-playing something they have seen elsewhere and this use of language enables them to relive the situation in a creative and imaginative way.

Children will often narrate their own play by speaking out loud and giving inanimate objects a voice. For example, they may have a rabbit puppet and a plastic carrot and be saying:

> Rabbit: Mmm, I'm very hungry.
>
> Carrot: Please don't eat me.
>
> Rabbit: But I love carrots.
>
> Carrot: But I want to play with you.
>
> Rabbit: OK, what shall we play?
>
> Carrot: Hide and seek?
>
> Rabbit: Yes, I'll count, 1, 2, 3 …

This is how children learn to work through problems such as initiating games with others.

When they concentrate on a single task

A child who is focused on a single task is developing many skills including creativity.

PAIRS ACTIVITY

Which creative skill? (10 minutes)

For each of the examples below, discuss which creative skills a child may be using.

- A 3 year old threading large beads onto a string.
- A 6 year old painting a picture of a daffodil in front of them.
- An 11 year old writing a short story about an imaginary world.

Consider the following skills: imagination, problem solving, creativity, exploring, experimenting, making sense of the world, language and vocabulary.

A child should not be disturbed when focused on a task; they may lose concentration and could stop their creativity. As children grow and develop, their ability to concentrate increases, they build on previous experiences and develop focus. This, in turn, supports their creativity.

When they do something new with the old and familiar

Young children often use one thing to represent another. This may be due to the absence of the object they want but it is also a part of their creative development.

Table 8.3 Fill in the blanks to show what a child could use to represent their desired object and add two ideas of your own

A child wants …	A child uses …	Options
A dog		• Dolls and teddies
A hat		• A cardboard box
A boat		• An upturned bucket
A cape		• Their arms
More friends		• A bowl
A chair		• A cushion
An aeroplane		• A piece of string
		• A table cloth

2.2 Promoting creativity

Children need to be allowed to explore equipment, materials and ideas

Some activities may have a planned outcome, but most should allow children to explore and experiment with what is available. Encouraging children to follow their ideas to their own conclusion will support the natural development of creativity.

Children should be given opportunities to use equipment, material and ideas in their own way, without correction

If children are told they are doing something wrong, it will stifle creativity. If the children in Figure 8.5 overleaf were told to take the cars back to the floor area then their imaginative play would have stopped and they probably would have lost interest in the activity.

A child taking a dinosaur for a walk in a buggy should not be told it is only meant for dolls as this will make the child feel as if they are wrong. The child is engaged in symbolic and imaginative play, which has a crucial role in the development of creativity.

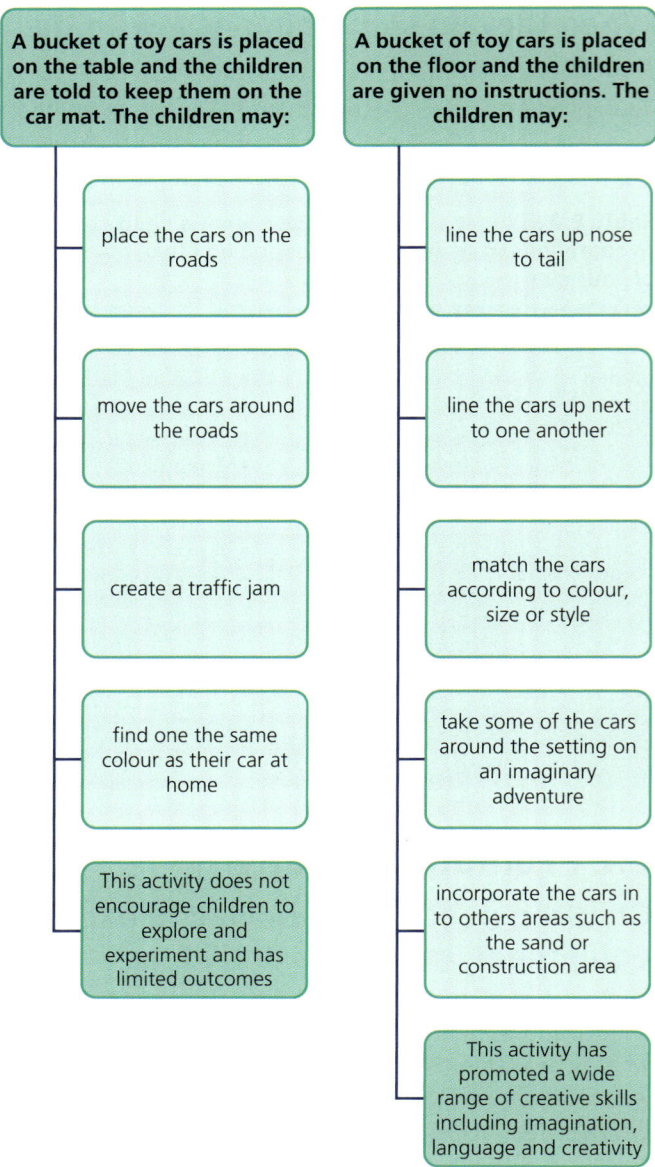

A bucket of toy cars is placed on the table and the children are told to keep them on the car mat. The children may:

- place the cars on the roads
- move the cars around the roads
- create a traffic jam
- find one the same colour as their car at home
- This activity does not encourage children to explore and experiment and has limited outcomes

A bucket of toy cars is placed on the floor and the children are given no instructions. The children may:

- line the cars up nose to tail
- line the cars up next to one another
- match the cars according to colour, size or style
- take some of the cars around the setting on an imaginary adventure
- incorporate the cars in to others areas such as the sand or construction area
- This activity has promoted a wide range of creative skills including imagination, language and creativity

▲ **Figure 8.5** Creating opportunities for children to explore and experiment

Children need to use this mastery to make new connections

When children are encouraged and allowed to use equipment and materials in their own way they can use these skills to make new connections, develop new skills and become competent in new things.

A child who has confidence in their own abilities is more likely to try things in a new way. If they have been allowed and encouraged to explore and experiment with materials and ideas, they are more likely to use this skill in later life. They will think about how they have done things in the past and use these ideas to make new connections, be creative and problem solve.

2.3 The theory behind the importance of play

Corinne and John Hutt

Dr Corinne Hutt (1934–79) began her career as a prison psychologist but then focused on children with autism; she worked with her husband John at the Park Hospital for children in Oxford.

Corinne and John Hutt were well known for their work on the study of the development of play, which was seen as influential at the time. They defined two general types of play that they described as **epistemic** and **ludic play**.

> 🔍 **INDEPENDENT RESEARCH ACTIVITY**
>
> **(45 minutes)**
>
> Research Corinne and John Hutt further and evaluate how both types of play support creativity. For each type of play describe at least one activity and discuss the opportunities for creativity and learning.
>
> Now choose one other play theorist, for example Montessori, Froebel, Piaget or Isaacs, and evaluate how they promote the importance of creativity.

> 🔑 **KEY TERMS**
>
> **Epistemic play** – acquiring knowledge through play. It is often associated with questions such as 'What does this object do?'
>
> **Ludic play** – a spontaneous type of play that draws on past experiences and often involves a range of symbolic or imaginary features. It can encourage a child to consider 'What can I do with this object?'

Figure 8.6 shows that both epistemic and ludic play support the need for children to explore and experiment with materials and ideas in different ways

Epistemic play

Focuses on children gaining knowledge through problem solving and exploring.

Children will already have an idea about what they want to do and epistemic play is when they work and play with objects and equipment to see what they do.

You play a crucial role in supporting a child's curiosity and getting involved in their play if asked.

For example, children may be playing with a set of large cardboard boxes and exploring and experimenting with them.

They may need your help to work out how to create their desired outcome but the child will be continually problem solving and building on previous knowledge.

Corinne Hutt believed that this type of play was beneficial because children learned more when focused on exploration and problem solving.

Ludic play

Can be seen as more free-flow, spontaneous and imaginative.

You are less involved during ludic play. Your role is observation and intervention if needed.

For example, children may be playing with a bag of assorted material scraps and one child uses a piece as a headscarf whilst another uses a piece as a cape.

The free-flow nature of this play will mean that the children can interchange their ideas and adapt their creative play accordingly.

Corinne Hutt did not feel that children were able to learn as much through ludic play and felt that free-flow play was not as important as other types of play, but some other theorists would disagree.

▲ **Figure 8.6** Epistemic and ludic play

2.4 The importance of using developmental stages

KEY TERMS

Developmental stages – the natural progression in which children grow and develop. Not all children will develop at the same rate, but most children will follow the same pattern of **milestones** in development.

Milestones – key points in development, for example when a baby sits, crawls or walks for the first time.

Understanding when different experiences are important

When planning creative activities, consider each child and young person's stage of development. When children feel confident and comfortable with familiar activities and experiences, you should introduce something different to stretch and challenge them. Engaging in the same creative activities day after day does not help them to develop new skills and ideas.

Table 8.4 National Curriculum subjects by key stages

Key stage 1 and 2	Key stage 3 and 4
English	English
Maths	Maths
Science	Science
Design and technology	History
History	Geography
Geography	Modern foreign languages
Art and design	Design and technology
Music	Art and design
Physical education (PE)	Music
Computing	Physical education (PE)
Ancient and modern foreign languages (KS2)	Citizenship
Schools must provide religious and sex education but parents can choose if their child attends	Computing
Schools will often offer: • Personal, social and health education (PSHE) • Citizenship • Modern foreign language (KS1)	Schools must provide religious and sex education but parents can choose if their child attends

Knowing where children may be heading next

Part of your role is to know when a child is ready to be challenged with a new activity or experience. You need to know where the child is in their own stage of development so that challenges can be provided to develop to the next stage.

For example, a 1 year old can be offered chubby crayons for a mark-making activity. The size and shape of the crayons make it easy for the baby to hold them in a fist-like grip. They will stab at the paper and soon learn that they will leave a mark. As the child becomes competent you can offer them paint on a chubby paint brush and then thinner crayons, pencils and brushes so that they slowly develop the grip required to hold a pen or pencil.

Developmental stages

Early Years Foundation Stage

The Early Years Foundation Stage (EYFS) is a statutory framework that sets out guidelines for care, learning and development, which must be followed by all providers of childcare for children from birth to 5 years.

The EYFS covers seven areas of learning and development, and states what children should know by the time they are 5:

- personal, social and emotional development
- physical development
- communication and language
- literacy
- mathematics
- understanding the world
- expressive arts and design.

It is your responsibility to know and follow the EYFS so that children have had a range of opportunities and experiences to support their development and readiness for school.

National Curriculum

The National Curriculum has been set by the government and ensures that all children of compulsory school age (5–16) are following the same range of subjects. It is broken down in to four key stages (KS):

- KS1 Year 1–2 Age 5–7
- KS2 Year 3–6 Age 7–11
- KS3 Year 7–9 Age 11–14
- KS4 Year 10–11 Age 14–16.

2.5 The links between creativity and areas of learning

Some areas of learning and development within the EYFS have obvious links to creativity, but all of the areas can promote creative development and creativity.

Table 8.5 Examples of creative activities and experiences and how they link to the EYFS

Area of learning	Links to creativity
Personal, social and emotional development	Expressing emotions and feelings through creative work, e.g. – Drama – Role play – Art work
Physical development	• Fine motor skills, e.g. – Threading – Painting – Gluing – Drawing – Small construction toys • Gross motor skills, e.g. – Outdoor role play involving running, jumping and chasing – Large construction toys
Communication and language	• Puppets • Role play
Literacy	• Story telling • Listening to stories
Mathematics	• Problem solving in construction • Puzzles • Matching and sorting
Understanding the world	• Small world toys, e.g. – Farm set – Zoo set – Dolls' house – Dinosaurs – Cars and planes • Bug hunts and life cycles
Expressive arts and design	• Music and movement • Dance • Musical instruments • Drama and role play • Messy play • Paint and glue • Technology, e.g. – Cameras – Paint packages

KNOW IT

1 Name one activity that could be described as epistemic play.

2 Name one activity that could be described as ludic play.

3 List the areas of learning and development within the EYFS.

4 Give three benefits of children experimenting with and exploring materials and ideas.

LO1&2 Assessment activities

Below are suggested assessment activities that have been directly linked to the pass and merit criteria in LO1&2 to help with assignment preparation; they include Top Tips on how to achieve best results.

Activity 1 – pass criteria *P1 P2 P3*

1 Explain five benefits of creativity.
2 Observe children in a nursery or school. Describe what they are doing to be creative and note down what factors support their creativity.

Activity 2 – merit criteria *M1 D1*

3 Choose two children of different ages and observe them during a creative activity. Consider:
a) their stage of development
b) what they are learning from the activity
c) how well suited the activity is to their stage of development
d) and justify any improvements you would make to the activity.

TOP TIPS
✔ Consider all activities, not just the obvious art-based ones.
✔ Look at what is provided for creativity as well as what children choose to use.
✔ Analyse what might happen if you did not consider developmental stages.

LO3 Understand the role of adults in promoting creativity for children and young people *P4 M2*

GETTING STARTED

(5 minutes)

Think about what is meant by being creative.

Write a list of at least three ways that you have been creative.

3.1 Interventionist and non-interventionist roles

> **🔑 KEY TERMS**
>
> **Interventionist role** – being actively involved in children and young people's play, creativity and learning.
> **Non-interventionist role** – not being actively involved in children and young people's play and creativity.

An interventionist's role

Adults working with children must decide when it is necessary to intervene in a child's play, creativity or learning. An **interventionist role** may be needed if a child is becoming frustrated with what they are doing.

If a child is left to struggle for too long they may become angry or give up. If you intervene at the right moment you can boost confidence and self-esteem and enable the child to problem solve and persevere.

A non-interventionist's role

If you take a **non-interventionist role** you are confident that the child will learn more by working things out for themselves rather than having someone offering advice or guidance. By leaving a child to be freely creative, their natural creativity can be developed. If you give them advice or instructions, their original ideas may be stifled.

3.2 Intervening sensitively

Creating conditions to inspire creativity

Children will play imaginatively with everything around them – a toddler may use a brick to represent a phone and a pre-schooler may encourage dolls and teddies to join in their role play. Older children may create imaginative scenarios in the park or playground, but they will all respond to structured creative experiences.

Spontaneous opportunities for creativity should be available and encouraged. You should also plan a range of experiences to develop and inspire creativity.

> ? **THINK ABOUT IT**
>
> Create a list of ideas to inspire creativity for the following age ranges:
>
> - under 5s
> - primary school children
> - young people.

Valuing all children's representations

Activities provided by adults may be interpreted differently by different children, e.g. a pile of bricks and animals may encourage one child to create stables and barns and another child to line up and sort the bricks and animals. Value each individual child or young person's representations; if a child felt that their contribution was not valued or good enough they may be reluctant to try again in the future.

Plan the physical environment

When planning creative activities or opportunities you need to consider the physical environment. For example, you would not organise a music and movement session in an area full of tables and chairs or an art activity where children cannot be messy. The physical environment available to you may determine the scale of your creative activity or experience but it should not limit creativity.

Look at the examples in Table 8.6. How does the planning support creativity in each situation?

Develop creativity through our interactions

Being empathetic

A child may feel disappointed with their creative work. Being told not to be silly and to just try again may harm their confidence. Listening to them talk about how they feel about their creation can support and encourage them and boost their confidence. By being empathetic you are respecting their feelings and not telling them how they should feel.

Nurturing curiosity

Children are naturally inquisitive; for example, when playing with paint they may be curious about what happens if they mix the colours. This should be encouraged and talked about, for example:

> I really like the patterns you are making with the white paint. Oh look, when you use the red on top, what happens?
>
> Pink!
>
> You have made a lovely pink colour. Well done!

Telling a child not to mix paint would not allow them to learn through experimentation and creativity.

Value process over product

Often the end product is seen as more important than the process of making it. Telling children how to produce identical celebration cards stifles creativity and could harm their self-worth. They may be nervous about using their own ideas in future because they are not the same as everyone else's.

Always value the process of being creative as much as what is actually created. A child may spend a long time at the clay table rolling bits of clay into small balls, lining them up and counting them. They may involve others by feeding them 'peas'. Once finished the child may discard their creations and move on to something else but doing this activity will have developed their fine motor skills, imagination, numeracy and patience.

Table 8.6 Planning the physical environment to support creativity

Activity	Space available	Planning required
Splatter painting with a group of 4 year olds	Messy play area with tables and chairs	• Move chairs to a safe place so that children can stand at the tables • Push tables together so the children have a larger surface area to work on • Check to see if anything around the area needs to be covered or moved
Small world play – farm set	Table top area with no space to move the furniture	• Gather some boxes and large sheets of material • Place the boxes on the tables to create hills and mounds • Lay the material over the boxes and carefully place the animals all around • Add shiny blue paper shapes to create ponds or lakes
A Year 7 group designing and creating a bridge made of cardboard tubes	A design and technology room with high tables and stools	• Encourage the group to plan on the table tops • Support each group to decide where they want to build their bridge • Safely move stools to create floor space where necessary

Recognising when to be silent, when to encourage, when to inspire and when to help

If a child is engaged in a creative activity, it is always best to wait to be invited to join in or give your opinion. If a child is constantly being asked 'What's that?' or 'What are you making?' then their creative ideas could be interrupted and they could lose focus or interest.

PAIRS ACTIVITY

To join in or not to join in? (10 minutes)

A 3 year old is playing with a box of construction bricks. They are building a tower and have got to the point where the structure is wobbling and may fall over. What would you do? Discuss with a partner:

1 How long you would watch before offering help?
2 The benefits of joining in and helping the child.
3 The consequences of offering help.
4 Possible learning opportunities for the child.
5 If you were to intervene, how would you approach the child and what would you say?

If you jump in too soon then the child will not learn through experimentation. If you leave it too long they may give up. You will get to know the children in your setting and be able to gauge the right thing to do. When you get your timing right you can inspire and help each child develop their skills and abilities.

3.3 The use of space and time

Creating the right environment to maximise creativity

The area in which children play and work should be inviting, stimulating and age and stage appropriate. A teenager would not feel comfortable painting at an easel designed for a 3 year old and a small child may feel overwhelmed in a space designed for teenagers.

Creativity can be developed and inspired by an exciting environment. A setting where equipment and materials are broken or incomplete will not stimulate children to explore, experiment and create.

For example, a group of 4 year olds find that a large black sheet has been draped over their setting's home corner. On the floor beneath they find torches, binoculars and hats, and tin foil and glow-in-the-dark stars hang from above.

- How might this inspire a child's imagination?
- Why would this have a different outcome if the objects had been placed haphazardly in a box and there was no sheet over the area?

Ensuring sufficient time

A child must be given time to be creative. They may become frustrated or angry if they are told to stop in the middle of their creation. If they do have to stop before they have finished, you need to handle this sensitively. Warn them that they will have to stop soon and encourage them to decide what to do with their creation until they can return to it. Young children will often forget about the project, but they must still be given the opportunity to return to it.

When planning an activity, be realistic about the time children will need to take part. No two children are the same, so it is impractical to, for example, allow 5 minutes per child. Some children will finish in 30 seconds and others may like to stay for the whole session to work at and develop their ideas.

3.4 The cycle of planning, implementing, observing, recording and assessing

Base planning on observation of needs and interests and building on previous experiences

Adults working with children observe them during their play in order to reflect on their learning. Some observations are carefully planned to assess specific areas of learning and development and other observations are spontaneous. All observations inform future planning to reflect each child's needs, interests and experiences.

GROUP ACTIVITY

What next? (5 minutes)

You are observing a group of 5 year olds outdoors. They are playing on the grass and notice a worm and a woodlouse. Two of the children shriek in horror and one child says they found a snake.

- What would you do if you were standing near the children at this time of discovery and exploration?
- How could you develop the children's understanding of the world around them?
- How could you plan an activity to further develop their creativity, imagination and understanding?

Relate planning to children's previous experiences

A group of children has discovered dry sand changes when water is added	
The children are asked what they would like to do next	They ask for watering cans, bottles, funnels and sieves

The children become curious about why the wet sand does not pour out of a bottle	
The children are offered spoons, spatulas and scrapers	The children discover they can dig the sand out of the bottles using the handle end of a wooden spoon

The children ask for containers with wider openings such as buckets, cups, tubs and boxes	
The children are encouraged to look around the setting to find their own equipment for the sand	You support the children's ideas but let them make all the decisions

▲ **Figure 8.7** Observing children and responding to curiosity, ideas and reactions

Involve children in planning and support child-initiated activities

Figure 8.8 also demonstrates how children can be involved in planning. In this example they showed an interest in the changing properties of sand and were encouraged to take this interest further and to develop their own ideas. **Child-initiated activities** allow children to take charge of what they want to do and to develop their own thoughts and ideas. The adult has responded to this and will have used appropriate language to extend and develop the children's learning as they planned together.

> 🔑 **KEY TERM**
>
> **Child-initiated activities** – enabling children to make decisions about their own activities and to lead the play or activity.

Organise materials, adults and children to allow time for exploration and play

Planning lets you organise your resources to produce the best outcome. A well-planned activity will encourage children to explore, experiment or to problem solve.

For example, for an activity using large wooden blocks in the outdoor play area, you need to organise:

- the outdoor space – make sure it is free and the weather is suitable
- the blocks – make sure they are accessible and available
- other adults – check availability to ensure the safety and welfare of the children
- the children – ensure they have enough time, building blocks and space to play.

Consider what children want to do or know next

One plan should follow the implementation and assessment of a previous plan.

Here is an example.

Planning next steps

- You carry out a butterfly painting activity.
- Children show curiosity about where butterflies come from.

- You plan to read the story of 'The Very Hungry Caterpillar'.
- You discuss the life cycle of a butterfly.
- You plan to create a wall display showing the life cycle.
- The children create pictures of eggs, caterpillars, chrysalis and butterflies.
- You discuss what the children would like to do next and record their ideas.
- You respond to their ideas and plan accordingly.

Afterwards you can assess the children's knowledge and plan activities to reinforce learning and understanding of the topic. This completes the cycle of planning, which requires you to plan, implement, observe, record and assess.

KNOW IT

1 Describe the difference between an interventionist and a non-interventionist role.
2 Give two benefits of involving children in planning.
3 Explain why the creative process is as important, if not more important, than the end product.

LO3 Assessment activity *P4 M2*

Below is a suggested assessment activity that has been directly linked to the pass and merit criteria in LO3 to help with assignment preparation; it includes Top Tips on how to achieve best results.

Create an information leaflet for new students to show the role of adults in the cycle of planning for creativity. Consider:

- how they can support creativity
- the importance of planning
- the benefits to creativity of observing, recording and assessing.

TOP TIPS

✔ Keep a diary of all of the times you promote creativity in one day.
✔ Ask to look at how the setting records their planning, observations and assessments.
✔ Consider what might happen if you did not plan effectively.

LO4 Be able to design and plan an activity/creative activity for use with a group of children or young people *P5 P6*

GETTING STARTED

Are you a planner? (5 minutes)

Do you like to plan everything you do or are you a spontaneous person? Consider:

- going on holiday
- having a night out
- buying a new outfit
- completing a set task
- going to the cinema.

4.1 Select and agree a suitable activity/creative activity

Group or individual

When designing and planning an activity, consider whether it is suited to group or individual work. Some are suitable in either situation.

Preferences of children or young people

When planning your activity, you should consider the preferences of the children in the setting. As you spend more time at the setting you will get to know the children and you can plan an activity that builds on their likes and interests.

Ability of children or young people

All children develop at their own rate and pace. Your plan should identify the suggested age range for your chosen activity but it must be suitable for all abilities within that age range and you should be able to adapt your plan accordingly.

Own ability

You should plan an activity that you will be confident to run and, while you might like to try something new, will run smoothly. Considering your own abilities when planning does not mean you have to do the same activity every time it just means that you have to be sure you are capable of completing the task.

Suitability to the children or young people's needs

It is essential you take individual needs into account when planning. Your plan should show how you could adapt the activity to suit individual needs where necessary.

'One-off' or ongoing programme

A one-off activity would involve you planning something that you only intend to do once. This could include a specific art or cooking activity. An ongoing programme of activities may involve an activity that is repeated, for example a music and movement or drama session.

Health and safety considerations

- Equipment: ensure that the equipment you are going to use is safe and suitable, e.g. age appropriate and no broken parts.
- Location: consider where you are going to carry out the activity, e.g. check the space is appropriate and safe for you, the children and those around you.

- Human resources: ensure you have enough adults to run the activity, e.g. if you are planning an outdoor activity you may need to involve another member of staff.
- Material resources: check that the resources, material and/or equipment are available, e.g. if you are planning a cooking activity you may need to buy some of the ingredients.
- Hazard identification: before running the activity you will need to be aware of anything that could be hazardous to you or the children, e.g. scissors, long paint brushes or anything that could be swallowed.
- Risk minimisation: ensure that any possible risks are minimized, e.g. scissors: children are closely monitored; long paint brush: children are shown how to hold it; choking hazard: children are not left unattended.
- Emergencies: it is your responsibility to know what to do in an emergency, e.g. if a child gets paint in their eye, keep them calm, call another member of staff and follow instructions.
- Legislation: all settings will follow health and safety legislation, and have health and safety policies and procedures, and you must adhere to these at all times, e.g. knowing your own role in the event of an accident or incident.

4.2 How to plan the activity/ creative activity

Most settings will have an activity planning sheet to help cover all areas of planning and ensure that everything has been considered before you carry out the activity.

There is no set format – Table 8.7 is an example of how all necessary criteria can be covered.

Table 8.7 An example activity planning sheet

ACTIVITY PLAN	
DATE:	TARGET CHILD/REN INITIALS:
DESCRIPTION OF ACTIVITY:	AREA/S OF LEARNING AND DEVELOPMENT:
AIM OF THE ACTIVITY: *What is the purpose of the activity?*	TIMESCALE: *How long will it take?*
LEARNING OBJECTIVES AND TARGETS: *What are the children expected to gain from the activity?*	
RESOURCES NEEDED: *List of resources needed to carry out the activity*	
INSTRUCTIONS: *Include clear instructions so that someone else could follow the plan*	
ACHIEVEMENT CRITERIA: *Identify how learning objectives and targets were or were not met*	
KEEPING SAFE: *What needs to be considered for health and safety during this activity?*	
INCLUSIVE PRACTICE/DIFFERENTIATION/LINKS TO EQUALITY AND DIVERSITY: *How will you meet all children's individual needs and ensure policies and procedures are followed?*	
COSTS: *Check with your supervisor before buying any resources. They may already have them or you may need to adapt your activity due to lack of funds*	

LO4 Assessment activity *P5 P6*

Below is a suggested assessment activity that has been directly linked to the pass criteria in LO4 to help with assignment preparation; it includes Top Tips on how to achieve best results.

Using Table 8.7, complete an activity plan for your chosen activity or creative activity. Consider:

- all elements of the plan including health and safety
- the children or young people in your setting
- the current topics or themes of the setting
- your role during the activity.

LO5 Be able to deliver and evaluate an activity/creative activity to a group of children or young people *P7 M3*

GETTING STARTED

Are you ready? (5 minutes)

You have 2 minutes to write down everything you need to consider when planning an activity. Compare your list with that of a partner.

5.1 Encourage children to participate

Disengaged children

Some children may choose not to join in an activity while others may not know how to join in. Be aware of them and give them every opportunity to take part if they want to but don't make them feel awkward or embarrassed. If they want to stand nearby and watch, this should be encouraged, and they should be allowed to join in at their own pace.

New activity

Children are naturally curious and if you plan and deliver an exciting and inviting new activity they may queue to join you. Your body language can affect how children will react to the new activity. If you look bored then children may not be keen to join you, but a smile and a busy table or activity area will encourage children to participate.

5.2 Monitor children's level of engagement

- Observe – observing children during an activity will enable you to judge how well it is going. If children are not completing the activity or are finishing in a few seconds then you will know that the activity is not engaging or challenging enough.
- Ask questions – asking open-ended questions will enable you to assess children's level of engagement.
- Adapt where appropriate – by observing and questioning the children you can decide whether you need to adapt the activity according to needs or interests (see LO1.5)

5.3 Obtain feedback

- From children and young people – children may suggest ways of doing the activity differently or you could ask them what they liked or disliked about it.
- From others involved – feedback from your supervisor or colleagues will support you to improve your own practice. Other adults in the setting will have experience of carrying out activities and you should take any feedback given as constructive support.

- During the activity – listening to or asking for feedback during the activity will help you to adapt it if it is not going according to plan.
- After the activity – feedback after an activity can give you the opportunity to reflect on how well it went and help you to decide how to do it next time.

5.4 Evaluate the success of the activity/creative activity

There are a number of questions you can ask yourself to evaluate your activity.

- Achievement of aim, objective and targets – did you achieve what you set out to achieve? If not, why not? Was the activity still a success?
- Own performance – how well do you think you did during the activity? Would you work differently next time? Why?
- Benefits to children or young people – what did the children gain from the activity?
- Relationships with the children – do you feel you worked well with all the children? Did you get to know the children better?
- How active support was provided – were you able to support all children so that they could join in to the best of their ability? How did you do this?
- Costs compared to alternative programmes – if applicable, do you think the activity could be carried out in a more economic way?

5.5 Identify possible improvements

Regardless of how well an activity went, you can always improve it.

Any issues need to be resolved by adapting your plan for next time, e.g. lack of preparation, more resources or time needed. Until you have run an activity it may be difficult to judge how to adapt it to individual needs. The activity could be at the wrong level or perhaps you needed to support participants more. All of these issues might cause you to rush and that, in turn, can impact on how you relate to the children.

The need for improvement is not a reflection on your ability; it is a natural and productive part of the planning process and ensures that everything runs

KNOW IT

1. Explain the importance of evaluating your planned activity.
2. Describe two ways to involve a disengaged child.
3. Name three ways of obtaining feedback.

smoothly and efficiently so that children achieve the best outcomes.

Read about it

Daly, M. (2006) *Understanding Early Years Theory in Practice*, Heinemann.

Macintyre, C. (2011) *Enhancing Learning Through Play*, Taylor & Francis Ltd.

Moyles, J. (2010) *The Excellence of Play*, Open University Press.

Pound, L. (2005) *How Children Learn: From Montessori to Vygotsky – Educational Theories Made Easy*, Step Forward Publishing.

Tassoni, P. and Hucker, K. (2005) *Planning Play and the Early Years*, Heinemann.

LO5 Assessment activity *P7 M3*

Below is a suggested assessment activity that has been directly linked to the pass and merit criteria in LO5 to help with assignment preparation; it includes Top Tips on how to achieve best results.

- Carry out the activity you planned above.
- Discuss the following to evaluate how well your activity went:
  - feedback from children
  - feedback from others
  - your thoughts during the activity
  - your reflection after the activity
  - what you would do differently next time.

TOP TIPS

- ✔ Persevere with your activity even if it is not going according to plan.
- ✔ Listen to those around you and adapt if necessary.
- ✔ Enjoy the activity.
- ✔ Keep a notebook and pen nearby so you can jot down ideas for improvements as you go along and identify things that are going well.

Unit 09

Supporting people with learning disabilities

ABOUT THIS UNIT

According to British Institute for Learning Difficulties (BILD), it is estimated that 1 in 198,000 people in England have a learning disability (2 per cent of the general population) so, if you want to work in health, social care and child care, you need to know how to support people with learning disabilities.

In this unit you will learn about the types and causes of learning disabilities and the differences between learning disabilities and specific learning difficulties. Potential difficulties for people with learning disabilities and ways of overcoming the difficulties will be explored. You will understand the support offered by services and practitioners as well as the methods of care. Legislation relating to learning disabilities will be examined.

LEARNING OUTCOMES

The topics, activities and suggested reading in this unit will help you to:

1 Know the types and causes of learning disabilities
2 Understand the difficulties that may be experienced by individuals with learning disabilities
3 Be able to support individuals with learning disabilities to plan their care and support

How will I be assessed?

You will be assessed through a series of assignments and tasks set and marked by your tutor.

How will I be graded?

You will be graded using the following criteria.

Learning outcome	Pass assessment criteria	Merit assessment criteria	Distinction assessment criteria
You will:	To achieve a **pass** you must demonstrate that you have met all the pass assessment criteria	To achieve a **merit** you must demonstrate that you have met all the pass and merit assessment criteria	To achieve a **distinction** you must demonstrate that you have met all the pass, merit and distinction assessment criteria
1 Know the types and causes of learning disabilities	**P1** Define the term learning disabilities		
	P2 Describe types of learning disabilities and their causes		
2 Understand the difficulties that may be experienced by individuals with learning disabilities	**P3** Explain the difficulties which may be experienced by individuals with learning disabilities	**M1** Assess the impact of difficulties on individuals with learning disabilities	**D1** Analyse ways to overcome difficulties experienced by individuals with learning difficulties
3 Be able to support individuals with learning disabilities to plan their care and support	**P4** Suggest services within the health and social care sector that can best support the needs of individuals with learning disabilities	**M2** Evaluate the impact of person-centred approaches on the quality of life of individuals with learning disabilities	
	P5 Explain the role of different practitioners in supporting individuals with learning disabilities in health and social care		

LO1 Know the types and causes of learning disabilities *P1 P2*

1.1 Definition of learning disabilities

GETTING STARTED

(15 minutes)

In pairs, come up with your definition of 'learning disabilities'. Share your ideas with the rest of the class. From all the different ideas decide on a final definition.

Table 9.1 Definitions of learning disabilities

	Definition	Source
MENCAP: a charity that supports people with learning disabilities	A reduced intellectual ability and difficulty with everyday activities – for example household tasks, socialising or managing money – which affects someone for their whole life.	www.mencap.org.uk
World Health Organization (WHO)	Characterised by impairment of skills across multiple developmental areas such as cognitive functioning and adaptive behaviour. Lower intelligence diminishes the ability to adapt to the daily demands of life.	www.who.int
Department of Health in England	A significantly reduced ability to understand new or complex information, to learn new skills (impaired intelligence) along with a reduced ability to cope independently (impaired social functioning). The onset of disability is considered to have started before adulthood, with a lasting effect on development. This definition includes **IQ** and functional aspects that make it distinct from the use of the term 'learning difficulties' which has a far wider application in education.	www.rcn.org.uk / Valuing People (2001)

All these definitions have a common theme of lack of intellectual ability and impaired ability to cope with the tasks of daily living.

Models of care for learning disabilities

In July 2015, NHS England, the Local Government Association (LGA), the Association of Directors of Adult Social Services (ADASS), the Care Quality Commission (CQC), Health Education England (HEE) and the Department of Health (DH) published a new draft national framework designed to improve the care of people with learning disabilities, shifting services away from hospital care and towards community-based settings. This new service model came from the Transforming Care for People with Learning Disabilities programme.

The service model sets out nine principles that define what 'good' services for people with learning disabilities and/or autism whose behaviour challenges should look like.

1 Providing more proactive, preventative care, with better identification of people at risk and early intervention.
2 Empowering people with a learning disability and/or autism, for instance through the expansion of personal budgets and personal health budgets and independent advocacy.
3 Supporting families to care for their children at home, and the provision of high-quality social care with appropriate skills.
4 Providing greater choice and security in housing.
5 Ensuring access to activities and services that enable people with a learning disability and/or autism to lead a fulfilling, purposeful life (such as education, leisure).
6 Ensuring access to mainstream health services (including mainstream mental health services in the community).
7 Providing specialist multi-disciplinary support in the community, including intensively when necessary to avoid admission to hospital.
8 Ensuring that services aimed at keeping people out of the criminal justice system are able to address

the needs of people with learning disabilities and/or autism, and that the right specialist services are in place in the community to support people with a learning disability and/or autism who pose a risk to others.
9 Providing high-quality hospital services that assess, treat and discharge people with a learning disability as quickly as possible.

(Source: www.england.nhs.uk)

Use and misuse of terms

Learning disability versus learning difficulty

There is confusion between the terms learning disabilities and learning difficulties as they are often used interchangeably.

Learning disability refers to a condition where an individual's ability to learn, understand and communicate is impaired.

Learning difficulty is often used in educational settings and refers to individuals who have specific problems with learning as a result of either medical, emotional or language problems but this does not affect the overall IQ of an individual and they do not have a significant general impairment in intelligence.

Various IQ classifications are used by health professionals to assess the presence and degree of learning disability. It is the only method of identifying the presence of learning disability in an individual, and the language associated with IQ scoring is now seen as outdated.

● 50–70 mild learning disability
● 35–50 moderate learning disability
● 20–35 severe learning disability
● below 20 profound learning disability.

(Source: British Institute of Learning Disabilities)

How and why terminology changes over time

Labels and terminology have changed over time as people realised that some names were offensive. The terms used within legislation were influenced by the language of the time. These may not have been seen as offensive at the time but became so because people used some of the terms as derogatory (to insult people). Individuals with disabilities became stereotyped with a negative image. Although it is important to know this historical context, only currently approved terms should be used in any setting.

Table 9.2 The changing language used for individuals with learning disabilities

Dates	Names called
1900–1920s	Mad, feeble minded, imbecile, fool, idiot
1913	Mentally deficient (Mental Deficiency Act)
1920s–1950s	Mentally defective
1944	Ineducable (unable to be educated) (1944 Education Act)
1950s	Subnormal, severely subnormal (1959 Mental Health Act)
1980	People with mental handicap
1985	People with learning difficulties (adopted by self-advocacy groups)
1990	Following NHS and Community Care Act, Department of Health's (DH) official term – people with learning disabilities

PAIRS ACTIVITY

(10 minutes)

Look at Table 9.2 and decide how many words would nowadays be considered insulting terms for individuals with learning difficulties. Discuss why there has been a shift away from these terms.

1.2 Types of learning disabilities

Down's syndrome

Down's syndrome is a genetic condition caused by the presence of an extra **chromosome** 21 in the body's cells. It is not a disease and is not usually inherited. Everyone born with Down's syndrome will have a degree of learning disability, but the level of disability will be different for each individual.

KEY TERM

Chromosomes – thread-like structures located inside the nucleus of animal and plant cells. Each chromosome is made of protein and a single molecule of deoxyribonucleic acid (DNA). Passed from parents to offspring, DNA contains the specific instructions that make each type of living creature unique.

CLASS DISCUSSION

(30 minutes)

Go to http://tinyurl.com/gtbb4we

Read the article about Seb's birth: does his mother's experience affect your view of having a Down's syndrome baby? For a completely different view go to http://tiryurl.com/h29kn95

Comment on the different viewpoints expressed in both articles. Remember that health and social care professionals need to be able to give care, support and advice without their personal views on these issues impacting on the advice and support they give.

Rett syndrome

Rett syndrome is a rare condition that affects the development of the brain. It can cause severe physical and mental disability that begins in early childhood. The condition affects approximately 1 in every 10–12,000 females and is rarely seen in males. Parents tend first to become aware of the condition when their child's development slows.

Williams syndrome

Williams syndrome (WS) is a genetic condition that is present at birth; it is characterised by medical problems, including cardiovascular disease, developmental delays and learning disabilities. Most people with Williams syndrome will have mild to severe learning disabilities and **cognitive** challenges.

KEY TERM

Cognitive – relating to the mental processes of perception, memory, judgement and reasoning.

Fragile X syndrome

Fragile X syndrome is a genetic condition and is the most common known cause of inherited learning disabilities it is also the most common known genetic cause of autism. It affects around 1 in 4000 males, as well as 1 in 6000 females. Learning disabilities occur in almost all boys with Fragile X, to differing degrees. Girls usually have milder learning disabilities than boys.

Learning disabilities with no known cause

Among people who have a mild learning disability, in about 50 per cent of cases no cause is identified.

In people with severe or profound learning disabilities, chromosomal abnormalities cause about 40 per cent of cases. Genetic factors account for 15 per cent, prenatal and perinatal problems 10 per cent, and postnatal issues a further 10 per cent. Cases which are of unknown cause are fewer, but still high at around 25 per cent (Chances4volunteering).

1.3 Causes of learning disabilities

Genetic

Inherited from parents

An inherited condition means that certain genes are passed from the parents that affect the brain development of the individual, for example in the case of Fragile X.

Presence of an extra or a missing chromosome

Chromosomes make up everyone's genetic blueprint and each individual usually has 46 chromosomes: 23 pairs. Sometimes there can be an abnormality in an individual's chromosomes, and this may lead to a learning disability. Every cell in the body has chromosomes containing genes that determine a person's unique characteristics. During conception, a child inherits one of each pair of chromosomes (and one of each pair of the genes they contain) from each parent. Sometimes a baby is born with too few or too many chromosomes, or with a damaged chromosome.

Metabolic

Our **metabolism** controls the chemical changes in the body. One metabolic disorder is phenylketonuria (PKU), which is a rare genetic condition that is present from birth (congenital). It is the lack of an enzyme that breaks down certain amino acids, which can be detected shortly after birth and controlled through diet. If it goes undetected then severe learning disabilities can result.

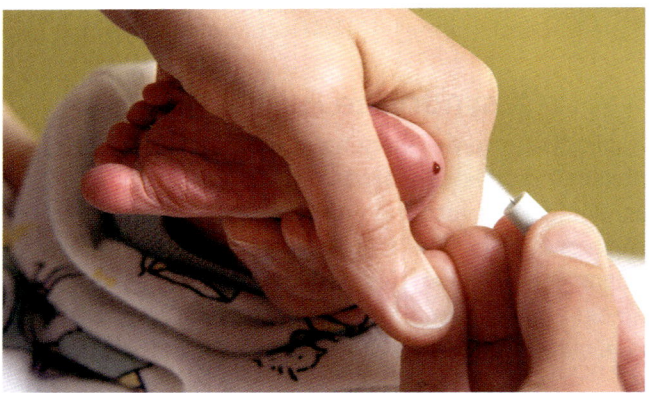

▲ **Figure 9.1** All newborn babies have a blood test to check for PKU

🔑 KEY TERM

Metabolism – the process the body uses to get or make energy from the food eaten. Food is made up of proteins, carbohydrates and fats. Chemicals in the digestive system break the food parts down into sugars and acids, the body's fuel.

Intra-uterine

This means something happened to the foetus while in the uterus. Pregnancy affects every physiological system in the body. Changes in the immune function and hormonal balance can make a pregnant woman more vulnerable to infection.

Lack of oxygen in the womb

Studies have found that lack of oxygen in the womb during foetal development leads to significant structural and functional brain injuries in the baby. It can also cause cerebral palsy.

Mother's illness during pregnancy

Some infections can be transmitted to babies through the placenta or during birth, and this may have serious consequences for the baby. The following infections can cause brain damage or learning difficulties:

- rubella
- chicken pox
- cytomegalovirus (one of the herpes group of viruses)
- toxoplasmosis.

GROUP ACTIVITY 👥

Research (30 minutes)

Divide into four groups and each research one of the mother's illnesses during pregnancy. Take turns presenting your findings to the other groups.

Mother's drug or alcohol use during pregnancy

If a pregnant woman drinks alcohol after the first three months of the pregnancy, it risks affecting the baby after they're born. The risks are greater the more she drinks. The effects include learning difficulties and behavioural problems.

Drinking heavily (more than six units a day) throughout pregnancy can cause the baby to develop foetal alcohol syndrome (FAS) (see also Unit 13, page 226). Children with FAS have:

- poor growth
- facial abnormalities
- learning and behavioural problems.

A foetus is very sensitive to drugs and cannot eliminate drugs as effectively as an adult can; therefore the chemicals can build up to high levels in the baby's system and cause permanent damage. Associated medical problems and birth defects include stroke, seizure, mental disability and learning disabilities.

Perinatal/neonatal (complications during or soon after birth)

A learning disability may result if the baby's oxygen supply is interrupted for a significant length of time during birth or if the baby is born significantly premature and becomes ill shortly after birth.

Postnatal

Some childhood infections can affect the brain, causing learning disability; the most common of these are encephalitis (inflammation of brain tissue) and meningitis (infection of the protective membranes that surround the brain and spinal cord). Social and environmental factors, such as poor housing conditions, poor diet and health care, malnutrition and lack of stimulation may lead to learning disability. Child abuse may also affect the brain as young children might be shaken by their parents which may lead to brain damage. Severe head injury, for example from a road accident, may result in learning disability.

1.4 Differences between learning disabilities and specific learning difficulties

Some physiological disabilities are not associated with learning disabilities.

Physiological conditions which may be misinterpreted as learning disabilities

- Cerebral palsy affects muscle control and movement. It is usually caused by an injury to the brain before, during or after birth. People with cerebral palsy may have difficulties in controlling muscles and movements as they grow and develop. This affects walking, speech and often swallowing.
- Like a learning disability, autism is a lifelong condition. Someone may have mild, moderate or severe autism, so it is now referred to as autism spectrum disorder (ASD). Autism is not a learning disability, but research suggests that around half of people with autism may also have a learning disability. Asperger's syndrome is a form of autism which also causes communication and emotional problems. However, people with Asperger's syndrome often have fewer problems with speaking and are less likely to have a learning disability.
- Global development delay refers to when a child takes longer to reach certain developmental milestones than other children their age.

Specific learning difficulties

Specific learning difficulties (or SpLDs), affect the way information is learned and processed. They are neurological (related to the nervous system rather than physiological), usually run in families and occur independently of intelligence. They can have significant impact on education, learning and on the acquisition of literacy skills.

Dyslexia

The most common SpLD, dyslexia, is usually hereditary. An individual with dyslexia may mix up letters within words and words within sentences while reading. They may also have difficulty with spelling words correctly while writing; letter reversals are common. Dyslexia affects the way information is processed, stored and retrieved, with problems of memory, speed of processing, time perception, organisation and sequencing.

Dyspraxia

Dyspraxia affects fine and/or gross motor co-ordination but the range of intellectual ability is in line with the general population. An individual's co-ordination difficulties may affect participation and functioning of everyday life skills in education, work and employment. Learning new skills at home, in education and work, such as driving a car, making a cake and using a computer may be difficult. There may be a range of other difficulties which can also have serious negative impacts on daily life. These include social emotional difficulties as well as problems with time management, planning and organisation.

Dyscalculia

Dyscalculia is a difficulty understanding mathematical concepts and symbols. It is characterised by an inability to understand simple number concepts and to master basic numeracy skills. There are likely to be difficulties dealing with numbers at basic levels; this includes learning number facts and procedures, telling the time, time keeping, understanding quantity, prices and money. Difficulties with numeracy and maths are also common with dyslexia.

Attention deficit hyperactivity disorder (ADHD)

Individuals with attention deficit hyperactivity disorder can exhibit signs such as inattention, restlessness, impulsivity, erratic, unpredictable and inappropriate behaviour, making inappropriate comments or interrupting excessively, and coming across unintentionally as aggressive. Frequently associated with dyslexia, individuals may have difficulty understanding when listening, expressing themselves clearly using speech, reading, remembering instructions, understanding spoken messages and staying focused.

KNOW IT

1 Describe one type of learning disability.
2 Discuss three of the principles from Transforming Care for People with Learning Disabilities.
3 Explain the difference between learning disability and learning difficulty.
4 Explain how the foetus can be affected by drinking alcohol during pregnancy.
5 Name three different types of SpLD.

LO1 Assessment activities

Below are suggested assessment activities that have been directly linked to the pass criteria in LO1 to help with assignment preparation; they include Top Tips on how to achieve best results.

Marsha has Down's syndrome and has a mild learning disability and is able to attend a mainstream school. Penny has Williams syndrome and has to attend a special school as she has a severe learning disability. Poppy has a learning difficulty and attends the same school as Marsha.

Activity 1 – pass criteria *P1*

Research and produce a definition of the term 'learning disabilities'.

Activity 2 – pass criteria *P2*

Create an information leaflet that describes Down's syndrome and Williams syndrome and their causes.

TOP TIPS ✔

✔ You need to provide a thorough definition from a variety of sources so ensure you research the term 'learning disability' on the Mencap, WHO and Department of Health websites.
✔ You must also research the models of care for learning disabilities, including use and misuse of terms (e.g. learning disability vs learning difficulty); how and why these may change over time).
✔ Ensure you describe both types of learning disabilities **and** their causes.

LO2 Understand the difficulties that may be experienced by individuals with learning disabilities *P3 M1 D1*

GETTING STARTED

(20 minutes)

Debbie has learning disabilities and lives independently. She shops at a local supermarket where she is familiar with its layout and the staff support her when she visits. The next nearest supermarket is a bus journey away. What difficulties might she experience if the supermarket closes for two weeks to be refurbished and to change its layout?

2.1 Potential difficulties and their impact

When studying this learning outcome, you may find it useful to refer to Unit 2 Equality, diversity and rights in health and social care, Unit 7 Safeguarding and Unit 12 Promote positive behaviour.

Communication

People who have a learning disability are aware of what goes on around them. However, their ability to understand and communicate may be limited, and they can find it hard to express themselves. Speech problems can make it even harder to make other people understand their feelings and needs.

Delayed language

Between 12 and 18 months, children begin to say words. Children learn language at different rates, but if they significantly miss language development milestones they are regarded as having a language delay. A language delay is when children have trouble:

- saying first words or learning words
- putting words together to make sentences
- building their vocabulary
- understanding words or sentences.

Language delays may result from a variety of underlying disorders, such as a learning disability, brain damage, dyslexia or cerebral palsy.

Difficulty in using language

Some children do not develop speech as easily as others or struggle to understand the meaning of words or gestures. These problems are examples of communication difficulty. Children with speech–language disabilities may experience difficulties with expressing ideas clearly. What the child says may be vague or hard to understand and they might use unspecific words such as 'stuff' or 'thing' to replace words they are unable to remember. They may use fillers such as 'um' to take up time as they attempt to remember a word.

Impaired speech

This is a condition in which the ability to produce speech sounds that are necessary to communicate is impaired. Speech impairments can be mild, such as occasionally mispronouncing some words, to severe, such as not being able to produce speech sounds at all. Impaired speech can significantly impact the ability to communicate. Speech impairments in childhood can have a negative influence on social development and at all stages of life can lead to social isolation, embarrassment and shame.

Understanding written information

Children with learning disabilities often have difficulty understanding written information. They lack the skills for understanding text and have poor word analysis. Some children read well, but when they are asked about what they have read they have little or no understanding of the words.

Environmental

People with learning disabilities are some of the most isolated and socially excluded people in society. However, since 2001 and the publishing of the government's white paper, Valuing People, there have been significant steps to give people with learning disabilities greater independence, rights and choices that can lead to equality and social inclusion. This ethos is also supported by the Disability Discrimination Act 2005 and the Human Rights Act 1998.

Transport

In 2007, Research for the Disability Rights Commission revealed that one in four individuals with learning difficulties felt that they lacked confidence in using public transport. They found that people with mental, rather than physical, impairments were among the most nervous and concerned about using public transport. There were a number of other fundamental re-occurring reasons why people with learning disabilities lack confidence and avoid using public transport.

The first barrier that individuals with learning disabilities feel they face is travel information as it is often presented in a way that is hard for many people with learning disabilities to understand. There is also a feeling that travel staff lack knowledge and appreciation for the problems faced by people with learning disabilities when using public transport.

In addition, there was also concern for personal safety; many people with learning disabilities lack confidence in using public transport services because they feel vulnerable to both attacks such as muggings, and other forms of harassment.

Living conditions

Many individuals with learning difficulties describe having no choice about where they live and who they live with. In 2011 Mencap commissioned a report into housing for people with learning disabilities – see Figure 9.2 for the results.

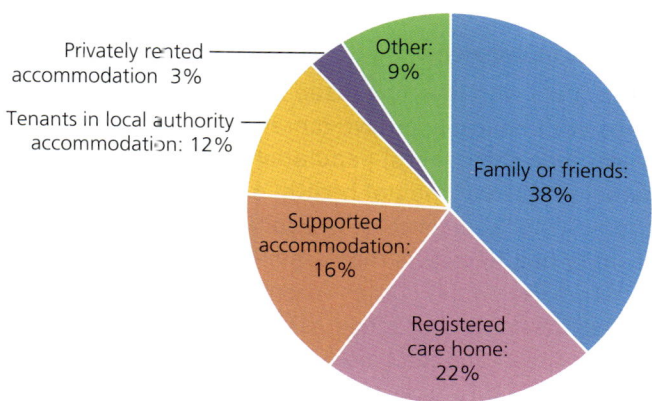

Privately rented accommodation 3%

Tenants in local authority accommodation: 12%

Other: 9%

Family or friends: 38%

Supported accommodation: 16%

Registered care home: 22%

▲ **Figure 9.2** Types of accommodation used by individuals with learning disabilities

Many people with a learning disability want to live a more independent life – something that requires housing arrangements that promote this. However, barriers to independence are the lack of suitable accommodation and the resources available to support them in the accommodation.

Most people with a learning disability who live with family and friends want greater independence, with around 70 per cent wanting to change their current housing arrangements to achieve this. Nearly 20 per cent of people with a learning disability known to local authorities live in accommodation that needs improvement. This includes one in three people living in registered care homes and one in four people living with family and friends.

Access to buildings

Sometimes individuals with learning disabilities also have a physical disability, and legislation in the Disability Discrimination Act states that reasonable adjustments should be made to buildings to make them accessible for individuals with disabilities, e.g. to have a ramp up to the front door instead of steps, to aid the use of wheelchairs.

Access to leisure

The government recognised the value of leisure activities for individuals with learning disabilities in Valuing People (Department of Health, 2001), which described day services in England as 'frequently failing to provide sufficiently flexible and individual support'. It stated that local authority leisure plans should address the needs of people with learning disabilities. The Department of Health green paper, Independence, Wellbeing and Choice (2005), made it clear that social care services are expected to help people to achieve access to leisure.

Access to services

Individuals with learning disabilities experience higher rates of ill health and have more complex health needs than the general population, including **epilepsy**, dental problems, mental health, and behavioural and nutritional disorders. In addition, access to primary health care is made more difficult because of communication difficulties when encountering health professionals, and practical issues such as long waiting times and lack of consultation time. This can result in a failure to access services such as men's and women's health screening, cervical screening, genetic screening, dental checks and health promotion. Basic health problems may be unidentified or regarded as part of the learning disability rather than a medical problem.

> ### 🔑 KEY TERM
>
> **Epilepsy** – a medical condition that affects the brain, causing seizures.

Access to information

Across public services there has been recognition that people with learning disabilities should be able to access information. People with learning disabilities need to be able to understand information if they are to have more choice and control over their lives and to become more active and equal citizens.

Easy Read is one way of making information more accessible. It:

- makes information easier to see
- uses easier-to-understand information
- uses simple words and pictures.

The main purpose of an Easy Read document is to tell people with learning disabilities what they need to know (see www.easy-read-online.co.uk).

Economic

Individuals with learning disabilities struggle with money as they are often in low-paid work, when they can manage to find employment.

Cost of leisure activities

Some local authorities encourage individuals with learning disabilities to take part in exercise classes, swimming or other activities such as sports and fitness, dancing or music and drama by keeping costs down. However, many individuals do not have the transport or the help to go, making the overall cost too high.

Some local authorities have a community outreach team that will help individuals with a learning disability to go out, make friends and enjoy activities in the community such as meals, day trips and trying out new activities. However, all of these have to be paid for and costs vary depending on the local authority and the duration of the activity. Obviously, one-to-one outreach activities will be a lot more expensive than group ones. Many people with learning difficulties find it difficult to spare the money for leisure activities as their benefits have been cut, which leaves them even more isolated if they cannot afford to go out.

Transport

Transport for people with learning disabilities is of vital importance. Good transport links open up access to services and activities within the local community. They also help people with learning disabilities to live more independently, giving them greater control over their lives; this is especially the case for those living in rural areas. Many people with learning disabilities do not drive so have to rely on public transport, which can be expensive.

Cost of care

Due to the range of different needs of individuals with learning disabilities, costs of care vary from individual to individual. Many are supported free of charge by parents and friends. However, there is still the physical and mental stress of looking after an individual with learning disabilities and they may need respite care to enable them to go on offering around-the-clock care.

The cost of care can be very expensive and the Independent Living Fund (ILF; now no longer operating) helped people with severe disabilities to lead independent lives in their community, instead of being placed in residential care. Recent changes in policy have given local councils the responsibility for assessing and allocating resources, rather than the centrally administered ILF.

The largest group of recipients – about a third – have severe learning disabilities, and the second largest group have cerebral palsy, but it is given to people with many different disabilities.

INDEPENDENT RESEARCH ACTIVITY

(15 minutes)

Research the community outreach team in your local authority. Is there a specific team for individuals with learning disabilities? What do they offer and how much do they charge?

Attitudes

After the huge success of the 2012 Paralympic Games, individuals with a disability of any type hoped that attitudes towards them would improve. Sadly, this has not been the case.

Prejudice

A survey carried out by Turning Point (a health and social care provider) in 2014 confirmed that individuals with learning difficulties face widespread prejudice among the general public. The poll of more than 1100 people also found that 23 per cent of the public expected people with a learning disability to live in a care home, while 8 per cent said they would expect them to be cared for in a secure hospital; 51 per cent of the 1100 people polled felt that 'learning disabled people were the most discriminated against group in society, ahead of gay people (44 per cent) and people from black and minority ethnic groups (44 per cent)'.

Stigma

Stigma is when people have negative beliefs, views or attitudes about individuals who belong to a certain group. Individuals with learning difficulties are part of a stigmatised group and this can have a negative impact on their psychological wellbeing.

Fear

Some individuals with learning difficulties are fearful of leaving their homes as they have come to expect name calling, staring, mocking, hitting and pushing as part of everyday life. They live in fear of victimisation. They are also targeted at home, perhaps with unpleasant things put through their letterbox.

Lack of understanding

A survey carried out in 2008 for Mencap asked more than 1600 people for an example of learning disability. Only 9 per cent of those surveyed were able to give a completely correct description. There is widespread confusion around what a learning disability is – 73 per cent of people gave examples that were wrong: 6 per cent thought blindness is a learning disability, 7 per cent named deafness, and 30 per cent dyslexia. Women had slightly more knowledge than men.

Discrimination

Many individuals with learning difficulties face discrimination throughout their lives. From the 2010 survey Opinion Matters for Turning Point, nine out of ten people (90 per cent) think that people with learning disabilities are discriminated against. One-third of people (33 per cent) think that people with learning disabilities cannot live independently or hold down a job. They are also discriminated against in the NHS with individuals with learning disabilities receiving poorer NHS care than other groups.

CLASSROOM DISCUSSION

(20 minutes)

Read the article at: http://tinyurl.com/z6n7z85

After all the equality legislation, such as the Disability Discrimination Act and Mental Capacity Act, discuss why people with learning difficulties still have problems accessing assessment and treatment for health problems.

Lack of choice

Individuals with learning difficulties are often not given choices as it is assumed that they cannot make choices. When an individual's choices lead to action this means they are controlling their own life even if they need a lot of help to make their choices happen.

In 2011, the National Development Team for inclusion (NDTi) published two reports (Supported Living – Making the Move and The Real Tenancy Test; www.ndti.org.uk/publications/ndti) to help address the problem of people with learning disabilities not getting equal access to housing or having their housing rights respected.

Despite more people with learning disabilities renting their own homes over the last ten years, the reports describe how people often lack real choice and control over where and how they live. Traditional forms of service provision, such as residential care, still dominate despite people saying they want more choice in housing.

There is a shortage of social housing and many private landlords do not want people with benefits in their houses and many will not want to adapt them. Some private landlords may also assume that people with learning difficulties will display challenging behaviour and cause damage.

Intellectual/cognitive

Individuals with a learning disability have a reduced intellectual capacity and may take longer to understand and process information, which disadvantages them when trying to access services and live in the wider community. Potential problems are described in Table 9.3.

Table 9.3 Effects on individuals of different categories of learning disability

Category of learning disability	Effect on individual
Mild	• Slower than typical in all areas of development • Able to learn practical life skills • Can read but has some difficulty in understanding and processing information
Moderate	• Noticeable developmental delays • Cannot communicate on complex levels • Difficulty in understanding and processing information
Severe	• Considerable delays in development • Can understand some speech but little ability to communicate or understand information
Profound	• Significant developmental delays • Extremely limited communication ability

Physical

Some people with learning disabilities have additional physical issues that affect their mobility.

Physical disability

A physical disability relates to total or partial loss of a person's bodily functions (e.g. walking, gross motor skills) and total or partial loss of a part of the body (e.g. a person with an amputation). People with physical disabilities have a physical impairment that

has a substantial and long-term effect on their ability to carry out their day-to-day activities. Someone with a moderate physical disability would have mobility problems, e.g. unable to manage stairs, and need aids or assistance to walk. Someone with a severe physical disability would be unable to walk and be dependent on a carer for mobility.

Problems with gait

Gait (the process of walking) and balance are intricate movements reliant on proper functioning from several areas of the body including the ears, eyes, brain and muscles. Problems with any of these areas can lead to walking difficulties, falls or injury if not addressed. Individuals with learning disabilities are more prone to falls because of gait instability and confusion.

Posture

For many, postural support can be critical in reducing pain, discomfort and creating the optimum situation for getting the best out of life and for a feeling of wellbeing. They cannot change their posture if they find themselves sitting uncomfortably, and are often incapable of communicating their discomfort. As a result, they are vulnerable to the adverse effects of poor positioning. For example, if they sit in the same position for a long time they may get pressure ulcers (an injury that affects areas of skin or underlying tissues). They may also slip down in a chair and put pressure on their spine.

Movement

A physical disability permanently prevents normal body movement and/or control. Some examples are given in Table 9.4. It is important to note that these conditions are not learning disabilities.

Table 9.4 Examples of physical conditions and their effect on movement; not all are related to learning disabilities

Physical	Effect on movement
Muscular dystrophy	Muscle fibres in the body gradually weaken over time, causing problems with movement
Acquired brain and spinal injuries	Permanent injuries to the brain, spinal cord or limbs that prevent proper movement in parts of the body
Spina bifida	Partial or full paralysis of the legs; little or no movement
Bone and joint deformities	Difficulty moving joints
Cerebral palsy	Depending on type and severity the individual may have difficulty moving body parts or the whole body; muscle weakness or tightness

Ways of overcoming potential difficulties

Financial assistance

There is a wide range of disability-related financial support, including benefits, tax credits, payments, grants and concessions available to support an individual who has disabilities. Each individual is assessed separately and they will be awarded benefits and so on depending on their situation. As well as benefits, an individual may be entitled to financial assistance with housing, housing adaptations or transport. There is also the opportunity of a personalised budget.

Advocacy

Advocacy means speaking up for someone. Individuals with learning disabilities may need an advocate because they are at risk of being ignored. Advocacy is about making things change because individuals' voices are heard and listened to. It is about making sure that they can make their own choices and have the chance to be as independent as they want to be. Advocacy is about putting an individual back in control of their own life.

Social inclusion

In the past, many individuals with learning disabilities relied on day centres for support. While this was useful, it added to the problem of social exclusion as individuals did not mix with the rest of the community. However, in the last decade the government has taken steps to encourage social inclusion and person-centred planning, as well as modernising day services to help encourage independent living and social skills for forming meaningful relationships with different groups of people.

Active participation

Active participation is person-centred by treating the person as an individual with their own thoughts and ideas. It recognises an individual's right to participate in everyday activities, relationships and life as independently as possible. The individual is an active partner in their own care or support rather than a passive recipient.

Empowerment

Empowerment gives an individual more power or control over their lives by giving them real choices and encouraging them to develop confidence in their own decision making. Empowering individuals means giving them all the information they need to make the right decision.

Positive images

A Mencap report called Changing Attitudes to Learning Disabilities recommends that the best way to have positive images of individuals with learning difficulties is for the public to have personal contact with them. For this to happen, people with a learning disability need to have equal participation in education, employment, social and leisure pursuits. This will challenge negative stereotypes. For children and young people, direct contact should be facilitated through inclusive activities and inclusive education. Positive portrayal in the media would also help so that individuals are not seen as weak, helpless and pitiable victims.

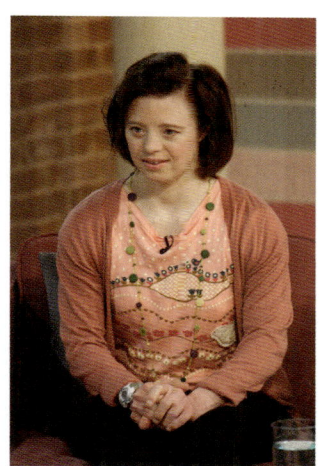

▲ **Figure 9.3** 'Upstairs, Downstairs' actress, Sarah Gordy, is a positive role model

Access to services and assessment

Most local authorities provide advice, support, assessment, treatment and therapies to support individuals with learning disabilities. Local authority teams include health and social care specialists such as social workers, social services assessment officers, community nurses, behaviour nurses, occupational therapists and physiotherapists. Psychologists, dieticians, and speech and language therapists can also offer the individual many types of support depending on their individual needs. See Figure 9.5 for more details of professionals' roles.

Accessible information

Mencap commissioned a guide in partnership with the Department of Health, as part of the programme of work set out in Valuing People Now, to ensure all individuals with learning disabilities were included. The guide was aimed at people commissioning support and services that would meet the communication needs of individuals with learning disabilities. However, it is also useful for family carers, professionals and people with a learning disability. The guide, called Make it Clear, explains what words to use, where to put the words on the page, how to use pictures, and the appropriate type of writing and paper to make the information accessible for individuals with learning disabilities (www.mencap.org.uk).

LO2 Assessment activity

Below is a suggested assessment activity that has been directly linked to the pass, merit and distinction criteria in LO2 to help with assignment preparation; it include Top Tips on how to achieve best results.

Dylan is 33 and lives in supported accommodation as he has a severe learning disability. He also has a physical disability and needs to use a wheelchair. Produce a presentation that:

● explains the difficulties which Dylan may experience. **P3**
● assesses the impact of the difficulties on Dylan. **M1**
● analyses the ways that Dylan could overcome the difficulties which he may face. **D1**

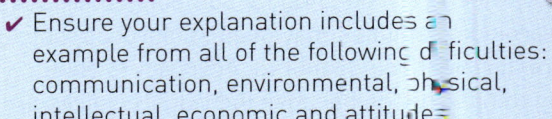

TOP TIPS

✔ Ensure your explanation includes an example from all of the following difficulties: communication, environmental, physical, intellectual, economic and attitudes
✔ Ensure you assess the impact of the difficulties you have named in the above task on Dylan.
✔ Remember you need to discuss the pros and cons of the ways Dylan could overcome the difficulties he faces and make reasoned comments.

LO3 Be able to support individuals with learning disabilities to plan their care and support *P4 P5 M2*

GETTING STARTED

(15 minutes)

Write down some of the clubs, groups and societies of which you have ever been a member. Write all the groups from your class on the whiteboard.

● Were individuals with learning disabilities in any of your groups?
● What percentage of the groups on the whiteboard had members who had a learning disability?
● Why do you think this was?

Read this Learning Outcome in conjunction with other units, including Unit 1 Building positive relationships in health and social care, Unit 6 Personalisation and a person-centred approach to care, Unit 12 Promote positive behaviour, Unit 13 Sexual health, reproduction and early development stages, and Unit 22 Psychology for health and social care.

3.1 Support services

Local Mencap

Mencap local groups support individuals with a learning disability and their families and carers in local communities. Each local group is different and its services can include anything from providing advice and information for family carers, running supported living services or organising social events.

Visit www.mencap.org.uk/findaservice/england to find out which services are on offer in your area.

Down's Syndrome Association (DSA)

Its aim is to help individuals with Down's syndrome to live full and rewarding lives. DSA runs a helpline and provides information about all aspects of living with Down's syndrome, including specialist advisers on benefits, education, health and social care. It advises new parents or anyone with questions as well as promotes and facilitates information exchange between members through various groups. DSA can advise on employment for people with Down's syndrome.

Phab clubs

Phab aims to promote and encourage individuals of all abilities to come together on equal terms, to achieve complete inclusion within the wider community. It supports a network of clubs for all age ranges, offering activities and holidays that members can share and enjoy together while promoting and encouraging self-confidence and independence in young people of all abilities. Phab helps to fund special residential breaks – inclusive experiences for disabled and non-disabled children and young people to share in a range of adventurous outdoor activities.

Residential care

Most residential homes for individuals with learning disabilities are individually designed and adapted to their needs. Often the residential care is provided in small units so that there is more of a family feel to them. If the individuals are assessed as being able to live independently they will be helped here to take their first steps to supported living.

Short-term breaks (respite care)

Respite is a short break for families caring for a relative with a disability or long-term mental or physical illness. Respite services for people with learning disabilities are provided after an individual assessment of need is carried out by a social worker or health professional. Respite provides a break for carers and for individuals with disabilities from their usual routines in order to improve the quality of their lives and support their relationship.

Special Educational Needs (SEN) provision in schools

While most children with a learning disability will get the support they need from their local nursery or school, some may still need a statutory assessment, and a legal document called a statement of special educational needs will be drawn up. This is a detailed record of the child's needs and the services that the local authority must provide for them. The process is often referred to as 'statementing'.

The support offered will depend on the needs of the individual; they may be offered one-to-one support in their normal class or be removed from the class to have individual one-to-one lessons.

Supported living

Supported living enables individuals to live in their own home instead of in residential care or with family. Individuals may also share with others. They may need support with some of the tasks shown in Table 9.5.

Table 9.5 Tasks needing support for supported living

Tasks	Examples of support
Household tasks	Washing up, ironing, cleaning
Personal care	Washing hair, cleaning teeth, showering
Maintaining a tenancy	Paying rent, water rates, electricity, gas
Taking medication	Ensuring pills are taken at the right time
Money management	Managing bills, budgeting
Building links with friends, family and the community	Going on visits to family and inviting them around for coffee/ phoning them; going to community events, e.g. coffee mornings
Social and leisure activities	Swimming, keep fit, going to classes of interest
Making healthy lifestyle choices	Shopping and cooking, encouraged to walk to shops

Employment services

In 2012, the Department of Health found that only 7 per cent of adults with learning disabilities were in some form of paid employment, the majority of which was part-time work, so many individuals with learning disabilities are not working. The most common tool used to support people with a learning disability is called supported employment. The personalised model uses a partnership strategy to enable people with disabilities to achieve sustainable long-term employment and to enable businesses to employ valuable workers.

3.2 Practitioners

Community learning disabilities teams

These teams consist of many different practitioners who have specialist training to work with individuals with learning disabilities. Examples are shown in Figure 9.5.

Unlike many of the professionals in the team, befrienders are often volunteers. They are caring and compassionate people who want to help adults with learning disabilities realise their full potential and help them to participate in activities in the community as other people do. They visit each individual weekly, typically for a 3-hour session, and work with them on a one-to-one basis, doing activities of the individual's choice. The activities are very varied: from exercise like walking, swimming, attending a gym or horse riding to visiting relatives or local visitor attractions, going shopping, or out for a meal. They might do some gardening together, or play darts or pool. For more information, go to www.befriender.co.uk.

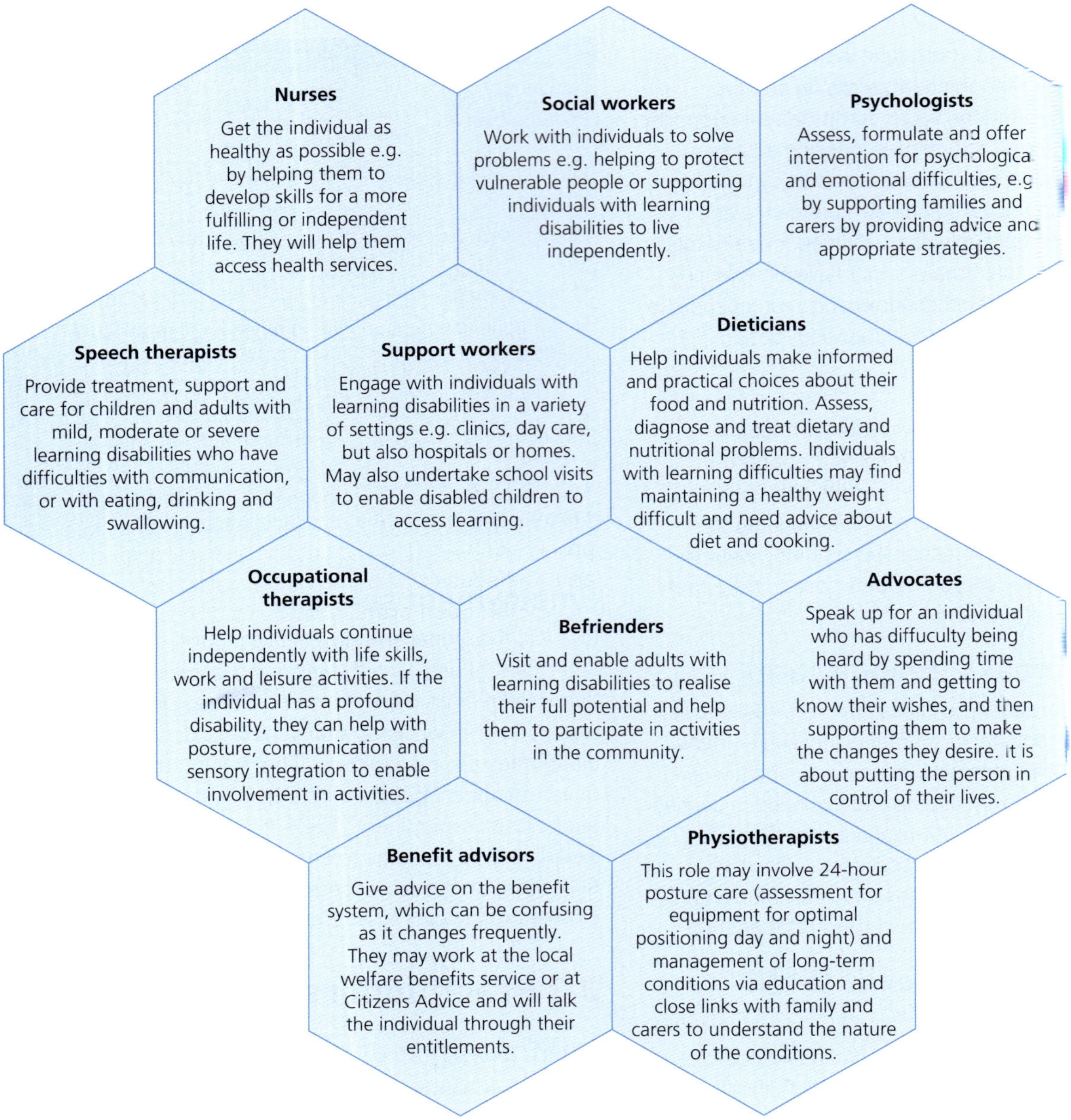

Nurses

Get the individual as healthy as possible e.g. by helping them to develop skills for a more fulfilling or independent life. They will help them access health services.

Social workers

Work with individuals to solve problems e.g. helping to protect vulnerable people or supporting individuals with learning disabilities to live independently.

Psychologists

Assess, formulate and offer intervention for psychological and emotional difficulties, e.g by supporting families and carers by providing advice and appropriate strategies.

Speech therapists

Provide treatment, support and care for children and adults with mild, moderate or severe learning disabilities who have difficulties with communication, or with eating, drinking and swallowing.

Support workers

Engage with individuals with learning disabilities in a variety of settings e.g. clinics, day care, but also hospitals or homes. May also undertake school visits to enable disabled children to access learning.

Dieticians

Help individuals make informed and practical choices about their food and nutrition. Assess, diagnose and treat dietary and nutritional problems. Individuals with learning difficulties may find maintaining a healthy weight difficult and need advice about diet and cooking.

Occupational therapists

Help individuals continue independently with life skills, work and leisure activities. If the individual has a profound disability, they can help with posture, communication and sensory integration to enable involvement in activities.

Befrienders

Visit and enable adults with learning disabilities to realise their full potential and help them to participate in activities in the community.

Advocates

Speak up for an individual who has difficulty being heard by spending time with them and getting to know their wishes, and then supporting them to make the changes they desire. It is about putting the person in control of their lives.

Benefit advisors

Give advice on the benefit system, which can be confusing as it changes frequently. They may work at the local welfare benefits service or at Citizens Advice and will talk the individual through their entitlements.

Physiotherapists

This role may involve 24-hour posture care (assessment for equipment for optimal positioning day and night) and management of long-term conditions via education and close links with family and carers to understand the nature of the conditions.

▲ **Figure 9.4** Examples of roles in community learning disability teams

3.3 Methods of care

Initial assessments

For the majority of individuals, the presence of a learning disability is diagnosed from birth or during the early development period of life, but even then their doctors probably will not be able to tell exactly how it will affect their development. The extent of the child's disability will become clearer as they reach the ages when they should be talking, walking or reading. At least if they have an initial assessment, the child's current needs can be assessed to work out what kind of support will help them, and they will be referred to a paediatrician.

Specialist assessments

Although some conditions are easy to diagnose, other parents may never receive a diagnosis, or may be told their child has 'global developmental delay', which indicates that the child will take more time to reach many developmental milestones. For some parents, getting a diagnosis can be a struggle, but the support of their health visitor and GP is often the first step to getting help. The GP should be able to refer them to a local paediatrician, a doctor who specialises in working with children who are ill or disabled, who will then be able to assess their condition or, if not, refer them to further specialist assistance.

Person-centred care plans

Person-centred care planning helps an individual plan all aspects of their life, ensuring that they remain central to the creation of any plan that will affect them. The individual remains in control of how these plans are made, who is to be involved in them, how they are to be recorded, and whose help they will need to make the plans happen. See Unit 6 for more information.

Individual learning plans

Also known as individual education plans (IEP), these plans are designed for children with special educational needs (SEN) to help them to get the most out of their education. An IEP builds on the curriculum that a child with learning disabilities is following and sets out the strategies being used to meet that child's specific needs.

An IEP is a teaching and learning plan and should set out targets and actions for the child that are different from those that are in place for the rest of the class. The IEP is not a legal document, which means that the local authority does not have to produce a plan or make sure that a child receives the support that is outlined in the plan. It informs the teacher of specific targets for the child and how these will be reached. The IEP allows staff to plan for progression, monitor the effectiveness of teaching, monitor the provision for additional support needs within the school, collaborate with parents and other members of staff and help the child become more involved in their own learning and work towards specific targets.

Education and health care (EHC)

The first stage of obtaining an EHC Plan is to carry out an EHC needs assessment with involvement from different professionals in education, health and social care. The local authority reviews the needs assessment and decides whether to issue an EHC plan or not. If they decide a plan is needed, it is drawn up by the local authority with the parent/young person's involvement. The parent/young person can specify the type of school placement they want and the local authority must then liaise with the school. The local authority has a legal duty to secure the educational provision detailed in the EHC plan. The local health care provider has a legal duty to arrange health care provision. The EHC plan specifies social care too, but there is no legal duty to provide this except for care provided under the Chronically Sick and Disabled Persons Act 1970.

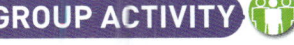 **GROUP ACTIVITY**

Interview with centre SENCO (30 minutes)

Invite your centre SENCO (special educational needs co-ordinator) to talk to your group about an IEP. Before the interview, prepare a list of questions you would like to ask them about how they would prepare an IEP for a fictional child. For example, one of the questions could be what should be in an IEP? Give a copy of the proposed questions to the SENCO in advance of the interview so they can prepare their answers and bring an IEP with them.

Multi-disciplinary approach

A multi-disciplinary approach involves a range of professionals from different specialities, from several organisations, working together to deliver comprehensive care for an individual. For example, a young person in a special school who has learning and physical disabilities may have a team consisting of their teacher, social worker, occupational therapist, psychologist, community nurse, physiotherapist and specialist doctor. These professionals will meet to review progress to date and to discuss and plan the best way forward for the individual. Each professional will suggest ways they can help to meet the plan.

> **? THINK ABOUT IT**
>
> ### Case study: Toby
>
> Toby is 15 and has Down's syndrome. He lives with his mum. He started to truant from school six months ago. He has been cautioned by the police for under-age drinking and for causing a disturbance. His mum has tried to reason with him but he takes no notice. Recently he was caught shoplifting alcohol from a local supermarket. He lashed out at the shop assistant who tried to stop him running off.
>
> Discuss which professionals could form a multi-disciplinary team to try to help Toby and his mum.

Safeguarding

Social care plays an important role in helping individuals with care and support needs to live full lives. This includes preventing abuse, minimising risk without taking control away from individuals, and responding proportionately if abuse or neglect has occurred. Local authorities, care providers, health services, housing providers and criminal justice agencies are all important safeguarding partners. The Care Act 2014 introduced new safeguarding duties for local authorities including: leading a multi-agency local adult safeguarding system; making or causing enquiries to be made where there is a safeguarding concern; hosting safeguarding adults boards; carrying out safeguarding adults reviews; and arranging for the provision of independent advocates. For more about safeguarding, see Unit 7 (page 133).

3.4 Legislation in relation to learning disabilities

NHS and Community Care Act 1990

This Act introduced a requirement for local authorities to help vulnerable adults remain in the community, preventing or delaying admission to institutional care. The Act requires local authorities to carry out assessments of people who 'appear to be in need' of community care services, and to arrange packages of care. Most social services departments operate a set of 'eligibility criteria' that define who is eligible for an assessment of need as well as support from services. The assessment process has largely been subsumed under the Single Assessment Process.

Mental Health Acts 1983 and 2007

One of the best-known functions of the 1983 Mental Health Act is the power to enforce the compulsory detention of a person with a 'mental disorder' (learning disability) when detention is necessary in the interests of their own health or safety or for the protection of others. In the 2007 Act amendments were made to:

- ensure patients receive the care they need to protect them and the wider public from harm
- support modernised services
- strengthen patient safeguards
- remedy Human Rights incompatibilities.

> 🔍 **INDEPENDENT RESEARCH ACTIVITY**
>
> **(30 minutes)**
>
> The 2007 Mental Health Act aimed to remedy human rights incompatibilities. What were these incompatibilities? Do you think they were remedied by the Act?
>
> The following resources may be useful:
>
> http://tinyurl.com/5s7sqoz
> http://tinyurl.com/7epfmqh
> http://tinyurl.com/hnbns4b

Mental Capacity Act 2005

The Act was introduced in response to concerns about the limited account taken of the voices and rights of adults who may 'lack capacity' to make informed decisions about our care and treatment (e.g. some individuals with learning disabilities but this may affect all of us at some time in our lives). This particularly applies to decisions about psychiatric treatment and the support of people in long-term care. The Mental Capacity Act clarifies, strengthens and protects the rights of people who wish to plan for becoming incapacitated, as well as the rights of those who currently lack capacity. It also clarifies the rights and duties of the carers and professionals who assist such individuals.

Anyone – a health or care professional, other professional, relative or carer – might need to decide whether the individual has the capacity to make a particular decision. In many cases that decision will be the responsibility of the family or carers. Where the decision to be made is more complex, a more formal assessment may be needed and this may involve doctors or other professionals. For example, where consent is needed for medical treatment or examination, a doctor or health care professional will decide whether or not individuals have the capacity to consent.

The Mental Capacity Act states that before anyone acts on behalf of someone who lacks capacity they must have a reasonable belief that the person lacks capacity.

Equality Act 2010

Equalities legislation has replaced anti-discrimination legislation. Anti-discriminatory practice is fundamental to the ethical basis of care provision and critical to the protection of people's dignity. The Equality Act protects those receiving care and the workers that provide it from being treated unfairly on the grounds of characteristics that are protected under the legislation. The 'protected characteristics' are:

- age
- disability
- gender reassignment
- pregnancy and maternity
- race – this includes ethnic or national origins, colour or nationality
- religion or belief – this includes lack of belief
- sex
- sexual orientation.

(Source: Government Equalities Office, 2010)

Human Rights Act 1998

The legal framework for human rights requires that health and social care workers, alongside other providers of public services, must respect the dignity of people using services. The ethics and values that underpin good practice in social care, such as autonomy, privacy and dignity, are at the core of human rights legislation. The Human Rights Act (HRA) applies to individuals with learning disabilities as equal citizens and has the potential to make a profound impact on their service provision, inclusion in society and quality of life.

In 2008 the Joint Committee on Human Rights issued a report, A Life Like Any Other? Human Rights of Adults with Learning Disabilities. This stated that the HRA provided a legal framework for service users to demand that they are treated with respect for their dignity'. The government accepted that it was the most vulnerable members of society, such as people with learning difficulties, who were most in need of protection of their rights under the HRA.

> ### ? THINK ABOUT IT
> Do you think the experience of couples with learning disabilities should be any different from any other couple who want to get married? Explain your reasons using the legislation to support your answer.

Children and Families Act 2014

This Act aimed to transform the system for children and young people with special educational needs (SEN) by placing families at the centre of decision making. It sets out requirements that education, health and care services should work together to provide joined-up support across all areas of a child's or young person's life. The Act replaced SEN statements with education, health and care (EHC) plans, and the system runs from birth to 25, rather than ending when a young person leaves school. The Act also introduced a 'local offer' of information for families covering the education, health and social care support available locally.

The Care Act 2014

The Care Act built on a range of existing legislation. It aims to involve the individual at the centre of their own care to meet their specific needs, thereby ensuring their wellbeing. According to the Act, the local authority has to:

- invest in preventative services and fully utilise existing community resources so problems do not escalate but are dealt with before too much intervention is needed
- establish an information and advice service covering new rights and entitlements
- facilitate a diverse, vibrant and sustainable market for care and support services that benefit the whole population
- work with the NHS and other key partners
- offer the individual a personal budget after assessment
- set up an adult safeguarding board.

3.5 Guidance

Guidance can be statutory (legally enforceable) or non-statutory. It provides advice and assistance on the procedures for putting provisions of law into action. Statutory guidance must be followed unless there is a valid reason not to.

The Code of Practice under the Mental Capacity Act 2005, for example, is statutory guidance. Non-statutory guidance is more advisory in nature and may be in a different form, for example a local authority leaflet. As a general rule, all guidance should be followed unless there are strong reasons not to do so.

Policies

All health and social care organisations working with individuals with disabilities have written policies in place in order to protect their staff as well as service users. These policies are based on legislation. They ensure that all staff working with individuals follow the same principles of care; for example, if there is an issue with safeguarding and the member of staff is unsure what to do then they can check the safeguarding policy for their organisation. Policies should be drawn up with the input of the individuals concerned so that they are empowered and feel they have a stake in the organisation.

Charters

Charters are a series of pledges giving organisations a clear framework for improving their practice. They help to define the quality of care that service users can expect from service providers. For example, go to the health charter website at http://tinyurl.com/p9kyjf3 or the social care one developed in partnership with the Voluntary Organisations Disability Group (VODG) at http://tinyurl.com/jt447pt.

Codes of practice

A code of practice is a set of written rules that explains how people working in a particular profession should behave. Most professional bodies have a code of practice that provides professionals with the advice and guidelines for delivering quality care, describing the standards of conduct and practice within which they should work. For example, the Health and Care Professions Council Standards of Conduct, Performance and Ethics (http://tinyurl.com/jwaje6u) is a list of statements that describe the standards of professional conduct and practice required of healthcare professionals.

Go to www.nmc.org.uk/standards/code to view the nursing and midwifery code of practice.

The white paper: Valuing People – A New Strategy for Learning Disabilities for the 21st Century

Valuing People (2001) sought to underpin the government's vision for people with learning disabilities by confirming four key principles of rights, independence, choice and inclusion.

Key elements were as follows:

- An end to long-stay hospitals.
- A five-year programme to modernise local council day services.
- A new national learning disability information centre and helpline in conjunction with Mencap.
- A national forum for people with learning disabilities.
- A learning disability task force.
- Specialist local services for people with severe and challenging behaviour, and integrated facilities for children with severe disabilities and complex needs.
- An extension of eligibility to direct payments, a scheme which allows service users to choose and purchase their own care.

Fair Access to Care Services

Fair Access to Care Services (FACS) guidelines were introduced by the government in 2003 as a means of providing local authorities with a common framework for determining individuals' eligibility for social care services and addressing inconsistencies in outcomes across the country.

The four bands of the FACS eligibility framework
Critical: when

- life is, or will be, threatened; and/or
- significant health problems have developed or will develop; and/or
- there is, or will be, little or no choice and control over vital aspects of the immediate environment; and/or
- serious abuse or neglect has occurred or will occur; and/or
- there is, or will be, an inability to carry out vital personal care or domestic routines; and/or
- vital involvement in work, education or learning cannot or will not be
- sustained; and/or
- vital social support systems and relationships cannot or will not be
- sustained; and/or
- vital family and other social roles and responsibilities cannot or will not be undertaken.

Substantial: when

- there is, or will be, only partial choice and control over the immediate environment; and/or
- abuse or neglect has occurred or will occur; and/or
- there is, or will be, an inability to carry out the majority of personal care or domestic routines; and/or
- involvement in many aspects of work, education or learning cannot or will not be sustained; and/or
- the majority of social support systems and relationships cannot or will not be sustained; and/or
- the majority of family and other social roles and responsibilities cannot or will not be undertaken.

Moderate: when

- there is, or will be, an inability to carry out several personal care or domestic routines; and/or
- involvement in several aspects of work, education or learning cannot or will not be sustained; and/or
- several social support systems and relationships cannot or will not be sustained; and/or
- several family and other social roles and responsibilities cannot or will not be undertaken.

Low: when

- there is, or will be, an inability to carry out one or two personal care or domestic routines; and/or
- involvement in one or two aspects of work, education or learning cannot or will not be sustained; and/or
- one or two social support systems and relationships cannot or will not sustained; and/or
- one or two family and other social roles and responsibilities cannot or will not be undertaken.

(Source: Department of Health, 2010)

Some local authorities will only offer help if the individual is in the critical or substantial categories, but this does vary across the country even though this system was meant to iron out inconsistencies in outcomes.

No Secrets 2000 on the protection of vulnerable adults

Local authorities are bound to follow No Secrets guidance unless under exceptional circumstances. It requires the identification of who is at risk and why. It requires local authorities to set up a multi-agency group led by social services but also involving NHS bodies and police to develop joint codes of practice and ways of working together. Multi-agencies should also develop policies for responding to allegations as well as carrying out investigations balancing confidentiality with information sharing.

Death by Indifference (Mencap 2007)

This report sets out why Mencap believes there is institutional discrimination within the NHS, and why individuals with a learning disability get worse health care than non-disabled people. It presents the stories of six people who they believe have died unnecessarily through doctors and nurses treating these individuals while failing to understand the medical needs or appreciate the seriousness of their conditions that led to their death.

KNOW IT

1 Explain how Mencap helps to support individuals with learning disabilities and their families.
2 Discuss the purpose and benefits of respite care.
3 Explain how an individual with learning disabilities could be enabled to live in their own home.
4 Explain what an occupational therapist does to assist an individual with learning disabilities.
5 Analyse how a person-centred care plan can support the human rights of individuals with learning disabilities.
6 Discuss how an IEP (Individual Education Plan) can help:
   a) the individual
   b) the teacher.
7 Explain what is meant by a multi-disciplinary approach.
8 Choose two pieces of legislation and assess the impact of both on an individual with learning disabilities.

L03 Assessment activity

Below is a suggested assessment activity that has been directly linked to the pass and merit criteria in L03 to help with assignment preparation; it includes Top Tips on how to achieve best results.

Chelsey is 15 and has Rett syndrome. As a result of this condition she has a severe learning disability as well as severe physical disabilities. She is cared for by her parents and lives at home with them and her two younger brothers. Research the services in your area and produce a leaflet for her parents that:

● suggests services within the health and social care sector that can best support the needs of Chelsey and her parents **P4**
● explains the role of different practitioners in supporting Chelsey and her parents **P5**
● evaluates the impact of the person-centred approach on Chelsey's quality of life. **M2**

TOP TIPS

✔ Ensure you research both the health and social care sectors, including statutory and voluntary, within your area.
✔ There is a long list of practitioners in the specifications which have to be included for this task so make sure you include them all.
✔ To evaluate the impact of person-centred approach on Chelsey's quality of life, you must evaluate the impact of the methods of care, the legislation in relation to learning disabilities and the guidance as directed in the specifications.

Read about it

British Institute for Learning Disabilities: www.bild.org.uk

Down's syndrome: www.downs-syndrome.org.uk

Cerebral palsy: www.scope.org.uk

Rett syndrome: www.nhs.uk/conditions/rett-syndrome/pages/introduction

Williams syndrome: www.williams-syndrome.org.uk

Fragile X: www.fragile.org.uk

Learning disabilities: www.learningdisabilities.org.uk

Specific learning difficulties: www.bdadyslexia.org.uk

Social inclusion: www.aboutlearningdisabilities.co.uk

Physical disability: www.firststopcareadvice.org.uk

Employment: www.learningdisabilities.org.uk

SENCO/supported living: www.mencap.org.uk

Phab clubs: phab.org.uk

Person-centred care plan: www.learningdisabilities.org.uk

IEP (Individual Learning Plan): www.specialeducationalneeds.co.uk

Opinion Matters Survey: www.improvinghealthandlives.org.uk/news

Charters: http://tinyurl.com/jt447pt

No Secrets: www.communitycare.co.uk

Unit 12

Promote positive behaviour

ABOUT THIS UNIT

Working together to promote positive behaviour with adults, young people and children is crucial for ensuring that they achieve their full potential and for creating a safe and secure environment where individuals' self-esteem, confidence and respect for others is valued and good behaviours and attitudes are promoted by and towards everyone.

In this unit you will learn about the different approaches that can be used for promoting positive behaviour, including why these are important and when they may be required. You will also learn more about how staff who work with adults, young people and children can manage challenging situations safely and in a positive way.

Being aware of the range of interventions that are used to promote positive behaviour, including the potential impact they may have on different individuals, will help you to further develop your knowledge and understanding of how to effectively de-escalate situations and manage behaviours. Finding out about the relevant legislation and guidance will help you to further develop your understanding of how interventions that are used in settings must also comply with these.

LEARNING OUTCOMES

The topics, activities and suggested reading in this unit will help you to:

1 Understand how to promote positive behaviour
2 Understand situations in which staff are required to use reactive and restrictive interventions
3 Understand interventions used to promote positive behaviour and the impact on the individual
4 Know relevant legislation and guidance related to promoting positive behaviour

How will I be assessed?

You will be assessed through a series of assignments and tasks set and marked by your tutor.

How will I be graded?

You will be graded using the following criteria.

Learning outcome	Pass assessment criteria	Merit assessment criteria	Distinction assessment criteria
You will:	To achieve a **pass** you must demonstrate that you have met all the pass assessment criteria	To achieve a **merit** you must demonstrate that you have met all the pass and merit assessment criteria	To achieve a **distinction** you must demonstrate that you have met all the pass, merit and distinction assessment criteria
1 Understand how to promote positive behaviour	**P1** Demonstrate a person-centred approach to promote positive behaviour	**M1** Assess how best practice could be evaluated in promoting positive behaviour	
	P2 Demonstrate best practice in promoting positive behaviour		
2 Understand situations in which staff are required to use reactive and restrictive interventions	**P3** Describe a situation where a reactive or restrictive intervention would be required	**M2** Assess how recognising stages of behaviour could promote positive behaviour	
3 Understand interventions used to promote positive behaviour and the impact on the individual	**P4** Demonstrate strategies that could be used to promote positive behaviour	**M3** Evaluate why restrictive interventions are used in only the most serious situations	**D1** Evaluate the impact of strategies used to promote positive behaviour on an individual's wellbeing
4 Know relevant legislation and guidance related to promoting positive behaviour	**P5** Describe legislation related to promoting positive behaviour		

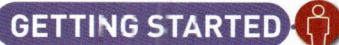

LO1 Understand how to promote positive behaviour *P1 P2 M1*

Positive behaviour (5 minutes)

Think about three things you have been praised for recently. Compare and discuss these with your peers.

1.1 Understand the contexts where the promotion of positive behaviour is required

Individuals express themselves and interact with others in many different ways and using a range of behaviours; some of these may be difficult to understand, whilst others may be unwanted. Promoting positive behaviour supports individuals' rights, promotes their wellbeing and recovery and keeps them and others safe. Figure 12.1 provides you with further information about the different contexts where the promotion of positive behaviour is required.

KEY TERMS

Acute psychiatric settings – residential and hospital settings that provide care with intensive medical and nursing support for individuals in periods of acute psychiatric illness or mental health needs.

Specialist assessment and treatment units – residential units that provide assessment and treatment in a therapeutic environment and are run by NHS Trusts and independent organisations.

Mental health units – hospital-based settings that provide specialised care and treatment to individuals with mental health needs.

Secure units – low, medium and high security facilities that provide specialised care and treatment to individuals with mental health needs and pose a risk to others.

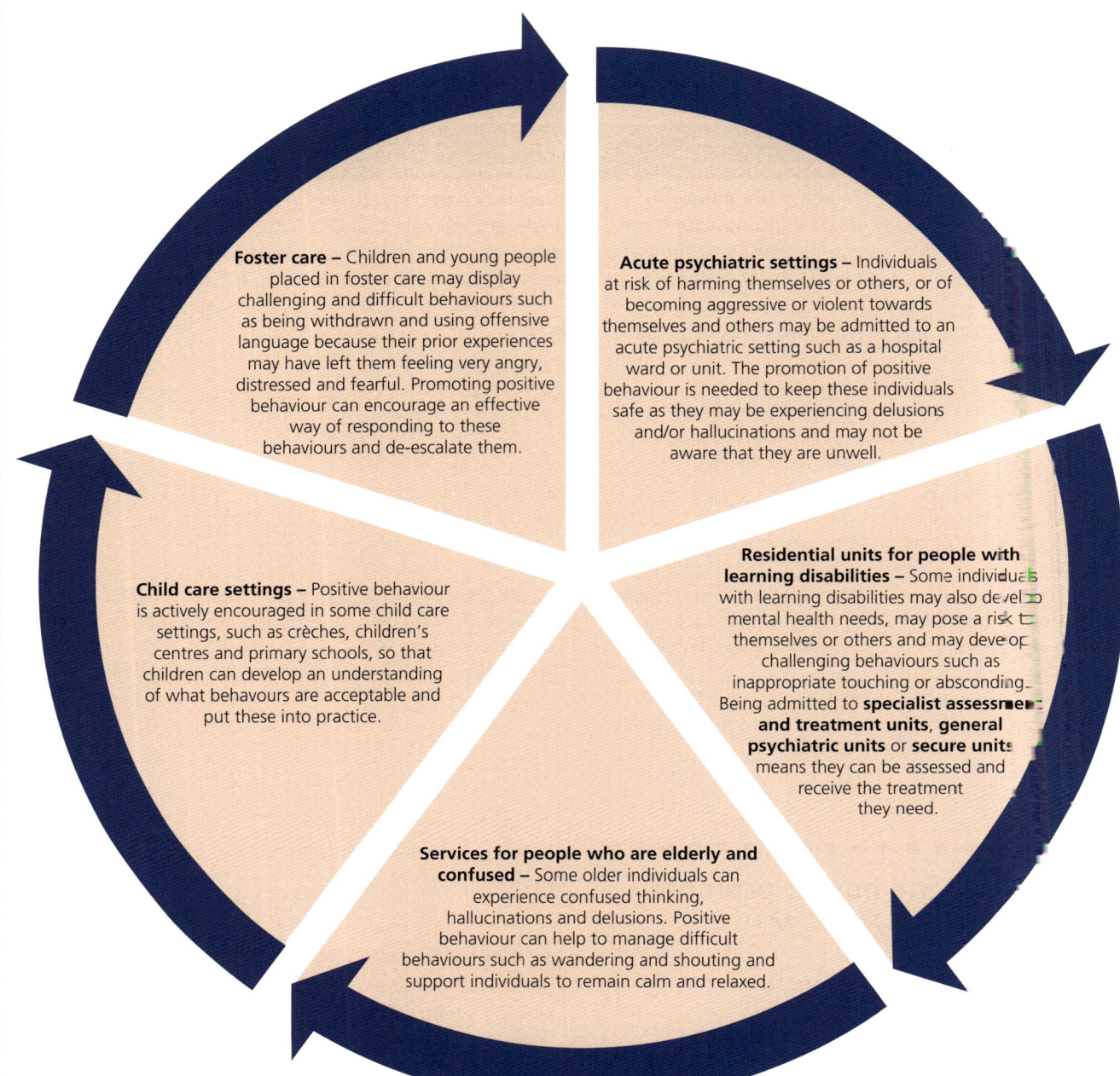

▲ **Figure 12.1** Settings and services that promote positive behaviour

1.2 Positive behavioural support

What does the term 'positive behavioural support' mean?

In February 2014, a programme led by the Local Government Association (LGA) and NHS England established the core principles that should be present across all education, health and social care services accessed by children, young people, adults and older people with learning disabilities and/or autism, who either display or are at risk of displaying behaviour that challenges. It refers to positive behavioural support as

being a way of working to increase individuals' quality of life and minimise the impact that behaviours that challenge may have on them and/or others.

'not a single intervention or therapy. It is a multi-component framework for delivering a range of evidence-based supports to increase quality of life and reduce the occurrence, severity or impact of behaviours that challenge.'

(Source: DOH, LGA and NHS England, Ensuring Quality Services, February 2014)

This was followed, in April 2014, with the Department of Health publishing the guidance Positive and Proactive Care: Reducing the Need for Restrictive Interventions. Both were in response to concerns over the inappropriate use of **restrictive interventions** such as those reported at Winterbourne View hospital rather than on preventative and proactive approaches to manage challenging behaviours across learning disability and mental health services and settings.

This guidance document defines positive behavioural support (PBS) as:

'a framework that seeks to understand the context and meaning of behaviour in order to inform the development of supportive environments and skills that can enhance a person's quality of life.'

(Source: DOH, Positive and Proactive Care: Reducing the Need for Restrictive Interventions, April 2014)

In addition, this guidance is used by the regulator, the Care Quality Commission (CQC), when assessing whether a health or social care provider is delivering safe and appropriate care and when determining the quality of care and treatment being provided.

1.3 Best practice in promoting positive behaviour

Best practice approaches can be effective both in terms of reducing the occurrence and impact of unwanted behaviours and supporting individuals to develop skills that can improve their quality of life.

Person-centred, values-based approaches

These can promote positive behaviour by:

- recognising individuals' unique needs, preferences, experiences, wishes and strengths
- improving their quality of life and wellbeing
- developing positive relationships between individuals, their carers, relatives and advocates, where individuals feel safe and are treated with compassion, dignity and respect
- empowering individuals to recognise their rights and be in control of their lives
- creating services and support that meet individuals' needs
- developing services and support that are flexible.

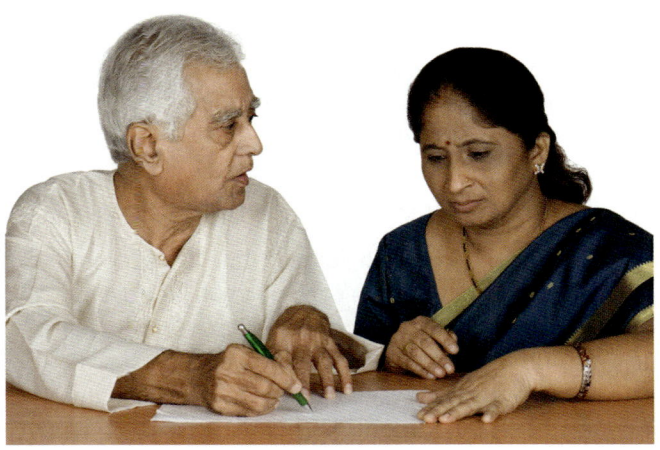

▲ **Figure 12.2** Involving individuals in their care, support and treatment

Assessment

This can promote positive behaviour by:

- early recognition of unwanted behaviours so that interventions and support can be planned, implemented and accessed by individuals, their carers, relatives or advocates

- early recognition of underlying risk factors in relation to an individual's personal and medical history, such as poverty, abuse, mental and physical health, the onset of conditions such as dementia that can increase the likelihood of unwanted behaviours so that interventions and support can be planned and put in place proactively and systematically
- identifying an individual's holistic needs, personal likes and dislikes through directly involving them, their carers, relatives or advocates so that interventions provided are specific to the individual
- developing an understanding of how, when and why the individual presents unwanted behaviours and their triggers so that the individual and others gain insight and begin to understand the support that is required.

1.4 Identifying patterns of behaviour

Precursor behaviours often precede unwanted behaviours. Those supporting individuals must be aware of these so that they can diffuse situations and

> 🔑 **KEY TERM**
>
> **Precursor behaviours** – changes in mood or behaviours that indicate that an individual is becoming anxious; these can be identified by those who know an individual well.

minimise or prevent challenging episodes.

Precursor behaviours will vary for different individuals and in different situations. They normally involve a change in the individual; this may be physically visible and include tense muscles, pacing up and down, sweating, a change in facial expressions and/or an increased breathing rate. Other changes may include the individual becoming withdrawn or talking or acting hurriedly.

Remember, each individual is unique and so precursor behaviours are also specific to each individual. Read through the observation report (Figure 12.3) completed by Sarah Miriaz, a senior residential worker for Andrew, a young man who has difficulty expressing himself due to his learning disabilities and dementia; note the

precursor behaviours that Sarah recognised, which helped to diffuse a potentially challenging situation from developing.

Observer: Sarah Miriaz

Individual observed: Andrew Boate

Date: 18/11/16

Time: 9.00am to 9.20am

Targeted behaviour: Pushing over furniture and/or hitting others when made to wait for a prolonged period.

9.00 am Andrew is sitting in a relaxed manner in the armchair by the main entrance waiting for his taxi to arrive to take him to his hospital appointment this morning.

9.05 am Saw Andrew pacing up and down the hallway and noticed some of his facial muscles twitching. Asked Andrew if he wanted a drink. Andrew turned away and stood facing the wall.

9.10 am Explained to Andrew that I had checked with the taxi company and that his taxi was on its way and would arrive in 10 minutes. Andrew shouted 'Thank you' in a very loud voice. His muscles looked tense, he was beginning to sweat and his breathing became rapid.

9.15 am I noted Andrew using prolonged eye contact with the support worker Mark who was sitting in the hallway waiting with him. I started talking to Andrew about his weekend away which he had told me about the day before. He said he enjoyed it and would like to go away again.

9.20 am Andrew's taxi arrives. He says good morning to the taxi driver and waves goodbye to me on his way out.

▲ **Figure 12.3** Example observation report

1.5 Understand the impact of the environment on behaviour

The social and physical environment can provoke unwanted behaviours that have an impact on individuals. Read through the two PowerPoint slides in Figure 12.4 developed by Max, the manager of an alcohol and drugs drop-in centre, as part of his training for a team of new volunteers. Note both the negative and positive ways that the environment can have an impact on individuals' behaviour.

The impact of the social environment

Issue	Possible solution(s)
Unfamiliar or new people (e.g. contractors or new staff)	
Contractors, new staff and visitors may make individuals feel anxious or withdraw from situations.	Recognising when this may happen and informing individuals about new people beforehand can help to reduce fears and/or irrational beliefs about their identity.
Dignity and respect	
Not finding out how to address an individual and not respecting their privacy can lead to them feeling frustrated and withdrawing from day-to-day activities.	Talking to the individual and finding out their preferences can help to reduce their frustration.
Activities and events	
Lack of meaningful activities or events can lead to individuals feeling bored and lacking self-worth.	Reduce boredom and increase stimulation by finding out what activities they would like to do and planning and developing these activities.
Routines	
Imposing routines and restricting individuals' autonomy can make them feel angry, frustrated and depressed.	Enabling them to make their own choices can increase self-worth and reduce their anger and depression.

The impact of the physical environment

Issue	Possible solution(s)
Noise	
Overcrowded and busy environments may make some individuals agitated or fearful.	Ensure the environment is calm, personal space and privacy are available and individuals can have time alone.
Temperature	
Environments that are too hot or too cold can make everyone uncomfortable.	Rooms and areas where the temperatures can be controlled are more likely to promote positive communications and behaviours.
Signage	
Inappropriate or unclear signage may lead to individuals feeling confused, disorientated and lost.	Clear signs and information will help individuals to feel reassured in their surroundings.
Lighting	
Poor or bright lighting can lead to individuals feeling tense or confused.	Ensuring lighting is adjusted and appropriate to each situation and individual can have a positive impact on individuals' moods and their interactions with others.

▶ **Figure 12.4** Understanding unwanted behaviours training

1.6 Understand the physiological aspects of behaviour

Physical factors as well as the environment can also have an impact on individuals' behaviours. Remember that these can be present for short or long periods and can be regular or infrequent. The effects of these physical factors on behaviour will be different and unique to each individual.

Table 12.1 provides you with more information about how physical factors can also be reasons for unwanted behaviour. Can you think of any other examples?

Table 12.1 Reasons for unwanted behaviour

Physical factor	Reasons why the factor can impact on behaviour
Pain	Not being able to understand the reasons for being in pain or the distress caused by being in pain may lead to individuals expressing this through unwanted behaviours.
Illness	A physical illness can affect an individual's emotional wellbeing and can impact on how an individual interacts with others; for example, an individual with a high temperature may behave differently to when they are well.

Physical factor	Reasons why the factor can impact on behaviour
Substance use	The repeated use of substances such as alcohol and drugs can lead to some individuals becoming addicted and showing unwanted behaviours due to these substances affecting their moods and highlighting feelings of anger, anxiety and unhappiness.
Epilepsy	Abnormal electrical activity in the brain caused by epilepsy can lead to the brain being damaged, which can in turn lead to unusual or unwanted behaviours such as physical aggression.
Diabetes	High levels of glucose in the blood caused by diabetes can lead to unusual or unwanted behaviours such as personality changes and unresponsiveness.
Dehydration	Dehydration can cause unwanted behaviours such as confusion, irrational thoughts and unresponsiveness.
Medication side-effects	Different medications can cause individuals to develop unwanted behaviours, i.e. **anti-psychotic medication** can lead to mood swings, irritability and aggression.

🔑 KEY TERMS

Anti-psychotic medication – a type of medication that is used to treat some mental health conditions.

1.7 Behavioural support plans

Support plans (or 'behavioural support plans') can be helpful for not only understanding and reducing unwanted behaviours, but also for enabling individuals to find alternatives to using such behaviours to express their needs. Everyone involved in an individual's care and support should be included when developing a behavioural support plan; wherever possible the individual and the individual's family, friends and any other people such as advocates who know the individual well must be involved. Behavioural support plans can also be produced in a format that meets the individual's needs and is easy to follow and understand.

Behaviour support plans provide those who work with individuals, such as carers, with clear information about:

- what should be done in response to unwanted behaviours
- how they should react in response to unwanted behaviours
- how to plan for safe, rapid and effective control of risky behaviour
- how to minimise the risk of unwanted behaviours escalating by using reactive strategies
- how to prevent unwanted behaviours by using proactive strategies.

Figure 12.5 describes Agnes' behavioural support plan; Agnes is 19 years of age and has an eating disorder.

MY LIFE, MY PLAN

My challenges:
Seeing others eating foods in front of me that I don't like
Fish, macaroni cheese, eggs and bananas.

The early behaviours I may show:
Scratching my neck, picking at my mouth, holding my stomach, pointing at my stomach, looking
tearful, looking scared, staring at the people or persons eating the foods I don't like.

The behaviour I may show if you do not notice my early behaviours:
Refusing to eat, throwing my plate of food on the floor (if I am eating), shouting out 'No' loudly, screaming 'It hurts'

How you can help me avoid these unwanted behaviours:
- Knowing and finding out from me the four foods that I don't like to see others eat in front of me.
- Ask me how I am feeling
- Talk to me about my favourite foods.
- Remind me how I enjoy cooking and how I won first prize for making an apple crumble when I was at school.
- Ask me if I want to leave the room; do not assume that I always want to as it will depend on what activity I am doing and how I am feeling.

How you can help me manage unwanted behaviours I show
- For the early behaviours I may show, you can reassure me that I will not be eating foods that I don't like and you can also talk to me about the hobbies or activities I have planned for the next few days as this will distract me
- If this does not work and my behaviours escalate, you can help me by remaining calm and moving away from me. It will also help me if you don't clear up any food spills until I've calmed down. When I have done so, I would prefer to do this.
- Afterwards, ask me whether I want to go for a walk with you or whether I prefer to go on my own.

▲ **Figure 12.5** Agnes' behavioural support plan

1.8 Strategies included within behavioural support plans

An effective behavioural support plan must include a good balance between primary, secondary and tertiary strategies that reflect and meet an individual's needs; remember what works for one individual may not work for another and so find out for every individual what strategies help, those that do not and in what situations.

Primary preventative strategies

These are ways that individuals can help to manage more effectively for themselves situations or aspects of their life that they may find challenging, such as an individual identifying ways that are effective in reducing their levels of anxiety and distress when in a busy or noisy environment, e.g. using visualisation, taking deep breaths, listening to music.

Secondary preventative strategies

These are useful for managing the onset of unwanted behaviours such as aggression, anxiety and distress and can prevent these behaviours from escalating and getting worse. Strategies can include de-escalation techniques, e.g. appearing calm; being at the same eye level and using respectful language when an individual is angry; diversion or distraction techniques, such as listening to the radio or talking about a favourite pastime when an individual is suffering pain; as well as disengagement activities such as mental and physical activities that promote wellbeing – talking with a friend or going for a run when an individual is depressed and likely to self-harm.

Tertiary strategies

These are useful for managing unwanted behaviours that have escalated and have as a result placed the individual and/or others in danger and/or at significant risk of harm. Reactive strategies may include the use of humour, engaging in a favourite activity or providing the individual with a private and safe place to have some quiet time on their own

Restrictive interventions are only used as the last resort and when there is significant risk of harm to the individual or others around them. These may include physically guiding an individual to move out of a busy public area or restricting an individual's movement so that they stop hurting themselves. It is also important that restrictive interventions are used for a minimum amount of time and alongside other strategies to help de-escalate and diffuse unwanted behaviours.

> **KNOW IT**
>
> 1 Name three settings where positive behaviour is promoted.
> 2 Define positive behavioural support.
> 3 Describe three person-centred approaches for promoting positive behaviour.
> 4 What are precursor behaviours?
> 5 Describe three ways that the environment can impact on behaviour.
> 6 What impact can pain and illness have on an individual's behaviour?
> 7 What is a behavioural support plan?
> 8 What is the difference between a primary and secondary preventative strategy?

● ●

L01 Assessment activities

Below are two suggested assessment activities that have been directly linked to the pass and merit criteria in LO1 to help with assignment preparation; they include Top Tips on how to achieve best results.

Choose one of the case scenarios below.

Scenario 1: Bella

Bella is 12 years of age, has been diagnosed with autism and was placed in foster care by the local authority following concerns that she was being abused at home by her mother's boyfriend. Her foster placement is at risk of breaking down because of her unwanted behaviours, which include swearing, kicking, destroying the furniture in her room and absconding in the middle of the night.

Scenario 2: Chris

Chris is 84 and is complaining of recurring stomach pains. His GP and hospital examinations have identified no medical problems. He lives in a residential care home and is now refusing food and is aggressive towards staff who encourage him to eat. He recently threw a bowl of hot soup over staff and is at risk of being asked to find alternative accommodation.

Activity 1 – pass criteria *P1 P2*

1 Using your chosen case scenario, demonstrate a person-centred approach to promote positive behaviour.

2 Using your chosen case scenario demonstrate best practice in promoting positive behaviour.

TOP TIPS
- ✔ Ensure you demonstrate a person-centred approach when promoting positive behaviour.
- ✔ Ensure you demonstrate best practice in the promotion of positive behaviour.
- ✔ Demonstrations can be achieved through the use of simulation and role play.

Activity 2 – merit criteria M1

Using your chosen case scenario, assess how best practice could be evaluated to determine its effectiveness in promoting positive behaviour.

TOP TIPS
- ✔ Ensure you provide an analysis, i.e. a detailed examination, of how best practice could be evaluated in promoting positive behaviour.
- ✔ Consider how to present your evidence, i.e. in an assignment, as a presentation to the rest of the group.
- ✔ Ensure you provide detailed evidence in relation to different ways of measuring the effectiveness of best practice in promoting positive behaviour, the strengths and weaknesses of different approaches.

LO2 Understand situations in which staff are required to use reactive and restrictive interventions *P3 M2*

GETTING STARTED

Reactions (5 minutes)

Can you think of an occasion when your behaviour got out of control? How did others react to your behaviour? How did you feel about their reaction?

2.1 Situations that require reactive and restrictive interventions

Reactive interventions are based on the information that is known about the individual and are in line with the individual's assessment and behaviour support plan. They involve identifying and responding to signs that unwanted behaviours may occur, with the aim of diffusing situations safely and quickly.

Restrictive interventions, by contrast, are used as the last resort or in an emergency situation; they can only be applied by trained professionals, in certain settings such as hospitals and when for example individuals are detained under the Mental Health Act.

Some more examples of situations where staff are required to use reactive and restrictive interventions are provided below.

Preventing someone from harming themselves

For example, an individual who has been diagnosed with Asperger's syndrome, lives at home with the support of carers and is one morning found repeatedly banging their head on the wall of their room.

Reactive interventions may include encouraging the individual to talk about how they are feeling or distracting them by talking about one of their favourite pastimes. As a last resort the individual's personal assistants may need to use physical restraint to prevent further self-harm. This may also include continuing to talk to the individual and explaining that restraint is going to be used, how and why.

Holding a person to receive a medical treatment in a planned situation

For example, an individual who has epilepsy and has an appointment at their local GP surgery to have a blood test to check the toxicity levels of the medications they are taking. They do not like needles and are anxious about hitting out at the person taking blood from them.

Reactive interventions could include the individual visiting their GP surgery before the appointment, the doctor explaining the treatment and why it is necessary, including talking through the consequences of not having the blood test done. The individual could also be encouraged to ask questions and share concerns. They could agree what they could do if they felt they were getting very tense and may hit out; this may include asking a personal assistant to accompany and sit next to them, and place their hand on the individual's arm, or guide them when leaving the room. As a last resort, restraint may have to be used.

Holding a person to receive a medical treatment in an emergency situation

For example, an individual who has dementia, has collapsed and requires life-saving heart surgery but becomes increasingly distressed at being treated by health professionals who are not known to them.

Reactive interventions could include explaining what is happening to the individual through visual and/or verbal cues. Staff could also refer to the individual's **advance care plan** (if there is one in place) and speak with the individual's family and/or those who know them well. As a last resort, if the individual continues to be distressed, medication could be used to encourage them to relax, thus reducing the risk of harm to the individual and others.

Self-defence

For example, a child who is deaf and blind becomes verbally aggressive while playing with other children in the play area and starts throwing furniture and toys at staff.

Reactive interventions could include talking calmly to the individual and supporting others in the play area to move to safety. As a last resort, if the unwanted behaviours continue, staff could remove items present in the individual's environment that could cause harm.

Escaping from violence

For example an individual who has abused alcohol and physically threatens a member of staff with a smashed bottle.

Reactive interventions could include speaking to the individual in a calm and non-confrontational manner and backing away from them. As a last resort, the individual may have to be physically restrained to prevent them causing any danger or harm to the staff member.

Protecting vulnerable people from violence

For example, an individual who lives in a shared flat, has learning disabilities and is being abused by their partner.

Reactive interventions may include reassuring the individual, listening to their feelings and fears as well as offering access to counselling services. As a last resort the individual may have to be moved from their flat into a safe and secure environment.

> **🔑 KEY TERM**
>
> **Advance care plan** – a plan to discuss and record in advance an individual's choices, decisions and wishes with respect to their care and treatment in case they are unable to express their preferences at a later stage.

2.2 Recognising stages of behaviour

Behaviour escalates in a number of stages or phases; knowing what these are and being able to recognise them can help staff to diffuse and/or de-escalate behaviours early on through the promotion of positive behaviour.

Table 12.2 provides you with more information about what each phase involves.

Table 12.2 The traffic light phases of behaviour

Phase	What it is	Actions required
The green 'proactive' phase	The individual is feeling calm and relaxed and is able to engage positively with you	Support the individual with maintaining these positive feelings Find out and reflect on the factors that are contributing to the individual feeling calm and relaxed
The amber 'active' phase	The individual's feelings change and they may start to feel anxious, agitated or distressed The individual may express this through unwanted behaviours	Support the individual to talk about how they felt when they were calm and relaxed Encourage them to use self-management techniques such as visualising being calm and relaxed, focusing on taking slow and deep breaths If this does not work then secondary strategies such as playing soft music and/or going for a walk may help
The red 'reactive' phase	The individual displays unwanted behaviour	Action needs to be taken quickly and in line with the individual's assessment and behaviour support plan to achieve safe and rapid control over the situation to prevent unnecessary distress and injury to the individual and others Tertiary strategies must be applied in the least restrictive way and in line with the principles of the Mental Capacity Act and the work setting's agreed ways of working
The blue 'post reactive' phase	Where the unwanted behaviour has stopped and the incident has come to an end The individual may express this by stating that they feel tired and by becoming calm and relaxed again as they were in the green proactive phase	Continue to monitor the individual, providing reassurance and remaining calm as not doing so may lead to their behaviour escalating again

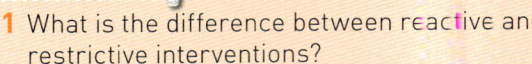

(20 minutes)

In small groups, discuss why it is important to recognise behaviours as early as possible. A group gets a point for every important reason they discuss. Then join together as a whole group to discuss the value of recognising behaviours.

KNOW IT

1 What is the difference between reactive and restrictive interventions?
2 Why is it important to recognise the different stages of challenging behaviours?
3 What does the green 'proactive' phase mean?

LO2 Assessment activities

Below are two suggested assessment activities that have been directly linked to the pass and merit criteria in LO2 to help with assignment preparation; they include Top Tips on how to achieve best results.

Activity 1 – pass criteria *P3*

Describe a situation where staff may be required to use a reactive or restrictive intervention. You can use one of the situations described in LO2.1 or you can use one of your own examples.

TOP TIPS ✔

✔ Ensure you detail information about one situation.
✔ Include details about the individual, the setting and the staff involved.
✔ Include detailed information with a clear rationale of the reasons why staff may be required to use a reactive or restrictive intervention.

Activity 2 – merit criteria *M2*

Using the situation you described in Activity 1, assess how recognising the different stages of behaviour could promote positive behaviour.

TOP TIPS ✔

✔ Ensure you provide an analysis, i.e. a detailed examination, of the importance of recognising the different stages of behaviour.
✔ Consider how best to present your evidence, e.g. in an assignment or as a presentation to the rest of the group.
✔ Ensure you provide detailed evidence in relation to the different stages of behaviour, how to recognise these and the strengths and weaknesses of doing so in terms of promoting positive behaviour.

LO3 Understand interventions used to promote positive behaviour and the impact on the individual *P4 M3 D1*

GETTING STARTED

The effects of positive behaviour (5 minutes)

Discuss how promoting positive behaviour makes you feel. Think about the effects that promoting positive behaviour has on others.

Behavioural outbursts, as you have found out, can be distressing and harmful to individuals and others, and can also be a source of stress for staff. Knowing more about the range of interventions that can be used to promote positive behaviour can improve the quality of individuals' lives and create safe and predictable environments for everyone.

3.1 Proactive interventions

Proactive interventions are used:

- to understand why unwanted behaviours may occur
- to understand the meaning of unwanted behaviours for the individual
- to prevent or reduce the likelihood of unwanted behaviours.

They involve the following.

Effective communication

Being aware of what you say and how you say it, including your body language and the words, pictures, signs and/or terminology you use, as this will effect how the communication is received and whether it is understood by the individual. Being aware of what an individual may be expressing through specific behaviours, vocal sounds or gestures is also important so that you can recognise early on how they are feeling and at what stage their behaviour is at. If you show compassion, empathy and understanding, the individual will feel valued that you are taking a genuine interest in who they are and be empowered to gain a better insight into their own behaviours.

Maintenance of good interpersonal relationships

Using person-centred approaches to work with the individual and others involved in their lives will enable you to find out more about the individual, their needs, preferences and wishes as well as build and maintain positive interactions and relationships (see Unit 1, page 14). Maintaining good interpersonal relationships will impact positively on an individual and can increase their self-esteem and promote their mental health and wellbeing.

Following any plan made to monitor and control behaviour

Discussing, agreeing and documenting a plan of support for the individual can help with monitoring and controlling behaviours that may be specific to the individual and/or that may be repeated. Observations of an individual carrying out their day-to-day activities and a behavioural intervention or support plan can help to promote positive behaviour by ensuring that staff who work with individuals understand their behaviours, both repeated and new behaviours, including:

- when they are occurring, times and locations
- with whom they are occurring
- how often
- how intense
- how long they last
- what needs to be put in place to both prevent these behaviours and manage them safely.

A decrease in the occurrence of unwanted behaviours will enable the individual to focus instead on their aspirations and have a positive outlook. In addition, others involved in their life, such as family and friends, may be more likely to engage with them and build positive relationships.

Recognising early triggers and being able to respond

Triggers are factors that can cause an individual's unwanted behaviours. These will vary for each individual but may be as a result of their environment, intervention, a condition or illness. Once these triggers have been recognised and documented, measures can be taken to avoid these. This will reduce or prevent unwanted behaviours and therefore minimise potential distress and harm.

There are many different methods of recording information about an individual's behaviour. A commonly used tool is known as the 'Antecedent, Behaviour and Consequence recording chart' (ABC chart). An example of the information that can be included on one is provided in Figure 12.6.

Name of individual:

Date, day, location and time of incident:

Specific behaviour targeted:

Details of antecedent events (what happened before the behaviour occurred?):
- What activity was the individual doing?
- What was happening in the environment?
- Who was present and what were they doing?
- Where were you and what were you doing?
- Had the individual requested something?
- Was something requested of the individual?
- Was there an unforeseen change to the individual's activities or environment?
- What was the individual expressing through their verbal behaviour?
- What was the individual expressing through their non-verbal behaviour?

Details of behaviour observed:
What did the individual do?

Details of consequent events (what happened after the behaviour occurred?):
- What happened after the behaviour occurred?
- What did you do in response to the behaviour?
- What were the individual's reactions to your response?
- Did anyone else present respond to the individual's behaviour?
- If yes, what did this person/people do and how did the individual react?
- Did anything change for the individual as a result of the behaviour?

Name of observer:

Signature:

▲ **Figure 12.6** An example of an ABC record chart

Prevention and early de-escalation

Proactive strategies that help to reduce behaviours can help staff to manage these and therefore directly improve the individual's quality of life. Effective communication where staff avoid confrontation and approach the individual in a calm and respectful way is the basis of all de-escalation strategies. It is also important to provide clear explanations and information when talking with the individual. Spending time with the individual, listening attentively and being non-judgemental are other important skills to have.

3.2 Reactive interventions

As you will have read in earlier sections in this unit, reactive interventions are those that are used by staff to promote positive behaviour once unforeseen challenging behaviours occur. Their purpose is to prevent the unwanted behaviours from getting worse by acting quickly. In this way the risk of any danger or harm to the individual and others in the environment will be minimised.

Reactive interventions are most effective when used:

- alongside proactive interventions
- after gathering information about the reasons for the unwanted behaviours, how and when these have occurred, e.g. through getting to know the individual, carrying out observations and completing ABC charts
- in line with the individual's behavioural support plan.

Reactive strategies are most effective when trained staff use a number of techniques that can include the following.

- Appearing calm: such as through neutral facial expressions, moving slowly, adopting a relaxed posture such as hands and arms in a relaxed, down position, speaking slowly and using a quiet tone of voice. This can have a positive impact on an individual by helping to reduce their distress or anger and making them feel happier and calmer.
- Being aware of the meaning behind the individual's body language can help staff recognise what phase of their behaviour the individual is in and what techniques to use to bring them back to the green 'proactive' phase. Staff must also be aware of their own body language and how this may be perceived by the individual; doing so may help de-escalate unwanted behaviours.
- Using distraction and redirection can be an effective technique to re-focus an individual's attention on a positive interaction, such as by talking about a topic that you know they are interested in or encouraging them to engage in an activity to promote relaxation and enjoyment. Depending on the individual, this could be a physical activity that requires high energy levels, such as going for a jog, or an activity such as listening to music that requires little energy.
- Moving away to give space: with some individuals who are displaying unwanted behaviours, it may be more effective for staff to move away or even the leave the area/room so that the individual can have some time on their own to calm down and reflect. Not doing so may make them feel more tense or they may feel that you are going to cause them pain or distress; their behaviours may escalate instead of de-escalate. For other individuals who are displaying unwanted behaviours it may be more effective for

staff to stay with them, providing reassurance and distracting them by talking to them. Moving away from the individual may cause them to feel rejected or that they are being ignored; this may in turn cause their behaviours to escalate rather than de-escalate.

INDEPENDENT RESEARCH ACTIVITY

Edward T Hall (60 minutes)

Conduct some independent research either on your own or in small groups and find out about Edward T Hall's theory of proxemics.

You may find the following link useful:

http://www.communicationstudies.com/communication-theories/proxemics

3.3 Restrictive interventions

All services that may have restrictive intervention plans for individuals must also have in place other proactive ways of reducing unwanted behaviours, because restrictive interventions must only be used as a last resort and by staff who have been trained to use them effectively. Restrictive interventions can take a variety of forms and can include the following.

- Physical restraint: 'any direct physical contact where the intervener's intention is to prevent, restrict, or subdue movement of the body, or part of the body of another person'.
- Mechanical restraint: 'the use of a device to prevent, restrict or subdue movement of a person's body, or part of the body, for the primary purpose of behavioural control'.
- Chemical restraint: 'the use of medication which is prescribed, and administered for the purpose of controlling or subduing disturbed/violent behaviour, where it is not prescribed for the treatment of a formally identified physical or mental illness'.
- Seclusion: 'the supervised confinement and isolation of a person, away from other users of services, in an area from which the person is prevented from leaving'.
- Long-term segregation: 'a situation where a person is prevented from mixing freely with other people who use a service'.

(Source: DOH, Positive and Proactive Care: Reducing the Need for Restrictive Interventions, April 2014)

The eight key principles that services using restrictive interventions must adhere to are outlined in Figure 12.7.

Physical restraint

This is an intervention that is used by staff as the last resort. As it is a time-limited intervention, staff must continue to use other techniques such as talking or distraction to calm the individual in an attempt to de-escalate the situation. Upholding an individual's dignity must also be taken into account when they are being physically restrained, such as by ensuring that their body is not exposed or by making the area surrounding them more private by asking others who may be present to leave or by screening off the area.

To ensure an individual's safety, **break away techniques** used by staff must *not* involve:

- preventing an individual from breathing
- covering an individual's mouth and/or nose
- applying pressure to an individual's neck, ribs or abdomen
- placing an individual in a face down position.

Maintaining an individual's safety and welfare throughout and after physical restraint is crucial and can be achieved by staff by closely observing them, e.g. by monitoring their breathing, pulse and appearance as well as their mental wellbeing so that any signs of physical deterioration or mental distress can be identified and help sought. If any of these signs are recognised during an intervention, the physical restraint must stop immediately so that the individual's health and wellbeing are not compromised.

> 🔑 **KEY TERM**
>
> **Break away techniques** – techniques that do not involve aggression or force, and aim to promote safety and mutual respect.

Mechanical restraint

This is an intervention that is used in exceptional circumstances by staff who work in high security units to manage extremely violent behaviours. For example, staff could support an individual who self-

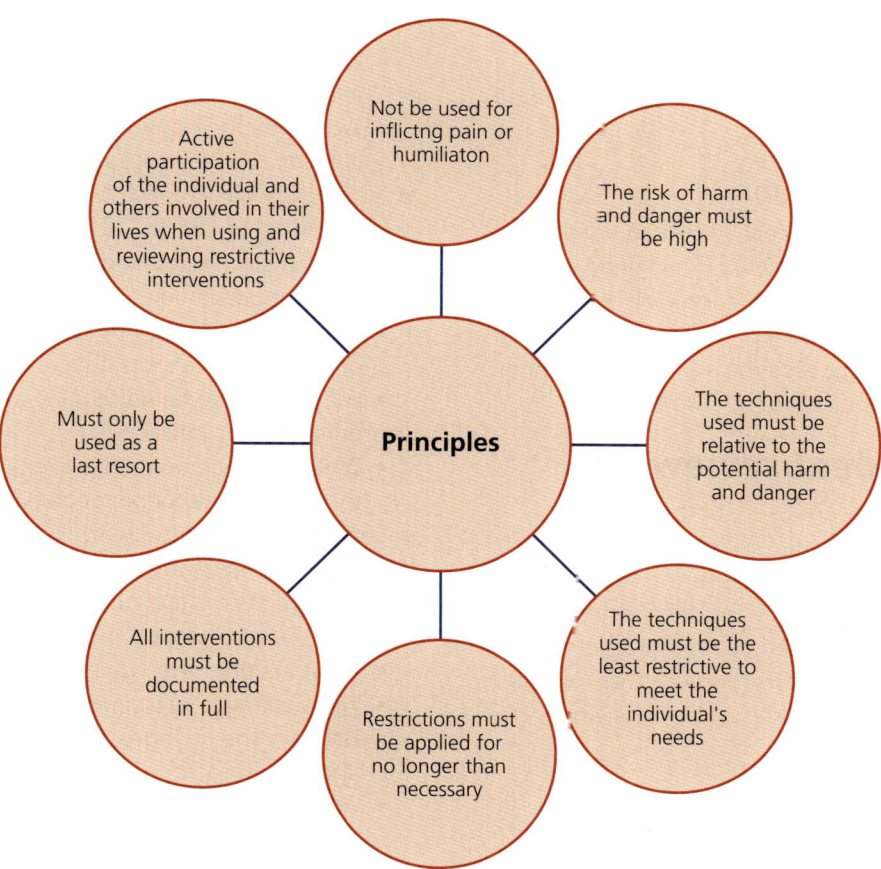

▲ **Figure 12.7** Restrictive interventions – key principles

Principles:
- Not be used for inflicting pain or humiliation
- The risk of harm and danger must be high
- The techniques used must be relative to the potential harm and danger
- The techniques used must be the least restrictive to meet the individual's needs
- Restrictions must be applied for no longer than necessary
- All interventions must be documented in full
- Must only be used as a last resort
- Active participation of the individual and others involved in their lives when using and reviewing restrictive interventions

harms by banging his head on the wall through using a mechanical restraint such as a cushioned helmet to prevent them from sustaining any serious injuries; this would be included as a planned mechanical restraint as part of the individual's behavioural support plan.

Chemical restraint

This is also an intervention that is used in exceptional circumstances by staff who are working with individuals displaying extremely aggressive or violent behaviours and may involve administering oral medication or an intramuscular injection. Chemical restraint must only be used when other interventions tried have not worked; again staff must be trained and carry out close observations of the individual's physical and mental wellbeing.

Seclusion

This is used as an intervention only when an individual has been detained under the Mental Health Act (see LO4, page 211). If staff use this intervention when an individual is not detained under the Mental Health Act (e.g. in an unforeseen emergency situation where the individual's behaviours become increasingly violent and are a danger to themselves or others) then it should be time limited and the individual must be assessed immediately for detention under the Mental Health Act.

Long-term segregation

This is an intervention used only by staff in hospital settings and only when an individual has been detained under the Mental Health Act. This intervention involves staff preventing individuals from interacting freely with others who may live or access the service, due to the risk of serious danger or harm to others.

3.4 Post-incident reviews

When any interventions are used, both staff and individuals should be provided with the opportunity to reflect on the incident, including sharing their feelings and discussing the effectiveness of the intervention used, whether it could be used again and whether it will be effective in different environments, as well as its impact on both the individual and others who were present.

Post-incident reviews or debriefs are also an opportunity for new learning, considering a change to practices and the development of strategies for individualised care if and when restrictive interventions are used again; this will also involve a review of the individual's behaviour support plan.

Christopher Johns' Model of Structured Reflection (2006) is a framework for reflective practice and continuous learning that is often used as the basis of post-incident reviews. It enables staff, individuals and others to do the following.

- DISCUSS THE INCIDENT
  - What happened?
  - When did it happen?
  - Why did it happen?
  - What factors contributed?
- REFLECT ON THE INCIDENT
  - How did I respond and why?
  - How did others respond and why?
  - Did I respond effectively?
  - What factors influenced how I responded?
  - Did others respond effectively?
  - What factors influenced how others responded?
  - How did I feel about the incident when it was happening and why?
  - What factors influenced how I was feeling?
  - How did others feel about the incident when it was happening and why?
  - What factors influenced how others were feeling?
  - What was the impact of my response on the individual, others present and myself?
  - What was the impact of others' response on the individual, others present and myself?
- AGREE ON WHAT COULD HAVE BEEN DONE DIFFERENTLY OR BETTER
  - How might I respond differently or better if the incident occurred again?
  - What would be the impact of responding differently or better on the individual, others and myself?
  - What needs to be done to be able to respond differently or better?
  - What could be done to prevent or reduce the risk of the incident happening again?
- DEVELOP LEARNING AND INSIGHT
  - How do I feel about the incident now and why?
  - How do others feel about the incident now and why?
  - What have I learned?
  - What insight have I gained?
  - What changes are going to be made and how?
  - How are the changes going to be communicated and monitored?
  - When and how are the changes going to be evaluated?

Reviewing incidents (20 minutes)

Think about an incident that you have read about or heard about that involves a vulnerable adult, child or young person. In small groups discuss why it is important to review incidents such as this after they have occurred. Ensure you provide as many reasons as you can for why it is important to do so for:

- individuals
- staff
- others who may have witnessed the incident.

Join together as a whole group to discuss and share your findings.

? THINK ABOUT IT

Case study: Janice

Janice is 45 years of age, has learning disabilities and lives in a residential care home. She has recently been admitted to hospital for a hernia operation. Janice has never stayed in hospital and is finding it difficult to settle in to her new and very different environment. Janice is visited every day in hospital by the staff who work in the residential care setting where she lives and her sister usually visits her on a Sunday.

The hospital staff have raised concerns over Janice displaying a number of behaviours including: refusing to eat, pulling out the catheter she wears during the night, taking off her clothes while talking with other patients and verbally abusing the other patients on the ward. Imagine you are Janice's sister and think about the following.

1 What impact is Janice's stay in hospital having on her?
2 What types of proactive interventions could be used with Janice to promote positive behaviours?
3 How can Janice be better supported when these behaviours occur?
4 How could the effectiveness of the interventions applied be assessed?

KNOW IT

1 What is the meaning of a proactive intervention?
2 How are both verbal and non-verbal communication used during reactive interventions?
3 What does the term 'physical restraint' mean?
4 What is the purpose of post-incident reviews?

LO3 Assessment activities

Below are suggested assessment activities that have been directly linked to the pass, merit and distinction criteria in LO3 to help with assignment preparation; they include Top Tips on how to achieve best results.

Activity 1 – pass criteria P4

Using one of the situations described in LO2.1, or using your own example, demonstrate strategies that could be used to promote positive behaviour.

TOP TIPS

✔ Ensure you demonstrate different strategies
✔ Ensure the strategies you demonstrate could be used to promote positive behaviour
✔ Demonstrations can be achieved through the use of simulation and role play

Activity 2 – merit criteria M3

Research the use of restrictive interventions. You will find the information available on Skills for Care's website useful, for example via http://tinyurl.com/zm6pud3

Evaluate why restrictive interventions are used in only the most serious situations.

TOP TIPS

✔ Ensure you provide an evaluation, i.e. a detailed examination, of the reasons why restrictive interventions are used in only the most serious situations.
✔ Consider how best to present your evidence, i.e. in an assignment or as a presentation to the rest of the group.
✔ Ensure you provide detailed evidence in relation to: what are restrictive interventions, how they are used, why they are used in only the most serious situations, their strengths and weaknesses.

Activity 3 – distinction criteria *D1*

Using the situation you described in Activity 1, imagine you are the individual's advocate and are supporting the individual at their care review to share their experience of the strategies used to promote positive behaviour.

Develop a presentation that evaluates the impact of strategies used to promote positive behaviour on the individual's wellbeing.

TOP TIPS

✔ Ensure you provide an evaluation, i.e. a detailed examination, of the impact of different strategies on an individual's physical and emotional wellbeing.
✔ Ensure your presentation reflects how you have involved the individual.
✔ Ensure you provide detailed evidence in relation to: the strengths and weaknesses of the strategies used in terms of their impact on the individual's physical and emotional wellbeing.

LO4 Know relevant legislation and guidance related to promoting positive behaviour *P5*

GETTING STARTED

Laws and guidance (5 minutes)

Discuss what laws are, how they are made in the UK and how they differ from guidance.

4.1 Legislation

Legislation is in place to ensure that positive behaviour is promoted with all adults, young people and children, by all those who live in, work in and visit health, social care and child care settings. Table 12.3 provides you with additional information about the key pieces of legislation that there are.

Table 12.3 Key legislation for promoting positive behaviour

Legislation	How it promotes positive behaviour in health, social care and child care settings
Mental Health Act 1983 (as amended by the Mental Health Act 2007)	A law that governs the admission, detention and treatment of individuals who have a mental illness, in hospital. It promotes positive behaviour by: • requiring that professionals seek individuals' consent to be assessed and treated in hospital • promoting individuals' and others' safety and wellbeing • promoting and protecting individuals and others from danger and harm • promoting the use of the least intrusive and restrictive interventions first • promoting person-centred values, i.e. dignity, respect, diversity • promoting the full involvement of individuals in all aspects of their care, support, treatment and recovery.
Mental Capacity Act 2005	A law that governs how individuals who lack capacity can be supported to make decisions for themselves and have decisions made in their best interests. It promotes positive behaviour by: • requiring that professionals do not assume an individual lacks capacity unless it has been established that this is the case • requiring that individuals are supported and enabled to make decisions • requiring that professionals only treat an individual as unable to make a decision when all possible options to enable the individual to do so have not been successful • requiring that professionals respect an individual's right to make mistakes and not treating individuals as unable to make decisions simply because the decision that has been made was not effective • requiring that decisions made by or on behalf of individuals are in their 'best interests' • promoting the use of the least intrusive and restrictive interventions first.

Legislation	How it promotes positive behaviour in health, social care and child care settings
Deprivation of Liberty Safeguards (under the Mental Capacity Act 2005) – DoLs	A law that governs how individuals who lack the mental capacity to consent to their treatment or care can be safeguarded. It promotes positive behaviour by: • preventing unreasonable decisions being made that restrict an individual's freedom • promoting an individual's right to have a representative • promoting an individual's right to challenge a decision that restricts their freedom • promoting an individual's right for deprivation of liberty to be reviewed and monitored regularly.
Section 3, Criminal Law Act 1967, Common Law	Section 3 of this law governs the common law rules on self-defence and requires that any force used must be reasonable. It promotes positive behaviour by: • ensuring that professionals that are required to use any kind of force only use force that is reasonable and necessary • requires professionals to only use physical force to remove the immediate threat of harm or danger away from themselves or others • requires professionals to stop using physical force when the immediate threat of harm or danger to themselves or others has been removed.
Health and Safety at Work Act 1974	A law that governs the key duties and responsibilities of all employers and employees in work settings including health, social care and child care settings. It promotes positive behaviour by: • promoting the health, safety and welfare of all individuals, employees, visitors and members of the general public • requiring employers to assess, manage, monitor and review health and safety risks that may exist • requiring employees to take responsibility for their own and others' health, safety and welfare at all times • requiring individuals to comply with the procedures in place across different settings for promoting their own and others' health, safety and welfare.
Human Rights Act 1998	A law that governs and protects individuals and others' human rights. It promotes positive behaviour by: • promoting individuals' rights including the right to life, prohibition of torture, inhumane or degrading treatment, the right to liberty and security, respect for private and family life, freedom of expression and prohibition of discrimination.
Equality Act 2010	A law that governs and protects individuals and others in society from direct discrimination, indirect discrimination, harassment and victimisation. It promotes positive behaviour by: • requiring that services including health, social care and child care services provide equality of access in relation to health care, support and treatment • requiring that health care services that are provided are free from direct discrimination, indirect discrimination, harassment and victimisation • requiring that reasonable adjustments are made by services when necessary so as to enable them to meet individuals' needs.
Police and Criminal Evidence Act 1984 (PACE)	A law that governs the powers of the police to protect the rights and freedoms of the public. It is accompanied by the PACE Codes of Conduct and includes police activities such as: stop and search, arrest, detention, investigation, identification and interviewing. It promotes positive behaviour by: • promoting individuals' rights during detention, treatment and questioning by police officers • requiring police officers to explain an individual's rights to them whilst being detained.

4.2 Guidance

'Investigations into abuses at Winterbourne View Hospital and Mind's Mental Health Crisis in Care: Physical Restraint in Crisis (2013) showed that restrictive interventions have not always been used only as a last resort in health and care. They have even been used to inflict pain, humiliate or punish. Restrictive interventions are often a major contribution to delaying recovery, and have been linked with causing serious trauma, both physical and psychological, to people who use services and staff. These interventions have been used too much, for too long and we must change this.'

(Source: DOH, Positive and Proactive Care: Reducing the Need for Restrictive Interventions, April 2014)

In April 2014, the Department of Health together with the Royal College of Nursing, Skills for Care and Skills for Health produced two key pieces of guidance: Positive and Proactive Care: Reducing the Need for Restrictive Interventions as well as A Positive and Proactive Workforce. Both pieces of guidance support the development of approaches and practices of delivering care and support that meet individuals' needs and enhance their quality of life so as to promote recovery and reduce the need for restrictive interventions.

Positive and Proactive Care: Reducing the Need for Restrictive Interventions (2014)

This aims to:

- encourage a culture across health and social care services that is committed to developing therapeutic environments to promote individuals' physical and emotional wellbeing
- encourage a culture across health and social care services where physical or restrictive interventions are only used as a last resort
- provide guidance on effective leadership and management of person-centred led approaches and interventions
- promote best practice principles (you read about these in LO3.3) across a range of health and social care settings so that these are used and applied consistently
- ensure that when restrictive interventions are used that this is done in a transparent, legal and ethical manner.

A Positive and Proactive Workforce (2014) A guide to workforce development for commissioners and employers seeking to minimise the use of restrictive practices in social care and health

This piece of guidance shares with Positive and Proactive Care six key principles that are required to deliver positive and proactive care.

- **Principle 1:** Compliance at all times with the relevant rights in the European Convention on Human Rights.
- **Principle 2:** Understanding people's behaviour by recognising individuals' unique needs, preferences, aspirations, experiences and strengths and enhancing their quality of life.
- **Principle 3:** Involvement and participation of individuals who have care and support needs, their families, carers and advocates in line with the person's wishes and confidentiality arrangements.
- **Principle 4:** Treatment of individuals who have care and support needs must reflect compassion, dignity and kindness.
- **Principal 5:** Services supporting individuals to balance safety from harm with freedom of choice.
- **Principal 6:** Positive relationships between professionals and the individuals they support must be protected and preserved.

GROUP ACTIVITY

Promoting positive behaviour legislation (60 minutes)

Work in small groups to discuss the reasons why three pieces of legislation and two pieces of guidance are relevant to promoting positive behaviour. Think about the impact they may have on individuals' lives. Record and present your findings to the rest of the groups.

KNOW IT

1 Identify three pieces of legislation that are related to promoting positive behaviour when working with individuals who display behaviours that challenge.
2 What does the Mental Capacity Act 2005 say in relation to promoting positive behaviour and who is it aimed at?
3 Name the six key principles shared between Positive and Proactive Care (2014) and A Positive and Proactive Workforce (2014).

LO4 Assessment activity *P5*

Below is a suggested assessment activity that has been directly linked to the pass criteria in LO4 to help with assignment preparation; it includes Top Tips on how to achieve best results.

Research the main pieces of legislation that are related to promoting positive behaviour.

Then produce an information fact sheet that describes each piece of legislation you've researched, including how it is related to promoting positive behaviour in individuals who display behaviours that are unwanted.

TOP TIPS
✔ Ensure you provide details about each piece of legislation.
✔ Include details about its purpose.
✔ Include detailed information about how it is related to promoting positive behaviour.

Read about it

Allen, D. (2011) *Reducing the Use of Restrictive Practices with People Who Have Intellectual Disabilities*, British Institute of Learning Disabilities.

DOH (2014) *Positive and Proactive Care: Reducing the Need for Restrictive Interventions*, TSO.

Emerson, E. and Einfeld, S.L. (2011) *Challenging Behaviour*, Cambridge University Press.

HM Government (2014) *Closing the Gap: Essential Priorities for Change in Mental Health*, TSO.

McGill, P. and MacDonald, A. (2013) Outcomes of staff training in positive behaviour support: a systematic review. *Journal of Developmental and Physical Disabilities*, 25(1): 17–33.

McGill, P., Bradshaw, J. and Hughes, A. (2006) Impact of extended education/training in positive behaviour support on staff knowledge, causal attributions and emotional responses. *Journal of Applied Research in Intellectual Disabilities*, 20(1): 41–51.

Mind (2012) *Mental Health Crisis Care: Physical Restraint in Crisis*, Mind.

NHS England and the Local Government Association (NHSE LGA) (2014) *Ensuring Quality Services* (EQS: Core principles for the commissioning of services for children, young people, adults and older adults with learning disabilities and/or autism who display or are at risk of displaying behaviour that challenges), TSO.

NHS England (NHSE) (2014) *Getting It Right for People with Learning Disabilities Going into Hospital Because of Mental Health Difficulties or Challenging Behaviours: What Families Need to Know*, TSO.

NHS Protect Guidance (2015) (updated version) *Meeting Needs and Reducing Distress: Guidance for the Prevention and Management of Clinically Related Challenging Behaviour in NHS Settings*, TSO.

Useful websites

Mencap: mencap.org.uk

Mind: mind.org.uk

The Challenging Behaviour Foundation: challengingbehaviour.org.uk

Rethink: www.rethink.org

Unit 13

Sexual health, reproduction and early development stages

ABOUT THIS UNIT

Health and wellbeing is of vital importance at all stages of life, even before a baby is conceived. This unit provides you with an overview of the factors influencing health and wellbeing through an understanding of reproduction and preconception, antenatal and postnatal care.

You will learn about sexual health and the types of contraception that are available. You will develop an understanding of the importance of prenatal health and the factors that could have an impact. The health and development of the foetus, stages of pregnancy and an overview of care and development of the baby in the first year of life are also explored.

LEARNING OUTCOMES

The topics, activities and suggested reading in this unit will help you to:

1 Understand sexual health and contraception
2 Understand the importance of prenatal health and the process of conception
3 Know the factors that could affect health in pregnancy and the success of the birth
4 Understand the stages of pregnancy and birth and the postnatal care of the mother
5 Understand the care and development of the baby in the first year of life

How will I be assessed?

You will be assessed through a series of assignments and tasks set and marked by your tutor.

How will I be graded?

You will be graded using the following criteria.

Learning outcome	Pass assessment criteria	Merit assessment criteria	Distinction assessment criteria
You will:	To achieve a **pass** you must demonstrate that you have met all the pass assessment criteria:	To achieve a **merit** you must demonstrate that you have met all the pass and merit assessment criteria:	To achieve a **distinction** you must demonstrate that you have met all the pass, merit and distinction assessment criteria:
1 Understand sexual health and contraception	**P1** Describe how sexually transmitted infections could affect the health and wellbeing of the individual	**M1** Analyse approaches that could be taken to promote sexual health	**D1** Evaluate the effectiveness of legislation in protecting the individual against unlawful and harmful intercourse
	P2 Summarise ways in which an individual may be protected against unlawful and harmful sexual intercourse		
	P3 Explain how a range of methods of contraception protect against pregnancy		
2 Understand the importance of prenatal health and the process of conception	**P4** Explain the process of conception	**M2** Assess ways in which individuals can ensure a healthy conception takes place	
3 Know the factors that could affect health in pregnancy and the success of the birth	**P5** Identify disabilities which occur *in utero*		
	P6 Describe factors that affect the health of the foetus		
4 Understand the stages of pregnancy and birth and the postnatal care of the mother	**P7** Describe the stages of gestation	**M3** Assess the importance of postnatal care of the mother	
	P8 Explain the birth process		
	P9 Identify support available to postnatal mothers		
5 Understand the care and development of the baby in the first year of life	**P10** Explain the expected pattern of development of the baby in its first year of life	**M4** Explain positive and negative factors influencing development in the first year of life	**D2** Analyse ways in which health and social care services could influence the care and development of the baby in its first year of life

L01 Understand sexual health and contraception *P1 P2 P3 M1 D1*

GETTING STARTED

What is 'consent'? (10 minutes)

In small groups, agree on a definition of what is meant by '**consent**' in a relationship. Each small group can then feed back to the whole group and decide on a whole group definition of 'consent'.

> 🔑 **KEY TERMS**
>
> **Consent** – permission for something to happen or agreement to do something.
>
> **Defendant** – someone accused of an offence.

1.1 Sexual consent

Sexual Offences Act 2003

Key aspects are that it:

- defines consent
- defines rape as the penetration by the penis of somebody's vagina, anus or mouth, without consent
- defines sexual assault as an intentional sexual touching without consent; it can include touching any part of the body, clothed or unclothed, by either a body part or an object
- classifies any sexual intercourse with a child aged 12 or younger as rape
- introduced 'risk of sexual harm' orders, specifically designed to protect children; these prohibit adults from engaging in inappropriate behaviour such as sexual conversations with children online
- created a number of offences:
  - Giving someone a substance without their consent and with the intention of overpowering them so that sexual activity can take place, e.g. drink spiking.
  - Befriending a child online and meeting or intending to meet them with the intention of abusing them (grooming).
  - 'Voyeurism' relating to those who observe others doing private acts without their knowledge, for sexual gratification.
  - 'Abuse of a position of trust towards a child'. This prohibits sexual contact between adults and children under 18 in schools, colleges and residential care.

The Act makes consent paramount when sexual acts occur between adults. It enshrines in law a clear definition of consent and the responsibility of **defendants** to show that they had reasonable grounds to believe that their sexual partner consented.

Statutory definition of consent

The Sexual Offences Act 2003, section 74, gives the statutory definition of consent. This is if a person:

> 'Agrees by choice and has the freedom and capacity to make that choice.'

For consent to be valid it must be voluntary and informed and the person consenting must have the capacity to make the decision. If, for example, the person is unconscious they do not have the 'capacity' to make a decision.

Legal age of consent

The age of consent (the age at which their consent to any form of sexual activity is legal) is 16 years. The age of consent is the same regardless of gender and whether the sexual activity is between people of the same or different gender.

Sex and relationship education (SRE) at school

Maintained secondary schools are required to deliver **SRE** for all pupils. There has to be sex education in science programmes of study at key stages 1 to 3. The requirements for academies, independent schools and free schools are slightly different, but most have an SRE programme. The topics covered include sexually transmitted infections, including **HIV/AIDS**. Maintained schools are also required to have a sex and relationships education policy.

> 🔑 **KEY TERMS**
>
> **SRE** – sex and relationship education.
>
> **HIV/AIDS** – a virus which attacks the immune system, and weakens the ability to fight infections and disease.

Current SRE education focuses on the importance of an individual taking responsibility for positively and actively gaining consent, promoting equality in relationships, and goes beyond simply teaching how to say 'no'. This reflects the Sexual Offences Act where the emphasis is on obtaining, rather than giving, consent.

1.2 Sexual health

The World Health Organization (WHO) defines sexual health as:

> 'a state of physical, mental and social wellbeing in relation to sexuality. It requires a positive and respectful approach to sexuality and sexual relationships, as well as the possibility of having pleasurable and safe sexual experiences, free of coercion, discrimination and violence'.

(WHO, 2006)

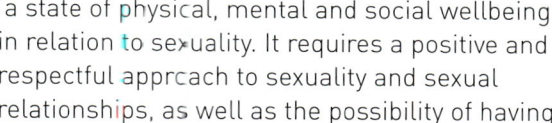

CLASSROOM DISCUSSION

Over to you … (20 minutes)

Discuss how the WHO definition encompasses the issues raised by the topics you have considered so far in LO1 of this unit.

Sexually transmitted infections (STIs)

Sexually transmitted infections (STIs) are infections or diseases that are passed on through unprotected sexual activity (sex without a condom). They spread through sexual contact. Left untreated STIs can cause

KEY TERMS

GUM clinic – a clinic specialising in genitourinary medicine.

HSV – herpes simplex virus.

Ectopic pregnancy – where the foetus develops outside the womb, usually in a fallopian tube.

Premature labour – when labour starts before the 37th week of pregnancy.

Septicaemia – a potentially life-threatening illness caused by an infection.

serious complications, such as infertility, and some may be fatal.

Nearly half a million people in the UK are diagnosed with an STI every year. STIs are easily spread because often there are no obvious symptoms to begin with. Younger adults are at greater risk as they are more likely to have unsafe sex with multiple sexual partners. Precautions such as wearing a condom and having regular tests can reduce the risk of STIs.

Examples of STIs are given in Table 13.1.

Table 13.1 Examples of sexually transmitted infections

STI	Symptoms and how health and wellbeing is affected	Diagnosis and treatment
Chlamydia	• Symptoms are not usually noticeable so most people do not know they are infected. • If symptoms occur, such as pain urinating and pain or bleeding during sex, it is usually 1–3 weeks after unprotected sex with an infected person. • Left untreated in women it can cause pelvic inflammatory disease (PID) which can lead to infertility. Men's testicles can become painful and swollen; if not treated fertility could be affected.	• A sample of cells is sent to a laboratory for analysis. Men usually provide a urine sample, while women provide a swab from their vagina or a urine sample. • Treated by antibiotics. • Sex should be avoided until the treatment is completed.
Bacterial vaginosis (BV)	• The balance of bacteria inside the vagina becomes disrupted. There is an unusual grey, watery vaginal discharge which may have a strong smell. • Scented or antiseptic bath liquids, vaginal deodorant and strong detergent may contribute to developing BV by upsetting the natural bacterial balance in the vagina. • It is not serious for most women except in pregnancy, when it may slightly increase the risk of premature birth or miscarriage.	• Any abnormal discharge should be checked by a GP or **GUM clinic**. A description of the discharge may be enough for diagnosis, or a test may be carried out on vaginal cells. • Treated by antibiotics, either tablets or a gel applied to the vagina for seven days. • Side effects of treatment include nausea and vomiting. Alcohol should be avoided.

STI	Symptoms and how health and wellbeing is affected	Diagnosis and treatment
Genital herpes	• Caused by the herpes simplex virus (HSV) which is highly contagious and spreads through skin-to-skin contact during sex. • Symptoms include blisters and sores around the genitals, vaginal discharge in women, pain when passing urine and general aches, pains and flu-like symptoms. • After the first infection the virus remains dormant in the body and can be reactivated, causing further outbreaks. • If herpes develops up to week 26 of pregnancy, there is an increased risk of miscarriage. After 26 weeks it could be passed on to the baby. A Caesarean section delivery prevents this.	• A sample of fluid is taken from a blister and tested for HSV. • For a first infection antiviral tablets are taken five times a day until there are no new sores or blisters. • The tablets can cause side effects such as sickness and headaches. • After more than six recurrent outbreaks in a year a long-term treatment plan involves taking antiviral tablets twice every day for 6–12 months.
Gonorrhoea	• A bacterial infection, easily passed through unprotected sex. • The infection can also be passed from a pregnant woman to her baby, and if untreated can cause blindness in a newborn baby. • Symptoms include a thick green or yellow discharge from the vagina or penis, pain when urinating and bleeding between periods. • Without treatment it can cause pelvic inflammatory disease (PID), which can lead to long-term pelvic pain, ectopic pregnancy and infertility. • It can cause miscarriage and premature labour. Men can experience a painful infection in the testicles and prostate gland which can lead to infertility. • In rare cases, if untreated, gonorrhoea can spread through the bloodstream to cause septicaemia, which is life-threatening.	• Tests involve a vaginal swab, or urine test for men. • Treatment involves an antibiotic injection in the buttocks or thigh, followed by an antibiotic tablet. • A further test is taken a week later to check if the infection has cleared.
Hepatitis	• Hepatitis B and C are infectious viruses, carried in the bloodstream and bodily fluids of an infected person. • They can be transmitted through unprotected sex. Mothers with hepatitis B can pass it to their babies during pregnancy or when giving birth. All pregnant women in the UK are offered a blood test to check if they are infected. • Symptoms are flu-like with loss of appetite, sickness and diarrhoea, jaundice and abdominal pain. It can be an acute infection that clears up in a few months or develop into a long-term chronic condition. A third of people with chronic hepatitis go on to develop liver disease, which can be very serious.	• If the infection is diagnosed in the early stages (acute hepatitis), blood tests will establish whether the body has produced antibodies to fight the virus. This may be repeated over many months as it takes time for antibodies to be produced. • A liver function test may also be carried out to check for damage. • The chronic disease can be treated with a combination of medicines that stop the virus multiplying to prevent cirrhosis and end-stage liver disease.
Pubic lice	• Tiny parasitic insects that live on coarse human body hair such as pubic hair. They are most commonly spread through sexual contact. • Symptoms include intense itching, inflammation and irritation caused by scratching. Black powder can be seen in underwear. Blue spots on the skin show where the lice are living (caused by lice bites) and small spots of blood also caused by lice bites.	• Can be treated at home with insecticide cream, lotion or shampoo. It will usually be applied once and then repeated after 3–7 days to kill any lice that have hatched since the first treatment. • Everyone the person has had close body contact with will need to be treated at the same time. Clothing, bedding and towels will require washing at 50°C or higher.

STI	Symptoms and how health and wellbeing is affected	Diagnosis and treatment

Syphilis	• A bacterial infection usually caught by having sex with an infected person. Pregnant women can pass the condition on to their unborn baby.
	• If untreated, syphilis can cause serious health problems for the mother and her baby, miscarriage or **stillbirth**. All pregnant women are offered a blood test to check for the infection. There are three stages of symptoms, as follows.
	  1 Primary – a painless, infectious sore on the genitals. This will disappear within 2–6 weeks. If it is not treated syphilis will move into the secondary stage.
	  2 Secondary – skin rash often on palms of hands and soles of feet, and sore throat, fever and swollen lymph glands. These symptoms may disappear in few weeks or come and go over a period of months.
	  3 Tertiary – years after the initial infection it may affect the brain, nerves, heart and eyes, causing strokes, dementia, paralysis, heart disease, blindness and deafness.
		• At a GUM clinic there will be a physical examination of the genitals. A blood test is taken and if sores are present a sample of the fluid will be taken.
		• Treatment of primary syphilis is a single dose of penicillin injected into the buttock.
		• Later stages require three injections at weekly intervals. Treatment of tertiary syphilis requires a longer course of antibiotics and may need intravenous treatment.
		• The earlier syphilis is diagnosed and treated the less chance of serious, potentially fatal, complications.

HIV/AIDS	• Most people infected with HIV experience a short, flu-like illness 2–6 weeks after infection, then will often not experience any symptoms for up to 10 years. However, the virus is active and causes progressive damage to the immune system. • Once the immune system becomes severely damaged, symptoms can include weight loss, chronic diarrhoea, night sweats, skin problems, recurrent infections and serious life-threatening illnesses. Earlier diagnosis and treatment of HIV can prevent these problems.	• The most common form of HIV test is a blood test. • If it is positive regular blood tests will monitor the progress of the HIV infection before starting treatment. If the number of cells important for fighting infection falls, whether or not there are any symptoms, treatment will start. • The treatment aims to reduce the level of HIV in the blood, allow the immune system to repair itself and prevent any HIV-related illnesses. • There is no cure, but treatments enable most people with the virus to live a long and healthy life, though there are side effects. • AIDS is the final stage of HIV infection, when the body can no longer fight life-threatening infections.

🔑 **KEY TERM**

Stillbirth – a baby that is not born alive after 24 weeks. It can be linked to placenta complications.

Personal safety

GROUP ACTIVITY

(20 minutes)

How well can you look after yourself? Following the link below, take the personal safety quiz.

http://tinyurl.com/h96k7us

Your whole class could take the quiz together, discussing your answers to reach a group consensus for each question.

Alcohol

• Too much alcohol can lead to risky behaviour.
• Alcohol might make unsafe sex more likely, which can result in an STI or an unwanted pregnancy.
• Alcohol can lead to being a victim of, or accused of, sexual assault.
• It is important to know your limits and drink sensibly, stopping when you know you have had enough.
• On a night out, alternate alcoholic drinks with soft drinks, drink more slowly and consume alcohol with food, or you could volunteer to drive and so not drink at all.

Nights out and transport

Safe transport home after a night out is essential. Having a plan is a good safety strategy. Before going out, think about how you are going to get home and find out the time of the last bus or train. Is there a friend you can travel home with? One friend might volunteer to be the driver and make sure everyone gets home safely. Alternatively, use a licensed taxi or a taxi marshalling scheme if there is one in your town. Always pre-book a minicab – never hail one off the street as the driver may not be licensed or vetted. The plan avoids having to accept a lift from a stranger, particularly one who warns you of the dangers of walking alone and then offers to accompany you.

Another strategy is to use a safety app, such as Lifeplug (www.lifeplug.net). In an emergency you unplug your earphones and your contacts will be notified via an SMS message of your location and that you need urgent help.

Social media – 'stranger danger'

Social media is an enjoyable and essential part of life today, but it can be dangerous, even fatal. Take as much care when meeting strangers online as you would face to face. Not everyone is who they say they are and you should never meet anyone you only know online without taking a trusted person with you.

Grooming

The Sexual Offences Act created the offence of 'grooming'. It is a crime to befriend a child or young person on the internet (or by any other method of communication) and meet or intend to meet the child with the intention of abusing them. The maximum sentence is 10 years' imprisonment. Risk of Sexual Harm Orders prohibit adults from engaging in inappropriate behaviour such as sexual conversations with children online. Vulnerable groups such as looked-after children (children in care) or those with learning disabilities are particularly at risk of sexual exploitation.

Child Exploitation and Online Protection centre (CEOP)

CEOP is a police-led child protection agency tackling sexual abuse on and offline. Its education service provides safety information and factsheets for children, young people, parents, carers and practitioners: www.thinkuknow.co.uk/parents. It also has a YouTube channel: www.youtube.co.uk/ceop.

Medical checks – self-care

Cervical screening test

Sometimes known as a 'smear test', this is a method of detecting abnormal cells on the cervix (entrance to the womb). Being screened regularly means any abnormal changes in the cells can be found at an early stage and if necessary treated to stop cancer developing.

Self-examination

Testicular cancer is the most common type to affect men aged between 15 and 49. Regular self-checking for lumps or changes in texture is recommended, as more than 96 per cent of men with early stage testicular cancer are cured.

Orchid, an organisation that focuses on male cancers, has a short video about how to carry out a testicle self-examination: http://www.yourprivates.org.uk/.

Women should check their breasts regularly; if there are any changes in size or shape of the breast or nipple, discharge, rash, lump or puckering of the skin they should see their GP. It is important to rule out breast cancer. Lots of women have breast lumps, and nine out of ten are not cancerous.

Tests for STIs

Sexual health or genitourinary medicine (GUM) clinics offer a range of services including tests for STIs. These can involve an examination of the genitals, giving a urine sample, having a blood sample taken, or a swab of the urethra, rectum, vagina or throat.

Anyone can go to GUM clinics regardless of their age. Some clinics hold sessions for particular groups of people, such as young people, gay men and lesbians. The clinics also offer treatment, free condoms, **contraception**, pregnancy testing and help for people who have been sexually assaulted.

1.3 Methods of contraception

> 🔑 **KEY TERM**
>
> **Contraception** – a method of deliberately preventing pregnancy.

Contraception (see Figure 13.1) enables someone to choose whether they want to start a family. However, barrier methods of contraception (male and female condoms) are the only types that help to protect against STIs.

Contraceptive pill

99% effective

- **Combined pill** – contains oestrogen and progestogen (female hormones) which prevent ovulation. Also makes it difficult for sperm to reach an egg or for an egg to implant in the womb lining. Has to be taken every day for 21 days, at the same time each day. There is then a seven-day break when a period-like bleed occurs.
- **Progesterone-only pill** – contains progestogen only. Works by thickening the mucus in the cervix, stopping the sperm reaching an egg. It can also stop ovulation. It is taken every day, at the same time, with no break between packs.

Female condom

99% effective

- Made from soft plastic, it is worn inside the vagina to prevent semen getting inside the uterus.
- Needs to be placed inside the vagina before there is any contact with the penis. Must be removed immediately after sex.
- Single use.

Male condom

98% effective

- Worn on the penis to prevent semen entering the vagina.
- Needs to be put on when the penis is erect and before it is in contact with the vagina.
- Single use.

Contraceptive implant

99% effective

- A 4 cm flexible tube, which is inserted under the skin of the upper arm by a trained professional such as doctor. It lasts for 3 years.
- By releasing progestogen into the body it stops ovulation each month.
- Thickens the mucus in the cervix, stopping the sperm reaching the egg, and thins the womb lining so an egg cannot implant.
- When it is removed fertility returns immediately.

Contraceptive injection

99% effective

- Lasts for 8, 12 or 13 weeks depending on the type.
- Releases progestogen into the bloodstream, preventing ovulation.
- Thickens the mucus in the cervix, stopping sperm reaching the egg, and thins the womb lining so an egg cannot implant.
- It can take up to one year for fertility to return after the injection wears off.

Contraceptive patch

99% effective

- A sticky patch, measuring 5×5 cm. It delivers hormones into the body through the skin, similar to a nicotine patch.
- Like the implant and injection, it prevents ovulation by thickening the cervical mucus and thinning the womb lining.
- Changed every week for 3 weeks, then a week without a patch.

Diaphragm/cap

92–96%, with spermicide

- A circular dome made of thin, soft silicone which is inserted into the vagina to cover the cervix, preventing sperm from entering the womb.
- A woman needs to be fitted for the correct size by a doctor or nurse.
- Used with spermicide, which kills sperm.
- Must be left in place for six hours after sex.
- Can be washed and reused.

Intrauterine device (IUD)

99% effective

- A small T-shaped plastic and copper device inserted into the womb.
- Needs to be fitted by a specially trained doctor or nurse. It lasts 5–10 years depending on the type.
- Stops the sperm and egg from surviving in the womb or **fallopian tubes**. It may also prevent a fertilised egg from implanting.

🔑 KEY TERM

Fallopian tube – there are two, one each side of the uterus. They connect the ovaries to the uterus.

221

99% effective	Intrauterine system (IUS)

- A small T-shaped plastic device inserted into the womb.
- Needs to be fitted by a specially trained doctor or nurse. It works for 3 or 5 years, depending on the type.
- Thickens the mucus in the cervix, stopping the sperm reaching the egg, and thins the womb lining so an egg cannot implant.
- It may also prevent ovulation.

Up to 99% but only 75% effective if mistakes are made	Natural family planning

- Involves plotting the times of the month when a woman is fertile.
- A woman has to keep a daily record of fertility signals, such as temperature and the fluids coming out of the cervix.
- It takes 3–6 menstrual cycles to learn the method.

▲ **Figure 13.1** Methods of contraception

PAIRS ACTIVITY

'Safer sex' – how much do I know? (15 minutes)

In pairs, follow the link below and then take the NHS sexual health self-assessment quiz 'Safer sex – how much do you know?'

http://tinyurl.com/lnfylbe

KNOW IT

1 State three key aspects of the Sexual Offences Act 2003.
2 What is meant by the term 'grooming'?
3 Give an example of how to stay safe on a night out.
4 Name four STIs.
5 Name a barrier method of contraception.
6 Give three examples of services provided by a GUM clinic.

LO1 Assessment activities

Below are suggested assessment activities that have been directly linked to the pass, merit and distinction criteria in LO1 to help with assignment preparation; they include Top Tips on how to achieve the best results.

The Health Promotion Unit and local hospital are planning to run a 'Health Week' at the community centre. The aim is to raise awareness in the community about sexual heath, pregnancy and birth, and baby care and development. You have been asked to take part in the health week by preparing materials to be used at a series of workshops during the event.

Activity 1 – pass criteria *P1 P2 P3*

Produce an information booklet for people to take away with them. The booklet should:

1 describe how sexually transmitted infections could affect the health and wellbeing of the individual
2 summarise ways in which an individual may be protected against unlawful and harmful sexual intercourse
3 explain how a range of methods of contraception protect against pregnancy.

Activity 2 – merit criteria *M1* and distinction criteria *D1*

The Health Promotion Unit have also asked you to produce a document for them which:

1 analyses approaches that could be taken to promote sexual health
2 evaluates the effectiveness of legislation in protecting the individual against unlawful and harmful intercourse.

TOP TIPS

✔ Think about how you will convey the information to the target audience.
✔ When analysing, discuss the pros and cons of approaches.
✔ When evaluating, make a qualitative judgement taking into account different factors and using available knowledge, experience and evidence.

LO2 Understand the importance of prenatal health and the process of conception *F4 M2*

🔑 KEY TERMS

Preconception health – consideration of health, fitness and lifestyle before trying to conceive a baby, to improve chances of becoming pregnant and to give the baby a good start.

Conception – occurs when the egg is fertilised by the sperm.

Neural tube defect – a condition that develops when the baby's spinal cord and spinal column do not form properly in the womb.

Ovaries – produce female hormones and produce 'ovum' also known as eggs.

GETTING STARTED 👤

Just relaxing? (10 minutes)

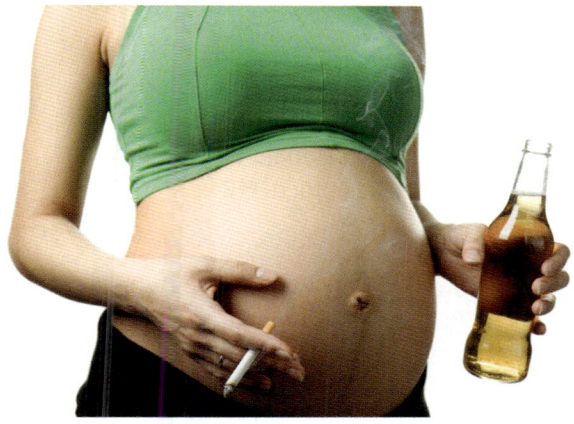

▲ **Figure 13.2** What do you think of this photo of a pregant woman?

Discuss your response to what she is doing; share your opinions with the rest of your class.

2.1 Factors which can affect conception

Maximising **preconception health**, for men and women, will create the best conditions for **conception** and development of a healthy baby.

Stopping smoking is one of the most important things to do in preparation for pregnancy. Smoking is linked to premature birth, low birthweight and miscarriage. It also reduces natural fertility for both men and women.

A woman trying to get pregnant should avoid drinking alcohol as it increases the risk of miscarriage and can cause serious health problems for the baby.

Regular exercise can help to prepare for the physically demanding pregnancy and birth. Being over- or underweight can reduce chances of conceiving.

Eating a healthy, balanced diet improves the level of nutrition and provides the best start for a pregnancy. Having decided to try and get pregnant, it is important to start taking folic acid straight away. Folic acid has been found to greatly reduce the risk of **neural tube defects** such as spina bifida.

Some prescribed medication and over-the-counter non-prescribed drugs like ibuprofen are not safe while trying to become pregnant or during pregnancy. A pharmacist can advise. Anyone taking illegal drugs needs advice and support to give them up. They should see their GP before trying to get pregnant for help in achieving a successful conception and healthy pregnancy.

The method of contraception used may affect how soon pregnancy is possible. It may take three months to a year for normal fertility to return after the contraceptive injection. It may take six months after taking the pill.

Some medical conditions can make conceiving difficult. Here are some examples.

- Polycystic ovary syndrome – a condition where the **ovaries** do not regularly release an egg (ovulate).
- Anorexia – a serious mental health condition. It is an eating disorder in which people keep their weight as low as possible. Over time, anorexia can lead to infertility.
- Amenorrhoea – when periods are absent due to an underlying medical condition, excessive exercise, excessive weight loss, or stress.

2.2 Process of conception

GETTING STARTED 👤

Conception (10 minutes)

Watch this clip of human fertilisation:

http://www.bbc.co.uk/education/clips/z6tkq6f

Figure 13.3 summarises the process of conception.

OVULATION
Approximately 14 days after menstruation, an ovum (egg) is released by one of the woman's ovaries and begins to travel down the fallopian tube.

↓

INTERCOURSE
Semen (sperm) is released (ejaculated) from the penis into the vagina. It travels up through the cervix and uterus and then into the fallopian tubes.

↓

FERTILISATION
Fertilisation takes place in the fallopian tube, the ovum is fertilised by one of the sperm and a baby is conceived.

▲ **Figure 13.3** The process of conception

In vitro fertilisation (IVF)

This is an assisted conception treatment. It happens outside the woman's body 'in vitro' which means 'in glass'. This refers to the glass dish that is used in the laboratory.

1 The woman takes medication to increase her egg production
2 A needle is inserted into her ovaries to collect the eggs.
3 In the laboratory the eggs are fertilised with sperm from her partner, or donated sperm.
4 Two to five days later one or two of the healthiest **embryos** are put back in the woman's womb.
5 There is a two-week wait before having a pregnancy test to see if the treatment has worked.

KEY TERM

Embryo – the fertilised egg divides to form a ball of cells called the embryo.

The success rate of IVF depends on the age of the woman and the cause of infertility.

L02 Assessment activity

Below is a suggested assessment activity that has been directly linked to the pass and merit criteria in LO2 to help with assignment preparation; it includes Top Tips on how to achieve the best results

Create a presentation with accompanying notes and materials for a workshop session for the community Health Week event.

The presentation should:

1 explain the process of conception. **P4**

The workshop materials should:

2 assess ways in which individuals can ensure a healthy conception takes place. **M2**

TOP TIPS

✔ Make sure you are explaining and not just describing. You will need to include relevant reasons, purposes and effects of the stages in the process of conception.

✔ Check that you have included a reasoned judgement or opinion on the importance of prenatal health to the process of conception.

LO3 Know the factors that could affect health in pregnancy and the success of the birth *P5 P6*

GETTING STARTED

What happened? (10 minutes)

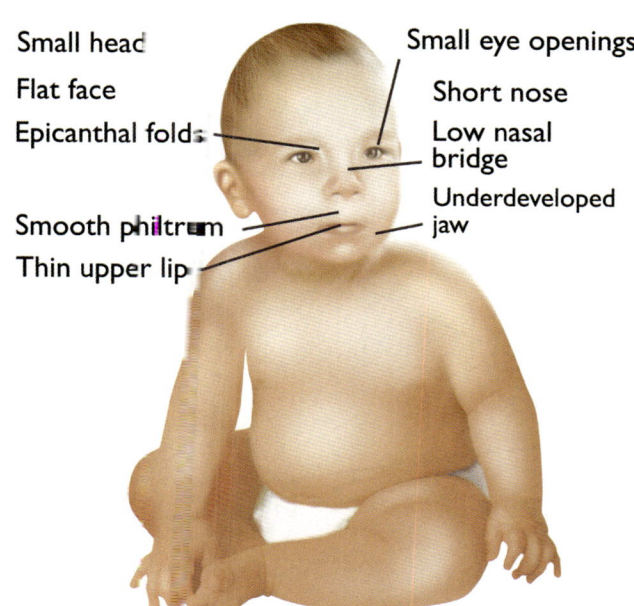

▲ **Figure 13.4** Look at the picture of the baby on which some physical defects have been noted.

Small head
Flat face
Epicanthal folds
Smooth philtrum
Thin upper lip
Small eye openings
Short nose
Low nasal bridge
Underdeveloped jaw

The baby has been affected by foetal alcohol syndrome. Discuss ways that a pregnant woman could avoid negatively affecting the development of the **foetus** during pregnancy.

3.1 Conditions *in utero*

Disabilities

At 18–21 weeks of pregnancy, a detailed ultrasound scan (anomaly scan) checks the baby for a range of physical abnormalities such as a cleft lip, diaphragmatic hernia and heart abnormalities. It also screens for conditions that develop *in utero*, such as those below.

Spina bifida

This is a condition where the neural tube, which eventually forms the spine, does not develop properly in the womb. The bones of the vertebrae do not fully close and in some cases the spinal cord is also affected. Severe forms can lead to weakness or paralysis of the legs, bowel or urinary incontinence, fluid on the brain and learning difficulties. The exact cause is unknown, but a lack of folic acid before and during the early stages of pregnancy can be a significant risk factor.

Down's syndrome

This is a genetic condition, caused by the baby having an extra copy of chromosome 21, which typically causes some level of learning disability and characteristic physical features such as eyes that slant upwards, small mouth with a protruding tongue, reduced muscle tone and below average weight and size at birth. Complications can include hearing and vision problems, heart disease, thyroid problems and recurrent infections such as pneumonia. The risk of having a baby with Down's syndrome increases with the age of the mother, from 1 in 1500 at 20 years old to 1 in 400 for a 40-year-old mother.

Foetal alcohol syndrome (FAS)

If a mother drinks alcohol, it can easily pass through the **placenta** into the baby's blood. Alcohol damages important cells in the baby's body that are necessary for growth and also disrupts the connection of nerve cells. This results in poor growth in the womb, a small head and jaw, and sometimes deformed limbs. Babies born with FAS are at greater risk of learning disorders and problems with thinking, speech and memory. They may develop mood, attention or behavioural problems such as **ADHD**, and may develop problems with the liver, heart, hearing or sight and have a weakened immune system. Some may only have mild symptoms, while others may be severely affected.

> **KEY TERMS**
>
> **Foetus** – from eight weeks after fertilisation until birth the embryo is called a foetus.
>
> **In utero** – something that occurs in the womb, before birth.
>
> **Placenta** – provides the foetus with oxygen and nourishment from the mother via the umbilical cord.
>
> **ADHD** – attention deficit hyperactivity disorder, symptoms include a short attention span, constant fidgeting and impulsive behaviour.

3.2 Factors which may affect the health of the foetus

Complications in pregnancy
Lack of oxygen to the foetus may result in the baby becoming distressed and being delivered by Caesarean section

Birth injury
Causes can include large babies, a long and difficult labour and breech birth position. Assisted delivery by forceps (large tongs) or ventouse (vacuum extraction) can cause bruising to the baby's head and face.

Alcohol
Large amounts of alcohol and binge drinking increase the risk of harm to the foetus, particularly in the first 3 months. There is no 'safe' level of alcohol use during pregnancy.

Access to antenatal care
A pregnant woman will have 7 to 10 antenatal appointments with a midwife, GP or at the hospital to identify and reduce any risks. She can raise any concerns. The baby's growth will be monitored throughout the pregnancy.

Genetic conditions
Inherited from parents e.g. cystic fibrosis, sickle cell anaemia, muscular dystrophy, haemophilia, thalassaemia and Huntingdon's disease. Genetic testing can identify potential conditions.

Stress
Unborn babies are exposed to their mother's stress hormones. This could affect the developing child and long-term stress can cause the mother to feel tired, depressed and more prone to illness. It is important that pregnant women are supported by their family, friends and employers.

Smoking/secondary smoking
Whether the mother smokes or experiences secondary (passive) smoking via others, there is an increased risk of pregnancy complications e.g. ectopic pregnancy, placental abruption, miscarriage, stillbirth and premature labour.

Factors which may affect the health of the foetus

Excessive exercise/ lack of exercise
Exercise can help to strengthen muscles and improve wellbeing. However, sport with a risk of falls such as horse riding, gymnastics and cycling, should be done with caution or avoided. To stay safe, drink plenty of water, don't exercise to exhaustion or when it is very hot, and stop if feeling unwell or in pain.

Use of prescribed/ non-prescribed drugs during pregnancy
Some medicines, including herbal, homeopathic or aromatherapy treatments, can harm the developing foetus so medication should always be checked by a pharmacist, midwife or doctor. Babies born to drug addicts can suffer withdrawal symptoms and may suffer long-term health issues.

Diet
The mother should eat healthily. Some foods need to be avoided as they might cause illness or harm the baby e.g. unpasteurised cheese and soft blue cheese can contain listeria, and raw or partly cooked eggs can carry toxoplasmosis – both can cause miscarriage or stillbirth. Shellfish should always be cooked to avoid food poisoning.

Vitamin B12 (folic acid)
Protects against neural tube defects such as spina bifida conditions in utero. The mother should take 400 mg every day before and during pregnancy and eat foods high in natural folic acid e.g. leafy green vegetables and brown rice.

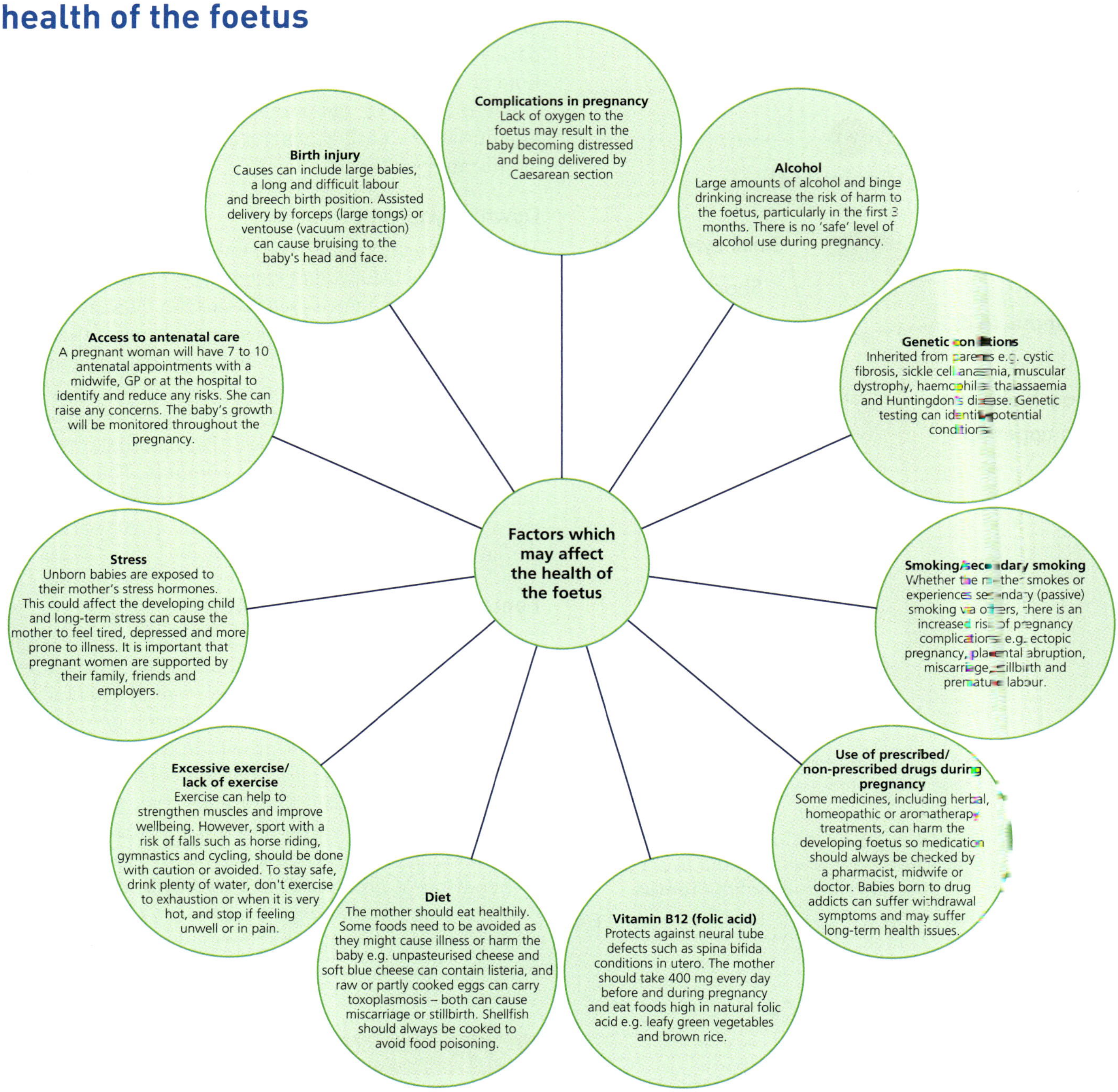

▲ **Figure 13.5** Factors which may affect the health of the foetus

---

🔍 INDEPENDENT RESEARCH ACTIVITY

Genetic conditions (30–40 minutes)

Access the NHS website to find out more detail about the conditions that can be inherited.

1 How is genetic testing carried out?
2 What are the benefits for prospective parents of having genetic counselling?

KNOW IT

1 Name three conditions *in utero* that can affect the health of the foetus.
2 Explain the effects of drinking alcohol when pregnant.
3 Describe features of a healthy diet when pregnant.
4 Give three reasons why attending antenatal care appointments is so important.

LO3 Assessment activity *P5 P6*

Below is a suggested assessment activity that has been directly linked to the pass criteria in LO3 to help with assignment preparation; it includes Top Tips on how to achieve the best results.

Produce a set of factsheets for visitors to the community Health Week event. The factsheets should include information that:

- identifies disabilities which occur *in utero*
- describes factors that affect the health of the foetus.

TOP TIPS

✔ Ensure that you have given both a name to and brief details of disabilities that occur *in utero*.
✔ Make sure you produce an account that includes all of the relevant details about factors that affect the health of the foetus.

LO4 Understand the stages of pregnancy and birth and the postnatal care of the mother *P7 P8 P9 M3*

GETTING STARTED

What is it really like? (10 minutes)

In preparation for studying LO4 on pregnancy, birth and postnatal care, encourage someone you (or your friends and family) know who is expecting a baby or has recently given birth, to share their experiences with you.

4.1 Gestation

This refers to the period of growth and development from when the ovum is fertilised, up to the birth of the baby. Gestation is divided into three trimesters.

Trimesters

First trimester 1–12 weeks

After fertilisation, the egg doubles its cells until, after five days, it has reached 16 cells. By the tenth day it forms a mass of cells called a blastocyst and has implanted into the uterus wall. The placenta, **umbilical cord** and **amniotic sac** develop. By week 10 the baby's organs, such as the heart and lungs, will have started forming. By week 12 the baby will be approximately 8 cm long. The eyes will be formed but closed, and the ears will have started forming. The brain will be growing rapidly so the head is much bigger than the body.

Second trimester 13–27 weeks

At this stage the organs mature and the skeleton starts to harden. The foetus will have bowel movements and the kidneys begin to pass small amounts of urine. By 20 weeks it is often possible to determine the sex of the baby. By the end of this trimester the baby has grown fingernails and teeth may have started growing under the gums.

Third trimester 28–40 weeks

The lungs mature throughout this trimester and the baby makes breathing movements, though the lungs do not work properly until birth. Eyes will open and close. The baby will kick and stretch and respond to sound. The baby will move into a head-down position ready for birth.

4.2 The birth process

The stages of birth

Stage 1 – neck of the uterus opens

- **Show** – the plug of mucus and blood that has acted as a seal for the cervix during pregnancy, comes away. This could be several days or a few hours before labour starts.
- **Rupture of the membranes** – the amniotic sac breaks and the fluid is released ('waters break').
- **Contractions** – hormones cause contractions where the muscles in the uterus tense and relax. To begin with the contractions gradually stretch and open the cervix; this can take several hours. When the cervix is 7–10 cm dilated, the contractions gradually get stronger and closer together.

Stage 2 – birth of the baby

Strong contractions push the baby's head lower and the mother will feel a strong urge to push. The baby moves further down the pelvis and when the head reaches the entrance to the vagina, called 'crowning', it is ready to be born. The head is born first, followed by the shoulders and rest of the body.

Stage 3 – delivery of placenta and membranes

The umbilical cord is clamped and cut. Then the placenta and membranes that held the baby in the uterus pass out of the body. This is usually assisted by an injection of oxytocin, which helps the uterus to expel the placenta and helps to reduce blood loss.

Pain relief

There are a number of different methods of pain relief available to help the mother to cope with labour. Some of the methods use drugs and others are drug free.

Table 13.2 lists examples of natural, drug-free pain relief methods.

Table 13.2 Natural pain relief during labour

Breathing & relaxation	Tension is reduced, making labour easier. Staying calm conserves energy and relaxes muscles. These techniques are taught in antenatal classes.
Water birth	Warm water in a birthing pool allows freedom of movement and lowers blood pressure. The partner can enter the pool and help.
TENS	Transcutaneous electrical nerve stimulation. An electrode pad is placed on the mother's back. A hand-held control produces a gentle electrical current which interferes with the passage of pain signals to the brain and helps the body to produce the hormone endorphin, which is a natural painkiller.

Table 13.3 lists examples of pain relief methods that use drugs.

Table 13.3 Pain relief using drugs

Entonox (gas and air)	A mixture of oxygen and nitrous oxide. Breathed through a mask or plastic mouthpiece. The mother can control her intake and it does not affect the baby.
Pethidine	A strong pain-killing drug which is injected. It relaxes the muscles but makes the mother very drowsy.
Epidural	Anaesthetic which is injected into the lower back. It completely blocks pain from the waist down. It has little effect on the baby but the mother may have a slightly longer labour as she cannot feel her contractions.

Methods of delivery including assisted delivery due to birth difficulties and complications

Delivery will either be vaginal or, if this is not possible, by Caesarean section.

> 🔑 **KEY TERM**
>
> **Breech position** – when the baby is 'bottom down' rather than head down in the uterus before birth.

Induction of labour

A mother can be helped to go into labour if there is a problem with the mother or baby and the baby needs to be born for safety reasons, or if the waters have broken and labour hasn't started within 24 hours. Some hospitals will induce if the pregnancy is overdue. Methods include a drip, a vaginal gel or rupturing the membranes

Assisted delivery

Sometimes labour does not go as planned and the mother may need help for the baby to be born safely. It could be that the baby is not getting enough oxygen, causing foetal distress; the baby could be in a difficult position in the uterus or the labour has been very long and the mother is exhausted. Delivery can be assisted in different ways.

- Forceps – large tongs with curved ends that fit around the baby's head. The doctor will pull gently while the mother pushes.
- Ventouse – (vacuum delivery) gentle suction is applied by a rubber cap placed on the baby's head
- Caesarean section – carried out if a vaginal delivery is not possible. It is a surgical operation where the baby is delivered through the mother's abdomen. Reasons could be severe foetal distress – the umbilical cord could be around the baby's neck, **breech position** baby or a very large baby, or if the mother is too ill to withstand labour.

Premature birth

A baby born before 37 weeks is a premature baby. A pre-term baby is likely to need special care as they may have problems with breathing, sucking and maintaining their own body temperature.

Miscarriage and stillbirth

A miscarriage is the loss of pregnancy during the first 23 weeks. The baby comes too early to survive on its own. The usual reason is that there is something wrong with either the baby's development or the cervix. A baby that is not born alive after 24 weeks is called stillborn. This most often happens due to placenta complications.

4.3 Postnatal care of the mother

The type and amount of **postnatal** care will depend on the individual mother and baby's circumstances. Usually a midwife will take care of the mother for the first 10 days following delivery, but if there has been a difficult or complicated birth this may be extended up to 28 days.

Statutory support

'Statutory' means the care to which a mother is entitled by law, support that it is her right to receive.

Midwife

- Cares for mother and baby for 10 days after the birth; care then transfers to the health visitor.
- Provides advice – breastfeeding, caring for baby.

Health visitor

- Responsible for the welfare of both the mother and baby.
- Visits the home, answers any questions and concerns.
- Checks baby is feeding well, gaining weight and developing well.
- Asks if mother has any physical or emotional needs.
- Looks for signs of **postnatal depression**.
- Offers advice and referral to specialist services if needed.

GP

- Will carry out the 6-week postnatal check.
- Chats about progress, how the mother is feeling.
- Checks uterus has gone down to pre-pregnancy size.
- Carries out 6–8 week developmental check of the baby.

Further detail of statutory NHS postnatal care can be found by using the following link:

http://tinyurl.com/hboveso

🔑 **KEY TERMS**

Postnatal – refers to the period after a woman has given birth, the first few weeks. 'Post' means after and 'natal' means birth.

Postnatal depression – a mental condition that some mothers develop after giving birth. It is a serious mental disorder that requires help and support.

Informal support

The mother's partner can help with general household tasks such as vacuuming and preparing meals, as well as changing nappies, sterilising bottles (if bottle fed), bathing the baby and screening visitors so they don't outstay their welcome when the mother needs rest. Family and friends can help as well, supporting the mother by shopping, collecting prescriptions or providing transport to the GP surgery. Simply being there to reassure her and to chat about any concerns is valuable support.

Other organisations

The NCT (National Childbirth Trust) provides information about all aspects of pregnancy, birth and care of a newborn. The NCT also runs antenatal classes in most areas.

Local mother and baby groups provide an opportunity to meet other new mothers, have a chat and share experiences and advice.

4.4 Types of support

- Information about diet, contraception and postnatal exercise can be easily accessed online using, for example, the NHS Choices website which covers all aspects of pregnancy, birth and child care.
- Friends and family can be an invaluable source of information drawn from their own experiences.
- Informal meetings of new mums can be very reassuring, whether face to face or via internet social networks.
- GP surgeries run mother and baby clinics that provide information about contraception and postnatal exercise
- The health visitor will be on the lookout for symptoms of postnatal depression and will also provide post-operative support following a Caesarean section.

KNOW IT 💡

1 Name the three stages of giving birth.
2 Give an example of natural pain relief when giving birth.
3 Describe one method used for an assisted birth.
4 Explain the role of the health visitor in postnatal care.
5 Describe ways a new father could support the mother in the first few weeks after the birth.

LO5 Understand the care and development of the baby in the first year of life *P10 M4 D2*

KEY TERM

Reflexes – inborn and involuntary movements, not voluntary movements.

5.1 Developmental stages

'Norms' and 'milestones' help to decide whether babies are progressing normally within the range of expected development. However, there are likely to be variations, with milestones not always achieved exactly at the expected age.

All aspects of development are linked, they do not occur in isolation, they are interrelated and one aspect of development will impact on another. For example, with emotional and cognitive development, a child who feels emotionally secure with familiar adults will want to communicate with them and in doing so gradually develops language skills.

Keeping a record

New parents are given a Personal Child Health Record (PCHR), called the 'red book' due its red cover. Parents can fill in details about their child; doctors and other health professionals record medical details such as immunisations, height and weight records. There is a milestones section to record the child's developmental progress.

Physical growth and appearance

A newborn baby weighs on average 3.5 kg, though this will vary considerably. Generally, smaller parents tend to have smaller babies and boys tend to be larger than girls.

The average length of a full-term baby is about 50 cm, with a head circumference on average of 35 cm. The head is very big when compared with the rest of the body; the arms and legs are short and plump. The abdomen is large.

On average, a baby doubles its birth weight in the first six months and trebles it by 1 year. The proportions of a child's body change with growth as some parts grow more quickly than others: at birth the head equals about 25 per cent of the length of the body, this percentage gradually decreases as the child gets older.

Physical movement and skills

Table 13.4 presents a summary of the physical movement and skills development of a baby from newborn to 1 year old.

Table 13.4 Physical movement and skills – newborn to 1 year

Age	Fine motor skills	Gross motor skills
Newborn	**Reflexes**: swallowing and sucking, grasp, rooting, startle, walking, falling.	
1 month	Opens hand and will grasp an adult's finger. Facial expressions – showing interest and excitement.	Can turn from side to back. May move head towards a bright light. Makes jerky, uncontrolled leg and arm movements.
3 months	Will move head to follow adult movements. Will watch hands and play with their fingers. Can hold a rattle briefly without dropping it.	Can lift head and chest when in the prone position (lying on their front). Can sit with back straight when held. Kicks vigorously with legs.

Age	Fine motor skills	Gross motor skills
6 months	Will reach and grab when a small toy is offered. Uses the whole hand (palmar grasp) to pass a toy from one hand to the other. Explores objects by putting them in mouth.	When held sitting or standing can do so with a straight back. Lying on back, can lift legs into vertical position, grasping feet with hands. Can change the angle of body to reach out for an object; can roll over.
9 months	Can grasp objects using finger and thumb in a pincer grasp. Continues to explore objects by putting them in mouth. Can release a toy from grasp by dropping it – cannot yet put it down. Imitates adult gestures.	Can sit up unsupported, with a straight back, for a short while. Can pull themselves into a standing position. Can stand by holding on to furniture. May take some steps when being held. Moves along the floor – bottom shuffling or crawling.
12 months	Can point at interesting objects with index finger. Can throw and drop toys deliberately. Builds with a few bricks. Can release a small object into another person's hand. May crawl upstairs or onto low items of furniture.	Is now mobile, can probably walk alone with feet wide apart or with one hand held. Can rise to a sitting position from lying down.

Cognitive function

Cognitive or intellectual, development is concerned with thought processes and thinking skills. From the start, babies develop concepts through their physical senses in order to understand their new environment.

Table 13.5 Cognitive development – newborn to 1 year

Age	Cognitive development
Newborn	Begins to develop concepts through the senses and growing understanding. Aware of physical sensations such as hunger and discomfort. Imitation of adults, for example facial expressions.
1 month	Recognises primary (main) carers. Repeats enjoyable movements. Turns to look at the face of someone speaking.
3 months	Shows an increasing interest in playthings and their surroundings. Recognises familiar situations. Shows an understanding of cause and effect by shaking a rattle to hear its noise.
6 months	Shows understanding of words such as 'bye-bye', 'mama', 'dada'. Raises arms to be picked up – demonstrating understanding of cause and effect, up and down.
9 months	Looks for fallen/dropped toys. Looks at small objects and reaches for them. Explores objects by touching, banging, shaking. Looks for a hidden object – knows it still exists though can't be seen.
12 months	When asked 'Where is the ball?' they will point to the ball. Uses trial and error to learn about objects. Begins to treat or use objects in an appropriate way, such as cuddle a soft toy and use a hairbrush. Enjoys looking at picture books.

Emotional development

Emotional development in a young child mostly occurs through socialisation, a process where the child learns knowledge, language and social skills from the people around them.

Table 13.6 Emotional development – newborn to 1 year

Age	Emotional development
Newborn	Expresses pleasure when being cuddled, fed or bathed.
1 month	Smiles at the carer. Can be described by a carer as developing a particular temperament or personality, such as lively and excitable or calm and placid.
3 months	Loves to receive attention and cuddles; smiles at familiar people. Stares intently at carer's face when feeding and shows enjoyment when being bathed.
6 months	Gets upset when main carer leaves. Cries and laughs when others do.
9 months	Prefers to be with a familiar adult and expresses fear of strangers by crying. Enjoys songs and rhymes with actions. Enjoys games such as 'peek-a-boo'.
12 months	May have comfort objects such as a blanket or soft toy. Shows affection for family members, likes to be with people they know. Waves goodbye.

Speech and communication

The ability to communicate develops through babies' interactions with others. Crying is a first method of communicating need and carers soon learn to differentiate between types of cry and what each means.

Table 13.7 Speech and communication development – newborn to 1 year

Age	Speech and communication
Newborn	Cries to indicate need. Hiccups, sneezes and burps. Imitates adults, for example facial expressions such as sticking their tongue out. Makes eye-to-eye contact.
1 month	Starts to make non-crying noises such as gurgling and cooing. Crying and other noises become more expressive. Looks attentively at the carer's face when being fed.
3 months	Beginnings of conversation, will exchange 'coos' with another person. Cries loudly to express a need. Smiles in response to being spoken to.
6 months	Imitates sounds and enjoys babbling. Makes a wide variety of different sounds – laughs, squeals, screams.
9 months	May say 'mum-mum', 'dad-dad' – repeats sounds, practising them. Copies sounds made by adults, for example animal noises, train noises. Follows simple instructions such as 'kiss granny'.
12 months	Imitates simple words. Language starts to become conversation. Babbling becomes more speech like and speaks two to six recognisable words.

5.2 Care and nutrition of the newborn to 1 year old

What does a baby need? (10 minutes)

Spend 5 minutes drawing a spider diagram of a baby's basic needs. Then share your thoughts with the rest of your class.

In order for babies to thrive, certain conditions need to be provided by parents or carers.

- The environment the child lives in will have a positive or negative influence on all aspects of their development. A warm, comfortable, safe and clean home will meet most of a child's physical needs and provides a healthy environment. If the home is cold, damp, unhygienic and unsafe the child may develop asthma or frequent coughs, colds, infections or may be injured. As a result, physical growth and development will be affected and the child may not progress as well intellectually or emotionally.
- The child should be protected by immunisations for diseases such as polio and meningitis. The full recommended schedule of vaccinations offered by the NHS can be found by following the link: http://tinyurl.com/j3nnvzw.
- Quality of nutrition from breast or bottle feeding through to weaning and eating solid food is essential for healthy physical development. Childhood obesity is an increasing problem and it is parents and carers who initially have most influence on a child's diet.
- Provision of adequate, clean and suitable clothing, having nappies changed as needed and being regularly bathed are all basic needs.
- Babies need stimulation and opportunities to play through which they learn about their world and people around them, develop communication skills and a sense of security. An attachment is a strong emotional bond with a carer, most often the mother or father.

CLASSROOM DISCUSSION

Baby bonding (20 minutes)

Watch the short clip 'Al – baby bonding' which is from the Channel 4 series 'One Born Every Minute':

http://tinyurl.com/jdwxbaw

- Discuss the ways that Al is bonding with his new son Ted.
- Consider how Al's bonding behaviour will benefit Ted's development.

Not all babies are loved and wanted. Research has shown that a lack of care, interest and attention has a profound impact on children who will lack self-esteem, feel insecure and unhappy and so may fail to thrive physically, emotionally, socially and intellectually.

RESEARCH ACTIVITY

Attachment theories (30 minutes)

Working in pairs or small groups use the internet or textbooks to find out about the attachment theories put forward by the psychologists John Bowlby and Mary Ainsworth.

These theories were put forward many years ago. Do you think they are still relevant today?

5.3 Health and social care and early years services

There are a range of services available to support parents and carers of babies and children. Some examples are described in Figure 13.6.

Service	Description
Child health monitoring	• Personal child health record. • Baby will be weighed regularly – once a month up to six months, every two months up to one year, then every three months. • Regular physical health checks, regular development checks.
Health visitor	• Advises on and offers support with breastfeeding. • Gives advice about diet and nutrition. • Monitors health and welfare of the mother. • See also LO4 (Postnatal care).
Child health clinics	• Run mother and baby, parent and toddler sessions. • Offer breastfeeding support clinics. • Run peer support groups. • Administer immunisations. • Health and development checks carried out.
Family nurse partnership	• A voluntary home-visiting programme for first-time mums under 19 years old. • A specially trained family nurse visits the young mum regularly. • Helps the mum to have a healthy pregnancy and plan her future.
Children's centres	• Linked to maternity services. • Provide advice and information e.g. parenting classes, benefits advice. • Full-day or temporary child care is available. • Support for children and parents with special needs.
Nurseries	• Provide care and education for children from birth to four or five years old. • Can be privately run, local authority run or attached to a primary school.

▲ **Figure 13.6** Health and social care and early years services

KNOW IT

1 What is the meaning of the phrase 'cognitive development'?
2 Give two examples of developmental milestones.
3 Name four essential needs of a newborn baby.
4 Give an example of how a parent or carer could start 'bonding' with their new baby.
5 Give two examples of services that could provide advice for a new mother.

Read about it

Fisher, A. *et al.* (2012) *Applied A2 Health & Social Care for OCR*, revised edition, Oxford.

Meggitt, C. (2012) *Child Development: An Illustrated Guide*, Pearson.

Minett, P. (2010) *Child Care and Development*, 6th edition, Hodder.

Moonie, N. *et al.* (2007) *Core Themes – Health and Social Care*, Heinemann.

LO5 Assessment activity *P10 M4 D2*

Below is a suggested assessment activity that has been directly linked to the pass, merit and distinction criteria in LO5 to help with assignment preparation; it includes Top Tips on how to achieve the best results.

Produce a 'toolkit' and information pack for the new parents visiting the Health Week event to take away with them. The pack should contain information that will enable them to understand how to care for and track the developmental progress of their baby in the first year of life.

The pack should include the following.

1 An explanation of the expected pattern of development of the baby in its first year of life.
2 An explanation of positive and negative factors influencing development in the first year of life.
3 An analysis of the ways in which health and social care services could influence the care and development of the baby in its first year of life.

TOP TIPS

✔ Think about your audience and how best to present the material.
✔ Make sure you have included all the relevant details, reasons for and effects of positive and negative influences on development in the first year of life.
✔ Ensure that your pack is professionally produced and contains no spelling errors.

Unit 14

The impact of long-term physiological conditions

ABOUT THIS UNIT

A long-term physiological condition is a health problem that is ongoing and needs to be controlled with medication or other therapies. There are many reasons why individuals may develop long-term physiological conditions and some are more serious than others. This unit will allow you to support individuals with long-term physiological conditions in planning their care and support. You will be introduced to the types, causes and effects on individuals of these conditions, and will learn about the day-to-day effects the conditions can have. There is a range of practitioners who care for and support individuals, and you will find out about their roles and the regulatory frameworks they work within. You will also be able to investigate the care and approaches available to those who are terminally ill.

This unit is relevant to anyone considering working in the health and social care professions. For more information about how the body works, and for definitions of some of the body's functions mentioned in this unit, see Unit 4 Anatomy and physiology for health and social care.

LEARNING OUTCOMES

The topics, activities and suggested reading in this unit will help you to:

1 Know what long-term physiological conditions are; their causes and symptoms
2 Understand effects of long-term physiological conditions
3 Be able to support individuals with long-term physiological conditions to plan their care and support
4 Know about end of life care

How will I be assessed?

You will be assessed through a series of assignments and tasks set and marked by your tutor.

How will I be graded?

You will be graded using the following criteria.

Learning outcome	Pass assessment criteria	Merit assessment criteria	Distinction assessment criteria
You will:	To achieve a **pass** you must demonstrate that you have met all the pass assessment criteria	To achieve a **merit** you must demonstrate that you have met all the pass and merit assessment criteria	To achieve a **distinction** you must demonstrate that you have met all the pass, merit and distinction assessment criteria
1 Know what long-term physiological conditions are; their causes and symptoms	**P1** Summarise types of long-term physiological conditions **P2** Describe known causes of long-term physiological conditions **P3** Describe possible symptoms of long-term physiological conditions	**M1** Provide biological explanations for symptoms of long-term physiological conditions	
2 Understand effects of long-term physiological conditions	**P4** Explain possible effects of two long-term physiological conditions on the daily lives of individuals **P5** Describe two possible ways of monitoring a long-term physical condition **P6** Describe treatment available for two long-term physiological conditions **P7** Explain two barriers to accessing treatment for long-term physiological conditions	**M2** Analyse the impact of current monitoring and treatment of long-term physiological conditions on an individual's life	**D1** Recommend ways of overcoming barriers encountered by individuals with long-term physiological conditions
3 Be able to support individuals with long-term physiological conditions to plan their care and support	**P8** Suggest services within the health and social care sector that can best support the needs of individuals with long-term physiological conditions **P9** Explain the purpose of local service provision for people with long-term physiological conditions **P10** Explain the importance of best practice when supporting individuals with long-term physiological conditions	**M3** Analyse local service provision available for an individual with a long-term physiological condition	**D2** Evaluate the impact of current frameworks on the support of individuals with long-term physiological conditions
4 Know about end of life care	**P11** Describe strategies and frameworks available to support individuals in the terminal stages of long-term physiological conditions	**M4** Describe moral and ethical conflicts surrounding end of life care	**D3** Summarise potential ethical and moral conflicts between individual choice and wider society

LO1 Know what long-term physiological conditions are; their causes and symptoms *P1 P2 P3 M1*

GETTING STARTED

(10 minutes)

What is chronic illness really like?

Talk to someone about their experience of a chronic illness. What surprises you?

1.1–1.4 Types, causes, symptoms and biological explanations of long-term physiological conditions

The tables that follow describe a range of long-term physiological conditions. Details of causes of the conditions are provided, which may relate to lifestyle choices, social influences, inheritance, birth injury or occupational causes. Also included in the tables are symptoms of the conditions, both observable and those experienced by the individual.

Chronic illness

A chronic illness or condition is one that is long lasting. It can be controlled but not cured.

Table 14.1 Asthma

Symptoms	Biological explanation
Recurring episodes of breathlessness; tightness of the chest and wheezing Asthma 'attacks'	Inflammation of the bronchi, which carry air in and out of the lungs, causing the bronchi to be more sensitive than normal Contact with something that irritates the lungs – known as a trigger (e.g. cigarette smoke, dust or pollen) – makes airways become narrow, the muscles around them tighten, and there is an increase in the production of sticky mucus (phlegm)
Cause: The exact cause of asthma is not known, but it is likely to be a combination of factors. It may be genetic, however a number of environmental and social factors are thought to play a role in the development of asthma; these include air pollution, chlorine in swimming pools and modern hygiene standards (known as the 'hygiene hypothesis'), where it is thought that modern hygiene standards have reduced our exposure to good and bad germs, which are known to help strengthen the immune system	

Table 14.2 COPD (chronic obstructive pulmonary disease)

Symptoms	Biological explanation
The term COPD covers a range of lung diseases, including chronic bronchitis, emphysema and chronic obstructive airways disease Shortness of breath, wheezing, yellow sputum, persistent cough and frequent chest infections are all symptoms	The airways of the lungs become inflamed and narrowed; as the air sacs get permanently damaged, it becomes increasingly difficult to breathe out There is currently no cure for COPD, but the sooner the condition is diagnosed and appropriate treatment begins, the less chance there is of severe lung damage
Cause: Smoking is the main cause of COPD and is thought to be responsible for around 90% of cases. Some cases of COPD are caused by certain types of fumes, dust and chemical exposure at work; there can also be a genetic tendency, but this is extremely rare	

Table 14.3 Heart disease

Symptoms	Biological explanation
Angina, heart attacks and heart failure are examples of heart disease Symptoms of angina can include chest pain, feeling of tightness in the chest, which may spread to the arms, neck and jaw; light-headedness, sweating, nausea and breathlessness can be signs of a heart attack	The walls of the arteries become blocked with fatty deposits, a process called atherosclerosis; when arteries become completely blocked it can cause a heart attack, which can permanently damage the heart muscle and if not treated straight away can be fatal Heart failure occurs when the heart becomes too weak to pump blood around the body; this can cause fluid to build up in the lungs, making it increasingly difficult to breathe
Cause: Coronary heart disease is usually caused by a build-up of fatty deposits on the walls of the arteries around the heart; risk of this developing is significantly increased by lifestyle factors such as smoking, lack of regular exercise, obesity, or having high cholesterol level, high blood pressure or diabetes	

Table 14.4 Liver disease

Symptoms	Biological explanation
Alcohol-related liver disease: nausea, weight loss, vomiting blood, loss of appetite, jaundice, swelling of legs/ankles/feet and abdomen, very itchy skin, confusion, memory problems, insomnia	Cirrhosis is scarring of the liver caused by continuous, long-term liver damage; scar tissue replaces healthy tissue – this prevents the liver from working properly and can lead to liver failure
Haemochromatosis: fatigue, joint pain, erectile dysfunction, absent periods, jaundice, enlargement of the liver, noticeable to the touch, and diabetes are some of the symptoms	A faulty gene allows your body to absorb excess amounts of iron from food; as a result, iron builds up over time and is usually deposited in the liver, pancreas, joints, heart or endocrine glands
Non-alcoholic fatty liver disease: build-up of fat in the liver cells	Build-up of fat in the liver cells. The liver can become inflamed leading over time to scar tissue forming around the liver and nearby blood vessels; this leads to cirrhosis and eventually liver failure
Cause: Alcohol misuse, regularly drinking large amounts of alcohol in a short time or drinking more than the recommended limits over many years Haemochromatosis is caused by a fault in a specific gene, known as HFE, which can be inherited Obesity is a cause of non-alcoholic fatty liver disease	

Table 14.5 Hepatitis B and C

Symptoms	Biological explanation
As for chronic liver disease (see Table 14.4)	Hep B: a highly infectious virus that is carried in the bloodstream and bodily fluids of an infected person; direct contact with the blood or bodily fluids of an infected person passes on the virus through the bloodstream
	Hep C: passed on through direct contact with infected blood
Cause: Liver infection passed on by the following means Hep B: a virus transmitted through unprotected sexual intercourse and infected blood Hep C: direct contact with infected blood from another person Both can be transmitted by sharing infected drug needles or razors, tattooing or body piercing with infected needles, and blood transfusions in countries where blood is not screened effectively for infection	

Neurological conditions

Neurological conditions are disorders of the nervous system.

Table 14.6 Motor neurone disease (MND)

Symptoms	Biological explanation
Weakened grip causing difficulties picking up or holding objects. Weakness at the shoulder, making lifting the arm above the shoulder difficult	Occurs when specialist nerve cells in the brain and spinal cord, called 'motor neurones', stop working properly; this is known as neurodegeneration
Tripping over a foot because of weakness at the ankle or hip	As motor neurones control muscle activity such as gripping, walking, speaking, swallowing and breathing, a person with MND will find these activities increasingly difficult and, eventually, impossible
Gradually the limbs become weaker and may progressively waste; the final stage is increasing body paralysis	
Cause: It is unclear why the motor neurones begin to lose function; it is believed that it is a combination of interrelated factors that ultimately affect either the motor neurones or the nerve cells that support them. Clumps of protein that develop inside motor neurones, affecting their function, are found in nearly all cases; in about 5% of cases there is a family history of the condition	

Table 14.7 Multiple sclerosis (MS)

Symptoms	Biological explanation
The main symptoms include fatigue, difficulty walking, numbness or tingling in different parts of the body, and muscle stiffness and spasms; there can be problems with balance and co-ordination, and in controlling the bladder, as well as blurred vision, and problems with thinking, learning and planning	The immune system attacks the myelin sheath in the brain and/or the spinal cord; this causes the myelin sheath to become inflamed in patches, which disrupts the messages travelling along the nerves. This disruption leads to the signs and symptoms of MS When the inflammation clears, scarring is left behind on the myelin sheath; this can eventually lead to permanent damage to the underlying nerves
Cause: It is thought that MS is caused partly by genes and partly by outside factors. Though not directly inherited, it is estimated that there is a 2–3% chance of developing it if you are related to someone with the condition. Those who smoke are about twice as likely to develop MS as non-smokers. Viral infections, in particular those caused by Epstein–Barr virus (such as glandular fever), might trigger the immune system. Low vitamin D levels may play a role in the condition, although it is not clear whether vitamin D supplements can help prevent MS	

Table 14.8 Alzheimer's disease

Symptoms	Biological explanation
The first symptoms are usually minor memory problems, such as forgetting recent conversations or events, and forgetting the names of places and objects Memory problems progressively become more severe, resulting in confusion, disorientation, and difficulty planning or making decisions Hallucinations, delusions and personality changes can develop	It involves a gradual loss of mental ability associated with the death of brain cells Scientists have found amyloid plaques (abnormal deposits of protein), and **neurofibrillary tangles** and imbalances in a chemical called acetylcholine in the brains of people with Alzheimer's; vascular damage is also common This all reduces the effectiveness of healthy neurons (nerve cells that carry messages to and from the brain), gradually destroying them Over time, this damage spreads to several areas of the brain; the first areas affected are responsible for memories
Cause: Age is a very significant factor in the development of Alzheimer's – the possibility of developing the condition doubles every five years after an individual reaches 65 years of age. There is a small increased risk if a close family member has the condition; several members of a family developing dementia over the generations can be caused by an inherited gene	

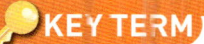 **KEY TERM**

Neurofibrillary tangles – twisted protein fibres in brain cells commonly recognised as a primary marker for Alzheimer's.

Table 14.9 Cerebral palsy

Symptoms	Biological explanation
Muscle stiffness or floppiness, muscle weakness, random and uncontrolled body movements, balance and co-ordination problems Repeated fits or seizures, drooling and swallowing difficulties Some people with the condition may have communication and learning difficulties	The white-matter part of the brain is responsible for communication between the movement and thought-processing sections of the brain. Brain damage can be caused in the womb or during labour by a reduction in the child's blood or oxygen supply, which damages the brain cells, with serious consequences as the white matter is responsible for transmitting signals from the brain to the muscles Abnormal development of the brain can lead to problems in transmitting information to muscles
Cause: Birth injury is thought to be a cause in about 10% of cases – this is where the baby is deprived of oxygen temporarily during a difficult or premature birth. Other causes can be an infection caught by the mother during pregnancy or mutated genes that affect the brain's development before birth	

Degenerative conditions

These are conditions that progress continually and cannot be cured as the individual's body increasingly deteriorates over a period of time. Motor neurone disease, multiple sclerosis, emphysema and coronary heart disease are examples. These are described above in the tables detailing chronic and neurological conditions. Further examples of degenerative conditions are described in the tables that follow

Table 14.10 Type II diabetes

Symptoms	Biological explanation
Feeling very thirsty, feeling very tired, urinating more often than usual, especially at night Unexplained weight loss, cuts or wounds that heal slowly, blurred vision Frequent episodes of thrush A common cause of vision loss and blindness, kidney failure and lower limb amputation	Insulin is a hormone produced by the pancreas, a large gland found behind the stomach; insulin controls the body's glucose levels by moving glucose from the blood into body cells, where it is converted into energy. Type II diabetes occurs when the body's production of insulin is insufficient to control glucose levels; this means that glucose stays in the blood and is not used as fuel for energy. Untreated diabetes can cause organ damage
Cause: Being overweight or obese is a risk factor; it has been found that fat around the abdomen releases chemicals that can upset the body's cardiovascular and metabolic systems Having a relative with Type II diabetes is also a risk factor – the closer the relative, the greater the risk. An individual's risk of developing diabetes increases with age; this may be because people gain weight and exercise less as they get older. It has been found that people of south Asian, Chinese or black African and African-Caribbean origin are more likely to develop diabetes	

Table 14.11 Osteoarthritis

Symptoms	Biological explanation
Joints become painful and stiff, most often in the knees, hips and small joints of the hands. There is joint tenderness and increased pain if the joint has not moved in a while. There can be a cracking noise or grating sensation of the joint, and a limited range of movement in the joint. Joints can appear more 'knobbly' than usual	General wear and tear of the joints is usually repaired by the body unnoticed, but with osteoarthritis the cartilage can be lost, bony growths develop and the area can become inflamed. Cartilage is a firm, rubbery material that covers the ends of the bones in normal joints. Its function is to reduce friction in the joints – it works as a 'shock absorber' and allows the joints to move smoothly. With osteoarthritis the cartilage becomes stiff, loses elasticity and may wear away over time. As the cartilage deteriorates, tendons and ligaments stretch and eventually the bones can rub against one another, causing pain
Cause: Though sometimes called 'wear and tear arthritis' it is not a normal part of ageing, but the risk of developing the condition increases as an individual gets older and in some cases it runs in families Being overweight or obese puts excess strain on the weight-bearing joints, so osteoarthritis can be more severe in obese people Osteoarthritis can develop in a joint damaged by an injury or operation; if the joint is not given enough time to heal after an operation or injury it may be affected by osteoarthritis in later life	

Table 14.12 Osteoporosis

Symptoms	Biological explanation
Often there are no obvious symptoms until a minor fall or a sudden impact causes a fracture; the most common fractures are of the wrist, hip and vertebrae (spinal bones) In some cases, a cough or sneeze can cause a rib fracture or partial collapse of a vertebrae, which can lead to curvature of the spine and loss of height	It is due to a loss of protein matrix from the bone resulting in a loss of bone density, weakening bones. Bones naturally become thinner with age, in particular in women, who lose bone rapidly in the first few years of the menopause; this is because the hormone oestrogen (which promotes bone formation) declines after the menopause
Cause: Losing bone density is a normal part of the ageing process, but in some cases it can lead to osteoporosis. Risk factors for developing the condition are a family history of the condition or of hip fractures, heavy drinking and smoking, having an eating disorder such as bulimia or anorexia, and long-term use of certain medications that affect bone strength, such as some of those used to treat breast and prostate cancer, or corticosteroids used for asthma and arthritis Other conditions can increase the risk of developing osteoporosis – for example, rheumatoid arthritis, coeliac or Crohn's disease, COPD and overactive thyroid gland. Women are at greater risk of developing the condition if they have an early menopause, a hysterectomy, or absent periods as result of over-exercising or too much dieting. Lifestyle factors such as diet and exercise can determine how healthy bones are	

Autoimmune conditions

An autoimmune condition is when the immune system, which fights infection, mistakes part of the body for a threat and attacks it. Multiple sclerosis is an autoimmune condition (see Table 14.6). Further examples are described in the tables that follow.

Table 14.13 Coeliac disease

Symptoms	Biological explanation
Indigestion, stomach pain, bloating, flatulence, diarrhoea or constipation, anaemia and loss of appetite Feeling tired all the time as a result of malnutrition Children not growing at the expected rate, and adults experiencing weight loss	The immune system mistakes gliadin, a substance found in gluten, as a threat to the body and so attacks it; this causes damage to the villi (tiny projections lining the small intestine); the antibodies cause the surface of the intestine to become inflamed and the villi are flattened so the body's ability to absorb nutrients is disrupted Villi normally help nutrients from food to be absorbed through the small intestine walls into the bloodstream. It is not a food allergy or a gluten intolerance. It is an autoimmune response where healthy substances are mistaken for harmful ones and the body produces antibodies against them
Cause: It often runs in families; if someone has a close relative with the condition their chance of developing it is higher. Research has shown that it is strongly associated with a number of genetic mutations that affect a group of genes (HLA-DQ genes), which are responsible for the development of the immune system. These mutated genes are, however, very common and so it is thought that environmental factors must trigger the condition in certain individuals. There is evidence that introducing gluten into a baby's diet before six months may increase their risk of developing the condition	

Table 14.14 Rheumatoid arthritis

Symptoms	Biological explanation
Symptoms vary from person to person; they may come and go, and change over time Throbbing pain and aching, stiff joints, which can swell and become hot and tender to touch Firm swellings called rheumatoid nodules can also develop under the skin around affected joints	The immune system mistakenly attacks the cells that line the joints The synovial membrane that lines and lubricates the joint becomes inflamed and sore; this inflammation gradually destroys the cartilage As scar tissue replaces the cartilage, the joint becomes misshapen and rigid
Cause: The exact cause of rheumatoid arthritis is not yet known. One theory is that a virus or infection triggers the condition. This causes an autoimmune response in which the body sends antibodies to the lining of the joints where they attack the tissue surrounding the joint. The risk of developing the condition may be increased by smoking and by hormones; it is more common in women due to their higher oestrogen levels. It could be inherited although this risk is thought to be low as genes play a very small role in the condition	

Table 14.15 Nephrotic syndrome

Symptoms	Biological explanation
Swelling of the body tissues (oedema) High levels of urine being passed A greater chance of catching infections due to the loss of antibodies that are proteins Blood clots can occur because, with this condition, proteins that help prevent clots are passed out with the urine	The kidneys do not work properly, causing large amounts of protein to leak into urine. Loss of protein through the kidneys (proteinuria) is due to an increase in permeability of the filtering membrane of the kidney (the glomerulus) due to kidney disease (glomerulonephritis); this leads to low protein levels in the blood (hypoalbuminemia), which causes water to be drawn into the soft tissues, causing oedema
Cause: It can occur as a result of kidney damage caused by another condition such as diabetes, sickle cell anaemia, and infections such as HIV, hepatitis or syphilis; it can also occur as a result of certain types of cancer, such as leukaemia, multiple myeloma or lymphoma	

Genetic conditions

Genes determine characteristics such as eye and hair colour, but can also increase the risk of a range of medical conditions. Many of these conditions occur as a result of a child inheriting a specific altered (mutated) version of a particular gene.

Table 14.16 Cystic fibrosis

Symptoms	Biological explanation
Lung problems: recurring chest infections, persistent inflammation of the airways, coughing, wheezing, shortness of breath Digestive system: diarrhoea, diabetes and malnutrition because the body struggles to digest and absorb nutrients; jaundice A serious bowel obstruction in the first few days of life (meconium ileus), which will require an operation to remove the blockage	The condition is present at birth due to a defect in a gene on chromosome 7 that controls the movement of salt and water in and out of the cells in the body. The protein produced by the gene causes mucus-secreting cells to make a very sticky type of mucus instead of a normal runny type. This, along with recurrent infections, results in a build-up of sticky mucus in the lungs and digestive system Over the years the lungs become increasingly damaged and may eventually stop working properly. Average life expectancy is reduced for people who have this condition, although it is rapidly increasing due to advances in understanding about treatments
Cause: Both parents must have a copy of the faulty (mutated) gene. If only one copy of the faulty gene is inherited, a child will be a carrier but will not have the condition themselves	

Table 14.17 Muscular dystrophy (MD)

Symptoms	Biological explanation
There are many different types of MD; all cause muscle weakness but the areas affected, and the severity of the symptoms, are different; some cause severe disability and many do not, however some are life limiting A progressive condition, it begins by affecting a particular group of muscles before affecting the muscles more widely A child with Duchenne muscular dystrophy (DMD) may have difficulty standing up, walking, running and jumping; they may learn to speak later than usual, and have behavioural or learning difficulties	Due to gene mutations, the cells that maintain an individual's muscles cannot do so, which can lead to muscle weakness and progressive disability An example type is Duchenne muscular dystrophy (DMD). This usually affects boys. If it does affect girls, the condition is usually milder. It is a life-limiting condition that causes progressive muscle weakness due to the breakdown and loss of muscle cells The individual lacks a single important protein in their muscle fibres called dystrophin By the ages of 8–12, the children are unable to walk, and by their late teens or early twenties the condition can become severe enough to limit life expectancy
Cause: In most cases, MD runs in families; it develops when a faulty gene is inherited from one or both parents. Depending on how it is inherited, the condition can be a: • recessive inherited disorder • dominant inherited disorder • sex-linked disorder The NHS choices website explains these types of inheritance in detail: www.nhs.uk/Conditions/Muscular-dystrophy/Pages/Causes.aspx	

Table 14.18 Phenylketonuria (PKU)

Symptoms	Biological explanation
No usual symptoms if treated early. The Guthrie test is carried out on all newborn babies to identify PKU; the condition can then be controlled by diet If untreated: learning disabilities, behavioural difficulties, epilepsy, brain damage	It is a genetic metabolic disorder that prevents the normal breakdown of protein because of a defective enzyme. Enzymes are proteins that control and speed up chemical reactions. Lack of the PAH enzyme means that a chemical named phenylalanine, which is found in some foods, cannot be properly processed by the body. Only a small quantity of phenylalanine is required to ensure normal growth. As it cannot be properly processed it accumulates in the body tissues and affects the normal development of the brain
Cause: It is a rare genetic condition that is present from birth. For the condition to develop, the baby would need to have inherited two mutated copies of the gene – one from the mother and one from the father. PKU will not develop if only one mutated gene is inherited, but the baby will be a carrier	

Table 14.18 Down's syndrome

Symptoms	Biological explanation
Babies may have reduced muscle tone (floppiness called hypotonia); eyes that slant upwards and outwards; a small mouth with a protruding tongue; a flat back of the head; below-average weight and length at birth	Usually, cells contain 46 chromosomes; in individuals with Down's syndrome, all or some of their cells contain 47 due to an extra copy of chromosome 21; this error occurs spontaneously – it is not a result of anything the parents have or haven't done
Individuals with Down's syndrome have a reduced life expectancy; they have learning and physical disabilities to varying extents	This added genetic material causes the physical and developmental characteristics associated with Down's syndrome
Cause: One extra copy of chromosome 21 in a baby's cells causes Down's syndrome. The main factor that increases the chance of a woman having a baby with Down's is her age – a woman who is 20 when she becomes pregnant has a risk of 1 in 1,500, at 30 a risk of 1 in 800, at 40 a risk of 1 in a 100 and, at 45, a risk of 1 in 50 or greater	

KNOW IT

1 What is meant by the term chronic illness?
2 Name two chronic illnesses.
3 What do the initials COPD stand for?
4 State a lifestyle and an occupational cause of COPD.
5 What causes an autoimmune condition?

L01 Assessment activity

Below is a suggested assessment activity that has been directly linked to the pass and merit criteria in L01 to help with assignment preparation; it includes Top Tips on how to achieve best results.

Activity 1 – pass criteria *P1 P2 P3 M1*

You have been asked to produce an information pack about the impact of two long-term physiological conditions. The pack is to be used by a local charity to train its volunteers who work with individuals diagnosed with long-term physiological conditions. The aim of the pack is to provide the volunteers with the knowledge and information they need to understand long-term conditions, and details of the type of support that is available and best practice to support individuals.

1 Write an introduction to the pack that provides a summary of different types of long-term physiological conditions. **P1**
2 Choose two different long-term physiological disorders and produce a description of their known causes. **P2**

3 Describe possible symptoms of two long-term physiological conditions and provide biological explanations for the symptoms. **P3 M1**

TOP TIPS

Each grading criteria has a 'command' word. It is very important that the coursework you produce does what the command word says. For example, if you produce a description when an evaluation is required your work will not meet the standard required by the grading criteria.

The command words in Unit 14 are as follows.

✔ **Summarise**: requires you to give a statement of the main points. You will provide an outline covering the key facts, features or aspects of long-term physiological conditions. **P1**
✔ **Describe**: requires you to give an account that includes all of the relevant details and characteristics of the causes and symptoms of two long-term physiological conditions. **P2**, **P3**
✔ **Explain**: requires more depth and detail than a description. You will include details of the biological reasons for symptoms of two long-term physiological conditions. **M1**

LO2 Understand effects of long-term physiological conditions *P4 P5 P6 P7 M2 D1*

(10 minutes)

Think about a time when you were ill – for example, with a cold or flu, a broken arm or nausea. Ask yourself the following questions.

- How did your normal daily life change while you were ill?
- Were there things you could not do for a while?
- Were there things you had to do differently?
- Did someone have to help you do things you normally do for yourself?
- Did you have to take a course of medication or have treatment of some kind? Did it have side effects?
- How did it affect your emotional, social and mental wellbeing?

Share your experiences with the group.

2.1 Daily effects

Long-term physiological conditions can have a profound impact on the physical, emotional, social and mental wellbeing of individuals, as they may require help and support with many aspects of daily living. It can become extremely difficult to maintain independence and carry on with daily routines and relationships. Some of the aspects of daily life affected are shown in Figure 14.1.

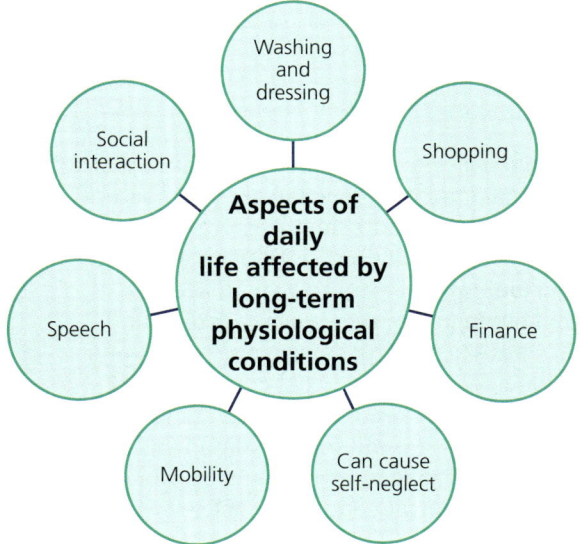

▲ **Figure 14.1** Aspects of daily life affected by long-term physiological conditions

The impact of being diagnosed with a long-term condition is to some extent condition-specific; however, a chronic illness, for example, may limit an individual's ability to carry on working, so they may have to give up their job. This can result in financial problems, and lead to worry, depression and/or worsening of their overall health and wellbeing. The family may have to assist the individual to carry out daily living activities such as washing and dressing, as well as provide emotional support. Over time this can lead to deterioration of family relationships. The individual may not ask for help because they don't want to be thought of as a burden on their family, and this could lead to self-neglect and a poor quality of life if they cannot do certain activities of daily living for themselves. It is a huge adjustment for an individual, and their family, to realise that they may not be able to fully look after themselves or live life as independently as they used to. They may also have to live with pain and fatigue or other symptoms that can be physically and mentally exhausting, having a negative effect on the individual's psychological wellbeing.

Further detailed information can be found in LO4 Unit 22 (page 296), which examines both the negative and positive impacts of requiring care.

? THINK ABOUT IT

What do you say?

Finola cares for her husband. He was an academic, a writer, a sportsman and a loving partner, but those parts of his life have now been lost as a result of the effects of a stroke. Now, Finola even has to speak for him.

Listen to Finola Marks' story using the following link: www.patientvoices.org.uk/flv/0542pv384.htm

Figure 14.2 shows a word cloud of Finola's story. It includes the words she used most frequently. Use some of the words from the cloud as headings to write an explanation of the impact her husband's condition has had on both their daily lives.

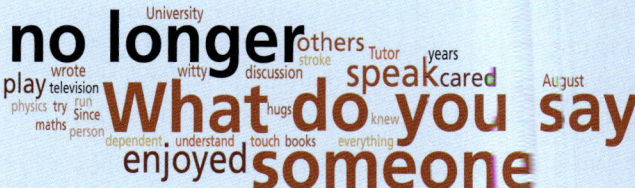

Figure 14.2 Finola's word cloud

Many other patients' and carers' stories about their experience of long-term conditions can be found on the Patient Voices website at: www.patientvoices.org.uk/stories.htm

2.2 Ways of monitoring

A variety of diagnostic techniques can be used to check, test and monitor an individual's body functions, and to diagnose and assess their condition.

Clinical observation

This is using diagnostic techniques to examine how an individual is functioning.

Body fluid tests

These involve taking samples of body fluids such as blood and spinal fluid. The samples are tested to detect dysfunction or chemical imbalance, to provide an indication of potential problems or the effectiveness of treatments. Blood tests are used if abnormal chemistry can be measured – for example, in diabetes – or to look for chemical markers of muscle weakness in motor neurone disease (MND). A lumbar puncture obtains spinal fluid that can be analysed for chemicals that are in the fluid that protects the brain and spinal cord. This test can detect a range of conditions, such as an inflammation of the nerves, damage to bones and problems with blood flow, as well as excluding other conditions.

Electrocardiogram (ECG)

An electrocardiogram is a test to check the rhythm and electrical activity of the heart. Sensors are attached to the skin and detect electrical signals produced by the heart each time it beats. The signals are recorded by a machine and then checked to see if there is anything unusual. An ECG can help to detect coronary heart disease where the blood supply is blocked or restricted by a build-up of fatty deposits.

X-rays

This diagnostic imaging technique gives a visual image of changes within a body system. Conditions such as arthritis, for example, can be seen in X-rays as erosions on the surface of bones.

MRI and CT scans

An **MRI scan** can – in the case of MND or Alzheimer's, for example – give a detailed image of the inside of the brain and spinal cord. It can take 15–90 minutes depending on the size of the area being scanned. The individual has to lie very still throughout the scan.

A **CT scan** is where several X-rays of the brain are taken at several different angles and a computer then puts the images together. A special dye has to be injected or taken as a drink before the scan. The scan takes 10–20 minutes, during which the individual has to lie very still.

Ultrasound

Ultrasound uses sound waves to examine internal organs and tissues such as the liver, kidneys and heart. A lubricating gel is used on the skin to allow smooth movement of a small hand-held probe, which is moved over the body part that is being examined.

Endoscopy

This procedure examines unusual symptoms such as difficulty swallowing and persistent abdominal pain. The inside of the body is examined using a long, flexible tube called an endoscope. The tube has a light and a video camera at one end. Endoscopes are inserted into the body through a natural opening such as the mouth or anus, or through a small surgical cut in the skin (keyhole). This can be uncomfortable so a local anaesthetic or sedative may be given. It takes around an hour to carry out.

Neurological assessment

For a condition such as MND, electromyography (EMG) is used to measure the electrical activity in the muscles to assess how well the motor neurones are working with the muscles. A nerve conduction test measures how quickly the nerves are conducting electrical signals.

Cognitive testing

This is used to help diagnose Alzheimer's, and to help assess its progression and severity. An individual's mental abilities may be tested and monitored using an MMSE (mini mental state examination). The MMSE tests a number of mental abilities, including memory, attention and language. This test involves, for example, memorising a list of objects, or naming the correct day of the week, month and year.

Spirometry

This test measures the breathing capacity of the lungs to diagnose and monitor a range of lung conditions, such as asthma, COPD and cystic fibrosis. It is also used as a standard check of general health for those with rheumatoid arthritis. The test measures the volume of air expired (breathed out) in total, and the force of the expiration in the first second of breathing out. The individual will have a clip on their nose, inhale and blow into a mouthpiece and then repeat this at least three times. The test takes between 30 and 90 minutes.

2.3 Treatment

A wide range of different types of treatment is available to address the symptoms experienced by those individuals with a long-term physiological condition. Some of the treatments involve medication or action that deals physically with symptoms. Other types of treatment may support the individual emotionally, helping improve their general sense of wellbeing and ability to cope with the changes the condition has caused. All the treatments aim to help the individual to maintain some independence and control over their lives, even if their long-term condition cannot be cured.

PAIRS ACTIVITY

(20 minutes)

Read 'Hip operation – Norman's Story', which can be accessed via the following link:

www.nhs.uk/Conditions/surgery/Pages/Normans-story.aspx

Work in pairs to discuss:

- how Norman coped with his need to have an operation
- the impact of the treatment on his osteoarthritis.

Drug therapy

Drugs can be administered in tablet or capsule form, or delivered directly into the bloodstream by intravenous drip or injection. Drugs may be used for a variety of reasons – for example, to kill pain, to replace missing chemicals such as insulin for diabetics, to get rid of fluid from heart failure or to slow the heart rate.

Surgery

Surgical treatment involves a surgeon cutting open the body and removing, replacing or repairing the damaged part. Examples are hip or knee replacements, angioplasty (inserting a stent to hold a blood vessel open) and a kidney or liver transplant. Where possible, **keyhole surgery** is used as it means a shorter hospital stay, faster recovery time, less pain and bleeding after the operation, and reduced scarring.

KEY TERM

Keyhole surgery – minimally invasive surgery. A laparoscope is inserted into a small incision and relays images of the inside of the abdomen or pelvis to a television monitor so that the surgeon can see the operation without exposing the area.

Physiotherapy

This helps restore or improve movement, mobility or function of the body. It consists of exercises, manipulation and massage on specific parts of the body or for movement of the whole body. It is used for a wide variety of conditions, including those relating to bones and joints, heart and circulation (such as, after a heart attack, the brain or nervous system), movement problems due to MS, and also lungs and breathing (such as COPD and cystic fibrosis). Massage is also used to improve quality of life for those with long-term conditions by reducing anxiety and improving sleep quality.

Complementary and alternative therapies (CAMs)

This term covers a range of treatments and medicines such as acupuncture, homeopathy, chiropractic, herbalism, meditation, colonic irrigation and aromatherapy. The NHS has recommended use of the Alexander Technique for Parkinson's disease, and acupuncture for persistent low back pain.

Occupational therapy

An occupational therapist will assess an individual to identify any difficulties they may be having with daily tasks such as dressing, bathing or shopping. The aim is to help the individual maintain their independence by providing equipment, adaptions to the home, or devices and strategies for doing an activity differently, to make tasks easier. For example, someone with rheumatoid arthritis may find it hard to prepare food or to get out of the bath, so a wide-handled vegetable peeler and grab rails in the bathroom could be provided to make such tasks easier.

Stem cells

These have the potential to make many copies of themselves (self-renewal) and to produce specialised cells (differentiation). Research is under way into specialised stem cells that could be used in the future to repair myelin sheath damage in MS and damage to the heart after a heart attack. Stem cell or bone marrow transplants are already used to treat conditions affecting the blood cells, such as leukaemia and lymphoma. A stem cell transplant involves destroying any unhealthy blood cells and replacing them with stem cells. This is a complicated procedure with significant risks and side effects, requiring preparatory treatment as well as a hospital stay and follow-up treatment for several weeks.

Physical activity

Exercise strengthens muscles and the cardiovascular system, and so helps prevent or reduce the impact of heart disease, diabetes and obesity. It also induces feelings of wellbeing, which can help mental health.

Counselling

Talking therapy allows an individual to talk about their problems and feelings in a safe and supportive environment. The counsellor will listen with empathy and will help an individual to deal with negative thoughts and feelings. See also CBT and in Unit 22, LO1, page 281.

Diet

Advice on a healthy diet (e.g. less fat, sugar and alcohol) may be appropriate for some conditions where weight loss is beneficial, such as arthritic knee or hip joints, coronary heart disease and diabetes. Coeliac disease requires the individual to follow a gluten-free diet. Other diseases may require vitamin or mineral supplements.

Further information about the impacts of treatment can be found in Unit 22, LO3, page 293.

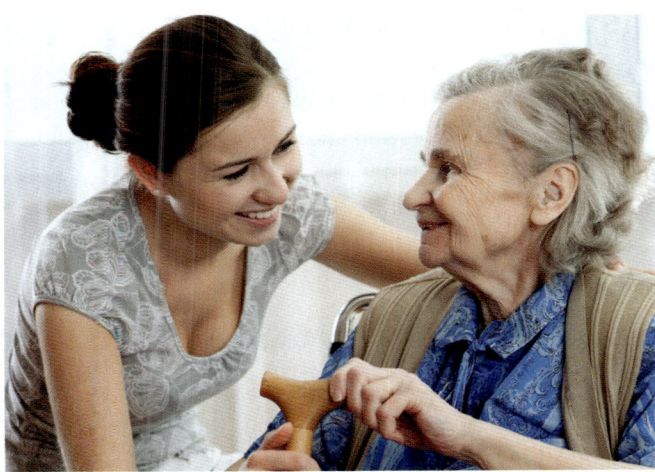

▲ **Figure 14.3** A person-centred approach is vital to effective care and support

2.4 Barriers to treatment

A barrier to treatment is something that prevents an individual receiving the treatment they need. Some examples of barriers are described below.

Resource availability; regional differences in service and provision

There are geographical variations in almost all aspects of care. Examples include variations in charges for disabled individuals' home care, NHS availability of the multiple sclerosis drug beta interferon, waiting times for NHS treatment, access to cancer screening programmes and availability of drugs for Alzheimer's disease.

Attitudes

Everyone has a different attitude to illness and nobody knows how they will react until they are faced with the possibility of having a long-term condition. In terms of attitudes being a barrier to treatment, some people may decide not to seek treatment because they are afraid that their suspicions that they have a long-term condition are correct, or they may feel that the condition or treatment has a stigma attached to it and they will be ashamed or think that people will treat them differently. Some individuals have a very stoic approach to life, 'get on with it' and try not to 'give in' to their symptoms, leaving it as long as possible before seeking medical support.

Culture

The society or groups to which the individual belongs may present barriers to treatment. For example, men may suffer from gender expectations that they should be tough and not make a fuss. A cultural expectation is that men do not talk about mental health, so some men don't behave proactively regarding their health in general and may avoid having the treatment they need. In some cultures, women will not accept treatment from a male practitioner. Jehovah's Witnesses do not allow blood transfusions.

Finances, travel and mobility

Attending regular specialist hospital appointments might involve time and cost. The individual may not have a car or may not be able to drive due to their condition. Public transport may not be frequent and may be expensive. The individual may need someone to accompany them if they have mobility problems, but there may be no one available. If treatment on the NHS is not available due to a long waiting list, the individual might not have the money to pay for private treatment. Being unable to work due to an illness reduces an individual's income as they may have to rely on state benefits. Further financial problems can result from delays in being assessed for benefits or receiving payments.

Occupational

Individuals may not want their employer to know that they are ill and so may not receive the treatment they need because they avoid taking time off work. Having some conditions may result in an individual losing their job if they are not allowed to do it with that particular condition. Individuals with long-term conditions may have to be medically assessed for fitness to drive – for example, those with heart conditions such as insulin-treated diabetes and unstable angina – and if, for example, an individual has symptoms such as fainting or loss of consciousness with their COPD. Some prescription medications can affect driving skills through drowsiness and impaired judgement.

Language and communication

Some minority ethnic groups may find it difficult to obtain treatment if they cannot find information in their own language. They may not speak English and so cannot explain what their symptoms are, and they may not know where to go for help. Other individuals may have difficulty communicating because of their condition – for example, a stroke or motor neurone disease can cause speech difficulties.

KNOW IT

1 Explain how the progression of an individual's COPD could be monitored.
2 What does MRI stand for?
3 What is MRI used for?
4 How could complementary therapies help an individual with a long-term physiological condition?

LO2 Assessment activities

Below are suggested assessment activities that have been directly linked to the pass, merit and distinction criteria in LO2 to help with assignment preparation. These are followed by Top Tips on how to achieve the best results.

Activity 1 – pass criteria *P4 P5 P6* merit criteria *M2*

For this task you will need to find two real-life case studies of individuals with the two long-term health conditions you focused on for LO1 Activity 1 (page 244). Use an authoritative source such as a charitable organisation's website or the NHS Choices website.

Write an additional section for the information pack you started for the previous activity. For each case study individual this section should provide:

- an explanation of the possible effects on their daily life of the long-term physiological condition **P4**
- a description of ways their long-term physical condition could be monitored **P5**
- a description of available treatments for their long-term physical condition **P6**
- an analysis of the impact on the individual's life of current monitoring and treatment of the long-term physiological condition. **M2**

TOP TIPS

- ✔ Make sure you include relevant reasons for the effects on daily life of the two long-term physiological conditions. **P4**
- ✔ Include all of the relevant details and characteristics of ways of monitoring and types of treatment available for two long-term physiological conditions. **P5**, **P6**
- ✔ Ensure you separate the information about monitoring and treatment to examine it methodically and in detail, in order to explain and interpret it. **M2**

Activity 2 – pass criteria *P7* distinction criteria *D1*

Based on your two case studies, produce a discussion document to be used at a staff meeting with the volunteers about barriers to accessing care. Your document should:

- explain two barriers to accessing treatment for the individuals in the case studies **P7**
- make recommendations for removing or minimising the barriers. **D1**

TOP TIPS

- ✔ Make sure you include relevant reasons for, and causes of, barriers to accessing treatment that apply to the condition and individual you have researched. (**P7**)
- ✔ Provide advice and suggestions based on the specific barriers you have identified. (**D1**)

LO3 Be able to support individuals with long-term physiological conditions to plan their care and support *P8 P9 P10 M3 D2*

3.1 Current frameworks

National Institute for Health and Care Excellence (NICE) guidance

This guidance aims to improve outcomes for individuals using the NHS and other public health and social care services. NICE considers whether a treatment benefits patients, will help the NHS meet its targets – for example, by improving cancer survival rates – and whether the treatment represents value for money or is cost effective. It also provides evidence-based guidelines on how particular conditions should be treated, and on how public health and social care services can best support people, as well as information services for those managing and providing health and social care.

NHS Outcomes Framework 2015–16

This sets out the five outcomes that will be used to hold NHS England to account for its performance. Indicators for measuring success are given for each of the following five outcomes:

1 preventing people from dying prematurely
2 enhancing quality of life for people with long-term conditions
3 helping people to recover from episodes of ill-health or following injury
4 ensuring people have a positive experience of care
5 treating and caring for people in a safe environment and protecting them from avoidable harm.

Full details can be found at: www.gov.uk/government/uploads/system/uploads/attachment_data/file/417894/At_a_glance_acc.pdf

Tackling High Blood Pressure action plan

This is a detailed national strategy for the prevention, detection and management of high blood pressure. A copy of the strategy can be accessed at: www.gov.uk/government/uploads/system/uploads/attachment_data/file/404881/Tackling_high_blood_pressure_-_FINAL.pdf

Living Well with Dementia: a national dementia strategy

This strategy outlines three key steps to improve the quality of life for people with dementia:

1 to ensure better knowledge about dementia and remove the stigma that surrounds it
2 to ensure that people with dementia are properly diagnosed
3 to develop a range of services for people with dementia and their carers, which fully meets their changing needs over time.

A copy of the strategy can be accessed at: www.gov.uk/government/uploads/system/uploads/attachment_data/file/168221/dh_094052.pdf

3.2 Local service provisions

● Hospital trusts provide secondary care. This means that an individual has to be referred by their GP to the hospital for treatment.
● Commissioning groups were introduced by the Health and Social Care Act 2012 to enable local areas to have more control over the care services provided so that they meet local needs. The commissioning groups are GP-led bodies that commission most health services. Commissioning is the process of planning, contracting and purchasing the specific health and social care services required by a local area.
● GP surgeries are providers of primary care. They are usually the first point of contact (other than accident and emergency departments) for individuals who require diagnosis, treatment or referral to a specialist.
● Social services carry out assessments and then plan and organise the provision of personal care, protection or support services for individuals with needs arising from illness, disability, old age or poverty.
● Domiciliary care agencies are care providers, often private companies, or sometimes local authorities, who provide care assistants to help individuals in their own homes. They assist with daily living activities such as getting in and out of bed, bathing and washing, and preparing meals.

3.3 Practitioners

During a long-term physiological condition an individual may receive care and support from a range of different practitioners. Some of these will provide practical help and advice on how to manage their condition on daily basis, while others will be health professionals who provide medication and treatment for the symptoms of the condition. Examples of practitioners are listed in Figure 14.4. Details of their roles can be found on the NHS Careers website: www.healthcareers.nhs.uk

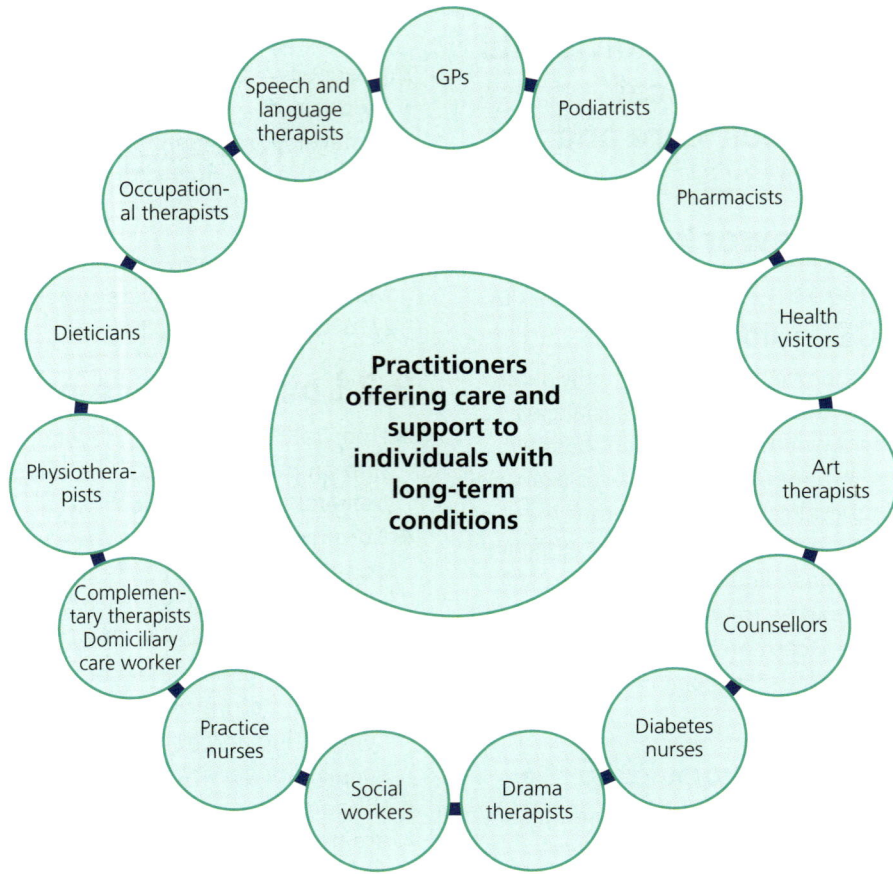

▲ **Figure 14.4** Examples of practitioners offering care and support to individuals with long-term physiological conditions

3.4 Third sector

The third sector includes voluntary and community organisations (both registered charities and other organisations such as associations, support groups, self-help groups and community groups), social enterprises and co-operatives. These organisations:

- are independent of the government
- are 'value driven', that is motivated by the desire to improve public welfare
- reinvest any profit in the organisation.

They aim to provide help and support for individuals and their families to cope with specific long-term physiological conditions. They provide information, advice and practical help – for example, from specialised care practitioners, hospice and respite care. They also provide opportunities for individuals with a long-term condition and their families to meet with others who have the same condition, to share their experiences.

GROUP ACTIVITY

(30 minutes)

Split into pairs or small groups. Each group should research a different third-sector organisation. Here are some links to a selection of third-sector organisations:

- www.dementiafriends.org.uk
- www.sueryder.org/how-we-help/care-services
- www.mariecurie.org.uk/who
- www.musculardystrophyuk.org
- www.mndassociation.org/life-with-mnd
- www.parkinsons.org.uk

Find out:

1 who the organisation supports
2 what type of support it offers
3 the benefits to individuals.

Share the information with the whole group.

3.5 Best practice to support individuals

Appropriate communication skills

Some examples are listed below, but more detailed information about using effective communication can be found in Unit 1, LO2 and LO4, pages 7 and 18.

- Empathy
- Tone
- Reflective listening
- Paraphrasing
- Use of SOLER, the key techniques for active listening
  - Squarely – how to position yourself in relation to the other person to show that you have a genuine interest
  - Open – how to maintain an open posture, e.g. uncrossed arms and legs to show that you are approachable)
  - Lean – the effects that leaning slightly towards the other person can have, e.g. to show you are interested
  - Eye contact – how and when to maintain eye contact to show that you are listening
  - Relax – the effects that being relaxed can have on the other person, e.g. to show that you have time for them

Removal of barriers to communication

- Avoiding technical language (see Unit 1, LO2.1 and 4.1)
- Inappropriate environmental conditions
- Assistive technology

Applying the values of care (respect, dignity, individual rights, confidentiality)

Detailed information about applying the values of care can be found in Unit 2, LO1.

Person-centred approaches

Legislation and national initiatives are focused on promoting and protecting the rights and needs of the individual. The values of care embed person-centred practice and ways of working to meet individual needs. This allows individuals using health, social care and child care services to say what is important to them, gives them more control and improves their quality of life. For more in-depth detail on person-centred care, see Unit 6, page 112.

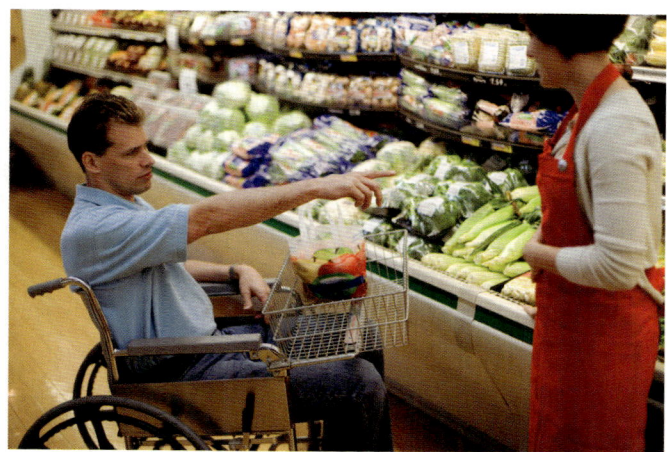

▲ Figure 14.5 Individuals with long-term physiological conditions can live independently in their community

KNOW IT

1 What are the five outcomes stated in the NHS Outcomes Framework 2015–16?
2 Produce a list of practitioners who may be involved in the care of an individual with cystic fibrosis. Describe their contribution to the individual's care.
3 Identify a third-sector organisation and explain the support it can provide for individuals with long-term physiological conditions.
4 Write a summary of using appropriate communication skills when caring for an individual who has Alzheimer's.
5 Why is a person-centred approach important?

LO3 Assessment activities

Below are suggested assessment activities that have been directly linked to the pass, merit and distinction criteria in LO3 to help with assignment preparation. These are followed by Top Tips on how to achieve the best results.

Activity 1 – pass criteria *P8 P9* merit criteria *M3* distinction criteria *D2*

Create a presentation, to be used for a training session for new volunteers. The presentation should be based on your previous case studies, and provide information about health and social care services that can support the individual's needs.

The presentation should:

- suggest local health and social care services to support the needs of the individuals and explain the purpose of that service provision **P8 P9**
- analyse the local service provision available for one of the individuals. **M3**

Produce a display for the training room noticeboard. The display should:

- provide an evaluation of the impact of one current framework on the support of individuals with a long-term physiological health condition. **D2**

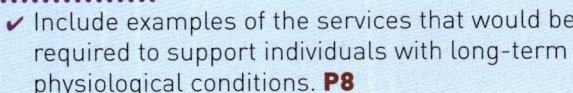

TOP TIPS
- ✔ Include examples of the services that would be required to support individuals with long-term physiological conditions. **P8**

- ✔ Make sure you give detailed reasons for, and purpose of, the services you have suggested for the individuals. **P9**
- ✔ Your analysis should examine in detail the local service provision available for one individual with a long-term physiological condition. **M3**
- ✔ Make a judgement, with reasons, about the impact of one current framework on the support of individuals with a long-term physiological health condition. Make sure you include different factors, which may be positives or negatives and strengths or weaknesses. **D2**
- ✔ Remember that your presentation needs to look professional and be suitable for the audience of volunteers.

Activity 2 – pass criteria *P10*

Write a script for a role play involving a volunteer and an individual with a long-term condition. The role play will be used as a demonstration to help give new volunteers an insight into best practice when working with an individual who has a long-term physiological condition. The role play script should be annotated to

- explain the importance of best practice when supporting individuals with a long-term physiological condition. **P10**

TOP TIP
- ✔ Think about how you can apply best practice when supporting the individual with a long-term physiological condition, including communication methods, choice of words, making appropriate suggestions and focusing on person-centred care.

LO4 Know about end of life care
P11 M4 D3

GETTING STARTED

(6 minutes)

Listen to this NHS 'Health Today' radio broadcast where Dr Richard Berman, consultant in palliative medicine, explains what is meant by **end of life care**: www.nhs.uk/video/Pages/health-today-radio-programme7-palliative-care.aspx

🔑 **KEY TERM**

End of life care – the care provided for individuals who are likely to die within the next 12 months.

4.1 End of life strategies and interventions

The following sections describe some examples of end of life strategies and interventions. There are many more on a local and regional level.

National End of Life Care Programme, Gold Standards Framework (GSF)

This approach is used to support the delivery of palliative care. If a patient with an advanced disease chooses 'comfort care' rather than 'curative' treatment, this is a trigger for **palliative care** to start. The GSF aims for every patient to have a 'good death' in the place of their choice (Thomas, 2003). The framework has five goals:

1 consistent high-quality care
2 alignment with the individual's preferences
3 pre-planning and anticipation of needs
4 improved staff confidence and teamwork
5 more home-based and less hospital-based care (NHS, GSF, 2010).

KEY TERM

Palliative care – an approach to providing care for individuals in the later stages of a terminal illness.

The GSF sets out seven standards of care to help achieve these goals. The standards are for: communication, co-ordination of care, control of symptoms, continuity of care out of hours, continued learning (promoting reflective learning), carer support, and care of the dying during the terminal phase.

A case study of the Gold Standards framework in action, as described by a GP, can be found on the Dying Matters website: www.dyingmatters.org/gp_page/dr-peter-nightingale-my-experience

NICE End of Life Care Quality Standard

This sets out how a high-quality end of life care service should be organised. End of life care is the care provided by the NHS for individuals who are likely to die within the next 12 months. The quality standard for end of life care is made up of 16 statements that describe high-quality care. The statements can be accessed on the NICE website: www.nice.org.uk/guidance/qs13/resources/end-of-life-care-for-adults-436888045

Commission on Assisted Dying

Members of the commission include a barrister, a former justice secretary and other experts, including doctors and a former president of the General Medical Council. It is funded by campaigners, one of whom was the author Sir Terry Pratchett who had Alzheimer's. The commission wants the law changed to allow assisted dying in certain circumstances: if the individual is over 18, is terminally ill and judged not to have more than 12 months to live. The individual must be making a voluntary choice and not be mentally impaired; they should be assessed by two doctors. Other countries, such as Switzerland, legally allow assisted dying.

CLASSROOM DISCUSSION

(30 minutes)

Divide into two groups. One group is to make the case FOR the right to die, the other group AGAINST the right to die. To help inform your class discussion, read the following articles.

- Assisted suicide: 'Strong case for legalisation': www.bbc.co.uk/news/health-16410118
- NHS website – arguments for and against euthanasia and assisted suicide: www.nhs.uk/Conditions/Euthanasiaandassistedsuicide/Pages/Arguments.aspx
- Q&A on assisted suicide: www.bbc.co.uk/news/health-16423206

Palliative care

This is defined by the World Health Organization as the 'active, total care of patients whose disease is not responsive to curative treatment. Control of pain, other symptoms and psychological, social and spiritual problems is paramount.' Many third-sector organisations, such as Marie Curie Cancer Care and Sue Ryder hospices and care centres, help to provide palliative care for individuals living with a terminal illness where a cure is not a possibility. The aim of palliative care is to help the individual and their family to achieve the best quality of life, offer a support system to help the family cope during an individual's illness, and provide support for the individual to live as actively as possible until their death.

Hospice care

This is personalised care provided by teams of professionals and also volunteers. Alongside taking care of the ill individual's physical needs they take a holistic approach, helping with their emotional, spiritual and social needs. They support carers, family members and close friends, both during an individual's illness and during bereavement. Hospices can provide a range of services in addition to pain and symptom control, such as complementary therapies, counselling, respite care, and practical and financial help. Most hospice care is provided by charitable organisations such as Marie Curie Cancer Care and Sue Ryder services.

Refusing treatment

Some people feel very strongly about treatments they do not want to have. For this to be legally recognised it is necessary for an 'Advance Decision to Refuse Treatment' order to be made under the guidance of a healthcare professional who is aware of the process. This is a legally binding document that must relate to specific treatments and circumstances, and will come into effect only if the individual has lost their capacity to make decisions. It is a voluntary process that should be initiated by the individual receiving care.

Advocacy

This is when a carer speaks on behalf of an individual unable to do so for themselves. This ensures the individual's views are put forward. Many charitable organisations, such as Age UK, will provide advocates for individuals with long-term physiological conditions. This can be towards the end of their life when support may be required to assist in decisions regarding issues such as continuing or withdrawing fluid and food intake or palliative care.

Euthanasia and assisted suicide

These are complex issues, with legal implications. Euthanasia in any form and assisted suicide is currently illegal in the UK. However, euthanasia is legal in the Netherlands, Belgium and Luxembourg. Assisted suicide is legal in Switzerland, Germany, Japan, Albania, Canada and in some US states.

Table 14.19 Terms used when discussing some end of life issues

Term	Definition
Active euthanasia	'A' performs an action that results in the death of 'B' Example: A doctor gives an injection of potassium chloride that results in the individual's death
Passive euthanasia	'A' allows 'B' to die. 'A' withholds life-prolonging treatment or withdraws life-prolonging treatment Example: A doctor withdraws treatment by switching off ventilator for an individual with end-stage motor neurone disease, who is unable to breathe
Voluntary euthanasia	When 'B' competently requests death himself, it is action that causes the death of 'B' at his request Example: An individual asks to be taken to a euthanasia clinic for a procedure that results in their death
Non-voluntary euthanasia	When 'B' is not competent to consent or object to euthanasia, it is the action that causes euthanasia Example: An individual in a coma receives an injection of potassium chloride with the intention to end their life in order to relieve suffering
Suicide	'B' kills himself Example: An individual takes an overdose of paracetamol with the intention to end their own life
Assisted suicide	'A' intentionally assists 'B' to kill himself Example: The wife of an individual who is bedbound leaves 40 paracetamol tablets by his bedside knowing that he will take them to commit suicide

(Source: adapted from Ministry of Ethics, 'End of life care' © www.MinistryofEthics.co.uk)

4.2 Regulatory frameworks

The government uses legislation to create regulatory arrangements for monitoring care organisations. It sets standards for service delivery and provides individuals with the right to access and receive care and support.

Suicide Act 1961

Suicide was considered a criminal offence until this act decriminalised it. Those individuals who attempt and fail to commit suicide are no longer prosecuted and sent to prison.

Human Rights Act 1998

This applies to all public authorities. A public authority is an organisation that has a public function, e.g. all kinds of care homes, hospitals and social services departments. Through a series of 'articles' this act sets out rights to which everyone is entitled. The rights most relevant to health and social care are:

- right to life
- right to respect, privacy and family life
- right to freedom from torture, inhuman or degrading treatment
- right to freedom from discrimination
- right to freedom of expression
- right to freedom of thought, conscience and religion.

GROUP ACTIVITY

(30 minutes)

Each group takes one of the human rights listed above and discusses practical examples of how health and social care settings could promote that particular human right while providing end of life care.

Share your ideas with the other groups, explaining how the law relates to supporting individuals' rights and the provision of quality end of life care.

Mental Capacity Act 2005

'Capacity' is the ability to make a decision. This act provides a legal framework that sets out key principles and safeguards to protect and empower those who are unable to make some of their own decisions, in particular regarding their end of life care. This includes individuals with Alzheimer's or who have had a stroke, for example. For more in-depth detail about this act, see Unit 2, page 32.

Care Act 2014

This act relates to those being assessed for or receiving social care, and their carers. It places a duty on local authorities to promote an individual's wellbeing. For more in-depth detail about this act, see Unit 2, page 36.

4.3 Ethics

Here are some examples of ethical issues relating to end of life care, where there is no clear 'right and wrong' action.

Palliative sedation

This is when an individual is given medication to make them unconscious and so unaware of pain. Many terminal illnesses can cause distressing and painful symptoms, and palliative sedation is a way of relieving suffering in the last hours of life. It is not intended to end an individual's life. Some critics, though, feel that it is a type of euthanasia because there is a risk it may shorten the individual's life. Others say that it is still ethical as long as it is in the best interests of the patient even though it has harmful side effects.

Food and fluid intake

Nutritional support can be given through a feeding tube, which can sustain life even when it is clear that there is zero prospect of the individual recovering from a terminal illness. The life-sustaining treatment is only prolonging the dying process. If an individual has made an advance decision outlining the care they want to receive or refuse, a decision will be made in their best interests based on their advance decision and treatment can be withdrawn. If there is no advance decision, and agreement cannot be reached, the case will go to the courts before any further action is taken.

Right to Die; assisted suicide; active and passive euthanasia; voluntary and non-voluntary euthanasia

See LO4.1, including the Classroom Discussion activity.

4.4 Morals

Here are some examples of moral issues relating to end of life care, when individual behaviours and beliefs may influence the outcome.

Societal views

- Doctors have an obligation to preserve human life, so many people believe that euthanasia is a violation of medical ethics.
- The doctor–patient relationship could be damaged if euthanasia became routine.
- Legalised euthanasia may discourage research into palliative treatments, and prevent cures and improvements from being developed.
- The 'slippery slope' argument is that euthanasia would lead to unintended changes to the way healthcare is approached, changes that we may come to regret. A concern is that once the NHS starts 'killing' patients a line has been crossed and a dangerous precedent set. Individuals who need constant care may feel pressurised to request euthanasia so they are no longer a burden on their family or on society with an NHS that is short of money and resources. Speeding up death could become routine, leading to a lack of compassion for elderly, disabled and terminally ill individuals.

Ulterior motives/manipulation

- An individual with a long-term physiological condition may feel pressured by their family into making a decision that is not right for them.
- An individual may be made to feel they are a burden on the family.

Religious views

- Followers of certain religions may believe that only God should choose when a human life ends, so they do not agree with extending life by using interventions such as feeding tubes or shortening life by assisted suicide.
- However, non-religious individuals may have similar beliefs based on the view that euthanasia and assisted suicide devalue life.

Eugenics

- This is the science of improving the quality of the human population by discouraging reproduction by those considered to have undesirable traits.

- Human genome editing is controversial; some think it is the first step towards 'genetically modified' babies.
- Once genetic changes have been made they will be irreversible and passed down future generations. This may lead to positive or negative results for humanity.
- However, one-year-old Layla Richards received a batch of immune cells that had had their DNA modified to seek out and destroy her abnormal leukaemia cells as well as being resistant to chemotherapy. Layla is well, and now back home with her family (source: www.nhs.uk/news/2015/11November/Pages/Gene-editing-breakthrough-in-treating-babys-leukaemia.aspx).

Personal wishes

A 'statement of wishes and preferences' allows an individual with a long-term physiological condition to have documented their wishes and preferences for future treatment. It may include where they would like to be cared for, what types of treatment they are prepared to have, and the reasons, beliefs and feelings behind their decisions. This should be taken into account when practitioners decide on an individual's future treatment options and it does have legal value under the Mental Capacity Act.

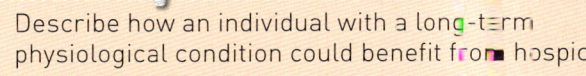

KNOW IT

1 Describe how an individual with a long-term physiological condition could benefit from hospice care.
2 What is palliative care?
3 What is the difference between passive and non-voluntary euthanasia?
4 How does the Mental Capacity Act protect the rights of individuals with long-term physiological conditions such as motor neurone disease?
5 State the meaning of 'eugenics'. Explain why eugenics is controversial.

LO4 Assessment activity

Below is a suggested assessment activity that has been directly linked to the pass, merit and distinction criteria in LO4 to help with assignment preparation. This is followed by Top Tips on how to achieve the best results.

Activity 1 – pass criteria *P11* merit criteria *M4* distinction criteria *D3*

Produce a handout for new volunteers about end of life care for individuals in the terminal stages of long-term physiological conditions. The handout should:

1 describe strategies and frameworks available to support individuals in the terminal stages of long-term physiological conditions. **P11**

2 describe moral and ethical conflicts surrounding end of life care. **M4**

3 summarise potential ethical and moral conflicts between individual choice and wider society. **D3**

TOP TIPS

✔ Describe in detail strategies and frameworks available to support individuals in the terminal stages of their illness. **P11**

✔ Give an account of the moral and ethical conflicts surrounding end of life care. **M4**

✔ Produce a summary that describes the main points about moral and ethical conflicts between individual choice and wider society. **D3**

✔ Remember, you must be objective when presenting different points of view, whatever your personal beliefs.

✔ You must provide a balanced summary that covers both the individual's and society's viewpoints.

Read about it

Fisher, A. et al. (2012) *Applied A2 Health & Social Care for OCR*, revised edition, Oxford.

Nicol, J. (2015) *Nursing Adults with Long Term Conditions* (Transforming Nursing Practice Series), Sage Publications.

Russell, L. and Roberts, C. (2014) *Introduction to Psychology for Health Carers*, CENGAGE Learning.

Thomas, K. (2003) *Caring for the Dying at Home: Companions on the Journey*, Radcliffe Medical Press.

Useful websites

BMA Quality and Outcomes Framework (QOF) guidance: www.bma.org.uk/qofguidance

Coeliac UK: www.coeliac.org.uk/home

Contact a Family – medical information: www.cafamily.org.uk/medical-information

Dying Matters: www.dyingmatters.org

Gold Standards Framework: www.goldstandardsframework.org.uk

Motor Neurone Disease Association: www.mndassociation.org

Muscular Dystrophy UK: www.musculardystrophyuk.org

National Kidney Federation: www.kidney.org.uk

National Osteoporosis Society: www.nos.org.uk/about-osteoporosis

NHS Health A–Z – Conditions and treatments: www.nhs.uk/conditions/Pages/hub.aspx

Patient Voices digital stories: www.patientvoices.org.uk/stories.htm

Unit 15

Promoting health and wellbeing

ABOUT THIS UNIT

Health and wellbeing are affected by lifestyle choices and these can have a positive or negative influence. People need to know all the facts so they can make an informed decision. Therefore, health education is vital to improve the health and wellbeing of an individual.

In this unit you will learn the reasons for maintaining a healthy lifestyle. You will be introduced to different health promotion strategies and examine government initiatives and legislation for a knowledgeable, healthy society. You will learn why local health improvement targets can differ from national targets and why health professionals may have different health messages depending on their target audience. Barriers that prevent individuals from changing their behaviour, despite receiving health advice, will be examined.

You will have the opportunity to plan, implement and evaluate your own health and wellbeing campaign.

LEARNING OUTCOMES

The topics, activities and suggested reading in this unit will help you to:

1 Understand reasons for maintaining a healthy lifestyle
2 Understand the use of strategies and campaigns and the roles of professionals in promoting health and wellbeing
3 Understand factors that influence responses to the promotion of health and wellbeing
4 Be able to implement and evaluate a campaign promoting health and wellbeing

How will I be assessed?

You will be assessed through a series of assignments and tasks set and marked by your tutor.

How will I be graded?

You will be graded using the following criteria.

Learning outcome	Pass assessment criteria	Merit assessment criteria	Distinction assessment criteria
You will:	To achieve a **pass** you must demonstrate that you have met all the pass assessment criteria	To achieve a **merit** you must demonstrate that you have met all the pass and merit assessment criteria	To achieve a **distinction** you must demonstrate that you have met all the pass, merit and distinction assessment criteria
1 Understand reasons for maintaining a healthy lifestyle	**P1** Describe the personal benefits of a healthy lifestyle	**M1** Analyse the impact on health of adverse lifestyle choices	
	P2 Explain the benefits to society of following a healthy lifestyle		
2 Understand the use of strategies and campaigns and the roles of professionals in promoting health and wellbeing	**P3** Explain health promotion strategies used by professionals when promoting health and wellbeing	**M2** Analyse the use of routine when promoting health and wellbeing	**D1** Evaluate the role of the media in promoting or influencing health and wellbeing
	P4 Describe the role of professionals in promoting health and wellbeing		
3 Understand factors that influence responses to the promotion of health and wellbeing	**P5** Explain possible barriers that prevent individuals from following advice on health and wellbeing	**M3** Discuss possible conflicts when promoting health and wellbeing	
4 Be able to implement and evaluate a campaign promoting health and wellbeing	**P6** Plan and carry out a small scale campaign promoting health and wellbeing		
	P7 Analyse the success of a campaign promoting health and wellbeing		

LO1 Understand reasons for maintaining a healthy lifestyle
P1 P2 M1

GETTING STARTED ·

(10 minutes)

Go to nhs.uk/Livewell/fitness/Pages/Whybeactive and follow the link for your age group. Do you do enough exercise each week to stay healthy?

1.1 Personal benefits of regular physical exercise

Physical

Weight loss

Combining exercise with a healthy diet is an effective way of losing weight. Weight is lost by creating a calorie deficit, burning more calories than the individual takes in, so undertaking activities that burn large numbers of calories is an excellent accompaniment to a calorie controlled diet.

Increased muscle mass and tone

Regular exercise tones muscles and helps create good posture, which puts less strain on muscles; poor posture causes many aches and pains. Muscle strength and tone, developed by regular exercise, will make daily tasks such as gardening and shopping easier. It will also help to prevent injury as good posture reduces the strain on muscles, **tendons** and **ligaments**. If muscles are not used, they will shrink.

> 🔑 **KEY TERMS**
>
> **Tendon** – a flexible but inelastic cord of strong fibrous collagen tissue attaching a muscle to a bone.
>
> **Ligament** – a short band of tough, flexible fibrous connective tissue which connects two bones or cartilages or holds together a joint.

Lower pulse rate

The pulse is how many times a minute the arteries expand and contract in response to the heart. It is identical to the heart rate. Individuals who are physically fit often have a low resting pulse rate and their pulse rate returns to normal quickly after exercise. This is because they have a large stroke volume (their heart can pump a lot of blood with each beat).

Larger heart

When exercising, the heart muscle contracts more often and more powerfully so it increases in size and strength. **Cardiac output** increases, so more blood is pumped out to the body by the heart. As a result, there is a lower resting heart rate with a quicker recovery time from exercise. The risk of heart disease is also reduced.

Increased lung efficiency

Aerobic exercise makes the lungs work harder as the body's need for oxygen is increased. The result is greater lung efficiency, which improves stamina and overall health. The stronger the lungs, the more oxygen the body has available and the easier it is for the body to recover and do what it needs to do to stay healthy. Lung capacity either shrinks or expands based on how active the individual is. Exerting energy in high-intensity sports, such as football, running, cycling, rowing, squash and hockey, pushes the body to the maximum and lungs will expand.

Increased bone density

While exercise is good for health, weight-bearing exercises are more beneficial in increasing bone density. These are exercises that individuals do while supporting their own weight (as opposed to sitting on a bike or swimming), for example using cross trainers, fast walking (outside or on a treadmill), **low-impact aerobics** and stair-step machines. Weight-bearing exercise is the keystone to an exercise-based programme for **osteoporosis**.

> 🔑 **KEY TERMS**
>
> **Cardiac output** – the amount of blood being pumped by the heart.
>
> **Aerobic exercise** – sustained, rhythmic activity that involves large muscle groups.
>
> **Low-impact aerobics** – slow and steady exercise, lessening the strain on joints.
>
> **Osteoporosis** – a condition that weakens bones, causing them to break and fracture easily.

Health

Reduced chance of developing obesity

Obesity is the state of being very overweight, with a body mass index of over 30. It is estimated to affect around one in four adults and around one in five children aged 10 to 11 in the UK (source: NHS website).

Obesity is generally caused by consuming more calories – particularly in fatty and sugary foods – than are burnt off through physical activity. The excess energy is stored by the body as fat. Obesity is an increasingly common problem because many modern lifestyles often involve eating excessive amounts of cheap, high-calorie food and spending a lot of time **sedentary** – sitting at desks, on sofas or in cars. Regular exercise reduces the chance of becoming obese.

> 🔑 **KEY TERM**
>
> **Sedentary** – inactive, not moving around a lot, tending to spend time sitting.

Reduced chance of developing Type II diabetes

See Unit 4, LO5.9 (page 82) for details about diabetes.

Regular exercise can help to lower blood sugar. The risk of developing Type II diabetes increases with age, perhaps because individuals tend to gain weight and exercise less as they get older. Maintaining a healthy weight by eating a balanced diet and exercising regularly can prevent or manage Type II diabetes.

Reduced chance of developing high blood pressure (hypertension)

This rarely has noticeable symptoms, but if left untreated it increases the risk of a heart attack, heart failure, kidney disease, stroke or dementia. Being active lowers the blood pressure by keeping the heart and blood vessels in good condition. Regular exercise can also help the individual to lose weight, which will also help lower their blood pressure.

Reduced chance of developing osteoporosis

This is a condition that weakens bones, making them fragile and more likely to break. Losing bone strength is a normal part of the ageing process, but for some individuals it can lead to osteoporosis and an increased risk of fractures

Psychological/emotional

Reduced stress

Exercise helps deplete stress hormones and releases mood-enhancing chemicals that help individuals to better cope with stress. Also, when taking part in exercise individuals are able to forget about their problems for a while and come back to face them feeling physically and mentally stronger.

Increased motivation

Exercise boosts energy as it can improve muscle strength and boost the individual's endurance levels. Exercise and physical activity deliver oxygen and nutrients to the tissues and help the cardiovascular system work more efficiently. Individuals have more energy and therefore more motivation to go about their daily lives and to try new things.

Reduction in depression

Exercise can help individuals with depression and prevent them becoming depressed in the first place. Exercise releases chemicals called endorphins that trigger a positive feeling in the body, usually accompanied by a positive and energising outlook on life.

Improved self-esteem and improved confidence

An individual who is successful in sticking with an exercise programme is likely to feel more confident about their physical ability to complete activities of daily living that involve a physical component, such as walking and lifting. Over time these feelings may extend to an individual's overall confidence as they experience enhanced body image and increased self-esteem.

Social

Increased social contact

Taking part in exercise allows an individual to catch up with existing friends and meet other people who also enjoy an active lifestyle. This common interest allows the individual to extend their social group. A team sport such as football or netball teaches co-operation and encourages players to bond. There is also the opportunity to appreciate others' efforts and receive praise from others in the team.

1.2 Personal benefits of healthy eating

Physical

Healthy skin

A varied diet with plenty of fruit, vegetables, whole grains and lean proteins can help the skin look healthy. The association between diet and acne is not clear but some research suggests that a diet rich in vitamin C and low in fats and processed or refined carbohydrates might promote healthy skin.

Improved immune system

A healthy diet plays a part in strengthening an individual's immune system, but an individual cannot just eat an orange or grapefruit and expect one quick burst of vitamin C to prevent a cold. A truly healthy immune system depends on a balanced mix of **vitamins** and **minerals** over time, plus normal sleep patterns and exercise.

Optimum organ function

Each body organ is adapted to perform a different function and make its own contribution to the body's overall health. Poor organ function and poor health can often be due to the body not getting the dietary substances it needs. (See Unit 4, LO3.5, page 72)

Weight loss

Eating a variety of foods can improve general health and wellbeing, as well help to manage weight. Individuals should follow a healthy eating plan such as the Eatwell Guide (Figure 15.1) and not starvation diets. Weight loss from a healthy plan will not be fast but it will be safer for the body as all essential nutrients will be provided.

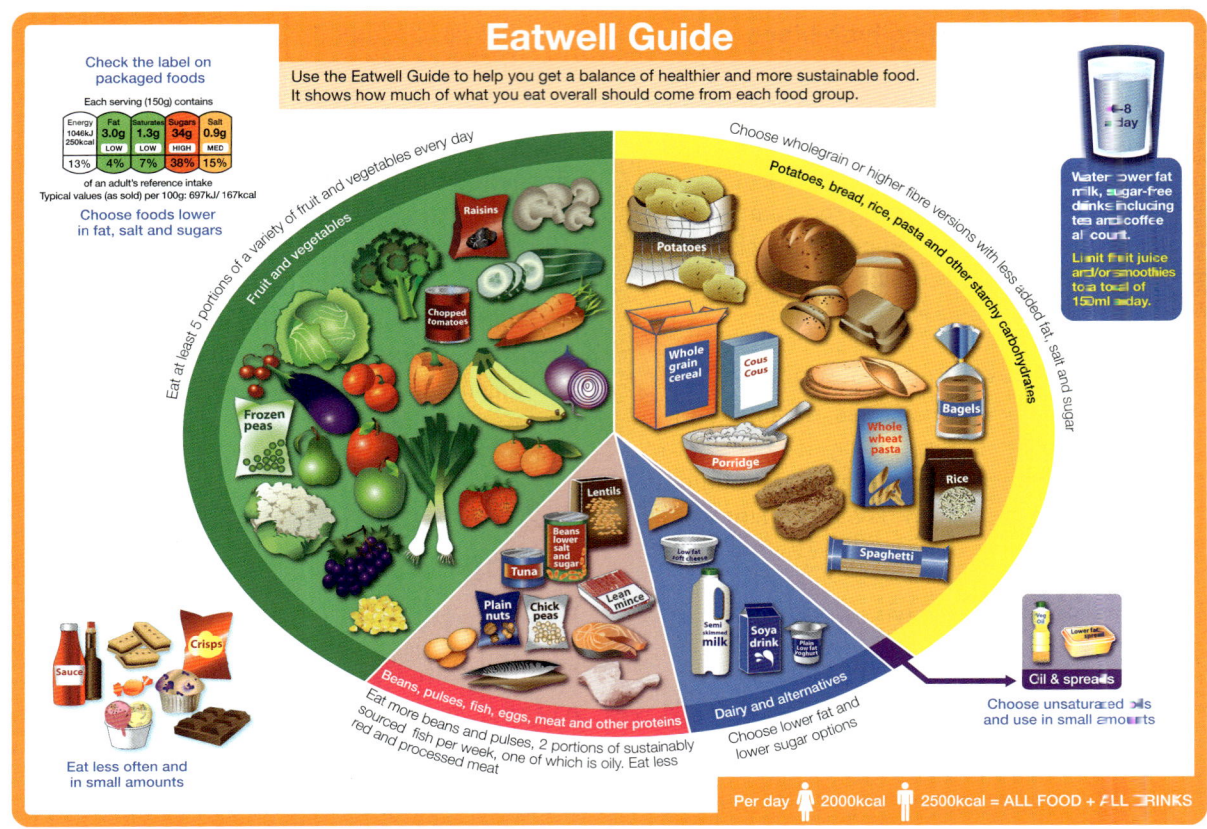

▲ **Figure 15.1** The Eatwell Guide shows the proportions of different types of food people should eat to have a healthy, balanced diet (Source: NHS)

🔑 **KEY TERMS**

Vitamins – a group of organic compounds that are essential for normal growth and nutrition, and are required in small quantities in the diet because they cannot be synthesised in the body.

Minerals – classed as micronutrients as they are needed in small quantities. They work with other nutrients so the body functions properly.

 PAIRS ACTIVITY

(20 minutes)

Examine Figure 15.1 and discuss with your partner whether you follow the suggested guidelines for a healthy diet. Explain why this simple diagram might help an individual who was struggling to remember which foods they should eat.

Health

Less chance of developing obesity

If individuals follow a healthy eating plan such as the Eatwell Guide they are less likely to become obese because they will be filling up with fruits and vegetables rather than high-fat, high-sugar foods that are full of empty calories.

Less chance of developing Type II diabetes

What an individual eats is the most important factor in preventing Type II diabetes. In a diet full of empty calories, quickly absorbed sugars and refined **carbohydrates**, cells slowly become resistant to the effects of insulin so blood sugar or **glucose** will remain at a high level. Over time, this can harm almost every organ in the body.

🔑 **KEY TERMS**

Carbohydrate – sugar and starches that provide energy for humans and animals.

Glucose – a simple sugar that is an energy source in living organisms and a component of many carbohydrates.

Less chance of developing high blood pressure

What an individual eats and drinks has an effect on their heart and blood pressure. The healthier their eating habits, the lower their blood pressure. If an individual does have high blood pressure, it is even more important to make healthy changes to their diet. A healthy diet can reduce the number of related medicines they need.

Less chance of developing osteoporosis

Eating a healthy, varied diet containing calcium and vitamin D can help prevent osteoporosis. Calcium maintains strong bones. Calcium-rich foods include leafy green vegetables, dried fruit, tofu and yoghurt. Vitamin D helps the body absorb calcium. It can be found in eggs, milk and oily fish.

Less chance of developing some cancers

Lifestyle factors, including the diet, can help to fight off cancer. Some foods actually increase the risk of cancer, while others support the body and strengthen the immune system Research shows that many cancer-related deaths are directly linked to lifestyle choices such as smoking, drinking, a lack of exercise and an unhealthy diet. Eating more fruit and vegetables can lower the risk of common cancers such as colon or breast cancer.

Improved fertility

It is now recognised by scientists that food and fertility are linked. If both parents-to-be stick to a healthy, balanced diet their chances of conceiving will be boosted.

Emotional

Improved self-esteem and confidence

Changing diet can help to reduce anxiety, boost mood, help the individual feel better about themselves and feel more confident. For example, eating carbohydrate-rich foods makes the brain receive more serotonin – a hormone that makes people feel positive, relaxed and confident. Foods or drinks high in sugar or caffeine, however, can cause mood fluctuations, which can leave them feeling lethargic, irritable and anxious. Some research also suggests that low levels of vitamins, minerals and essential fatty acids can affect mental health; for example, links have been seen between depression and low levels of **omega 3 oils**.

> 🔑 **KEY TERM**
>
> **Omega 3 oils** – well known for their health benefits and important for normal metabolism.

Improved concentration

The brain uses up about 20 per cent of the individual's daily calorie intake. Eating regularly – three healthy meals a day – is a good way to ensure the brain is supplied with sufficient high-quality nutrients to carry out its role. Good concentration depends on keeping the messages flowing freely between brain cells. These cells need oxygen from blood sugar to function.

1.3 Benefits to society of maintaining a healthy lifestyle

Table 15.1 Benefits to society of maintaining a healthy lifestyle

Benefits to society	Reason
Increased life expectancy	The average life expectancy for the UK has risen from 75.9 in 1990 to 81.3 in 2013 (source: *The Lancet*) because of an active lifestyle and a good diet. Individuals are able to work for longer and pass on their experience and knowledge to younger colleagues.
Reducing sickness and dependency	Those who have lived a healthy, active and busy life before retirement are more likely to stay fit, well and independent afterwards. This will save the state money for medication, hospital beds and social care.
Reducing cost of care	Healthy individuals are less likely to need expensive hospital treatment or need as much medication, e.g. statins to reduce cholesterol levels. They will not need to have a carer in their own home or to live in a retirement home.
Controlling communicable disease	People with healthy immune systems are less likely to catch a **communicable disease** such as influenza as their bodies will be able to fight it off.

> 🔑 **KEY TERM**
>
> **Communicable disease** – an illness spread through fluid exchange, for example sneezing or coughing, or contact with a carrier.

1.4 Adverse lifestyle choices

These are lifestyle choices that have a harmful or detrimental effect on an individual's health.

Smoking

Cigarette smoking is the greatest single cause of illness and premature death in the UK.

Smoking deaths are mainly due to cancers, **chronic obstructive pulmonary disease** (COPD) and heart disease. It increases the risk of **cardiovascular disease**, which includes **stroke** and heart attack, and leads to a build-up of fatty material (atheroma), which narrows arteries. The carbon monoxide in tobacco smoke reduces the amount of oxygen in the blood so the heart has to pump harder to supply the body with oxygen. Exercise is difficult as the individual becomes short of breath. The nicotine in cigarettes stimulates the body to produce adrenaline, which makes the heart beat faster and raises the blood pressure, making the heart work harder. Blood is more likely to clot, which increases the risk of a heart attack or stroke (source: British Heart Foundation).

🔑 KEY TERMS

Chronic obstructive pulmonary disease (COPD) – a collection of lung diseases.

Cardiovascular disease – a disease of the heart or blood vessels.

Stroke – a serious and life-threatening medical condition that occurs when blood supply to part of the brain is cut off.

Pancreatitis – a medical condition where the pancreas becomes inflamed over a short period of time.

Alcohol

When an individual drinks an alcoholic drink, the alcohol quickly enters the bloodstream, gets broken down and distributed throughout the body, affecting the brain and other tissues.

Alcohol can have an adverse effect on all of the body systems. Health risks include:

- cancers such as mouth, throat, oesophagus, larynx, breast and liver
- stroke
- heart disease
- liver disease
- **pancreatitis**
- reduced fertility
- diabetes
- depression and anxiety.

There is no guaranteed safe level of drinking, but the more individuals drink, the greater the health risks.

Drug use

Drugs are chemicals. Different drugs, because of their chemical structures, can affect the body in different ways. Some drugs can change the body and brain,

sometimes permanently. More deaths, illnesses and disabilities stem from substance abuse than from any other preventable health condition. Individuals who live with substance dependence have a higher risk of all bad outcomes, including unintentional injuries, accidents, domestic violence, medical problems and death.

Legal highs

According to FRANK (www.talktofrank.com), legal highs contain one or more chemical substances that produce similar effects to illegal drugs like cocaine, cannabis and ecstasy. In fact, many substances in legal highs have already been made illegal. They cannot be sold for human consumption so are often sold as incense, salts or plant food to get round the law. The packaging may have a list of ingredients but the individual cannot be sure that this is what the product will contain.

These new substances are not yet controlled under the Misuse of Drugs Act 1971 and there is not enough research on them to know about their potency, adverse effects from human consumption or when used with other substances or alcohol. However, many legal highs have been linked to poisoning, emergency hospital admissions, including into mental health services, and deaths.

Unprotected sex

Unprotected sex can have permanent and lifelong consequences because of the health consequences of a sexually transmitted infection (STI). Human immunodeficiency virus or HIV can also be spread during unprotected sex. The more an individual has unprotected sex with others, the more chance one of them might have HIV and the greater chance the virus will be passed on. There is no cure for HIV, but there are treatments; AIDS is the final stage of HIV infection, when the body can no longer fight life-threatening infections.

Unprotected sex can also cause pregnancy, which can lead to health issues in some women.

Overexposure to UV light

The most common form of UV light is UVA. In addition to natural sunlight, common sources of UVA include tanning beds and lamps. At low levels, UVA tans the skin and triggers the formation of beneficial vitamin D. Overexposure to UVA, however, can suppress the immune function, cause abnormal skin toughening and lead to cataracts. Potential consequences of UVB overexposure include sunburn, cataracts and the onset of skin cancer. Normally, the ozone layer in the atmosphere prevents substantial amounts of UVB from reaching the planet's surface, but the depletion of atmospheric ozone may increase the effects of UVB and increase the risk of skin cancer.

? THINK ABOUT IT (15 MINUTES)

Why do you think some people ignore advice about the dangers of using sun beds?

KNOW IT

1 Explain two physical benefits of regular physical exercise.
2 Explain two emotional benefits of regular physical exercise.
3 Explain two health benefits of healthy eating.
4 Discuss three benefits to society of maintaining a healthy lifestyle.
5 Describe the effects of two adverse lifestyle choices.

LO1 Assessment activities

Below are suggested assessment activities that have been directly linked to the pass and merit criteria in LO1 to help with assignment preparation; they include Top Tips on how to achieve best results.

Baz is a 26-year-old man who is careful about his food intake and has a healthy BMI. He does not smoke or drink alcohol. He goes to the gym three times a week and runs on the other four days. He also plays basketball and socialises with friends from the team.

His brother Max neglects his physical health. He eats a lot of takeaways and goes to parties instead of taking exercise. He often binge drinks and smokes but says it is only a social habit and he could give up any time. He likes to have a tan so uses his sunbed four times a week. Max boasts about the number of sexual partners he has.

Activity 1 – pass criteria *P1*

Describe the benefits of Baz's lifestyle.

Activity 2 – pass criteria *P2*

Explain how Baz's lifestyle benefits society.

Activity 3 – merit criteria *M1*

Analyse the impact on Max's health of his chosen lifestyle.

TOP TIPS

✔ Think about what is meant by a healthy lifestyle in terms of diet, exercise, drinking and smoking.
✔ When analysing, remember to separate what you have found out into different sections.

LO2 Understand the use of strategies and campaigns and the roles of professionals in promoting health and wellbeing *P3 P4 M2 D1*

GETTING STARTED

(20 minutes)

Are there any health promotion campaigns that have influenced you?

Why did you notice them?

2.1 Health promotion strategies

Behaviour change models

The health belief model (HBM)

This was developed to understand the failure of individuals to adopt disease prevention strategies or screening tests for the early detection of disease. It suggests that an individual's belief in a personal threat of an illness or disease, together with their belief in the effectiveness of the recommended health behaviour or action, will predict the likelihood of the person adopting the behaviour.

Ultimately, an individual's course of action often depends on the individual's perceptions of the benefits and barriers related to health behaviour. There are six constructs of the HBM (see Figure 15.2).

The Stages of Change Model

Also known as the Trans Theoretical Model (TTM), the Stages of Change Model is a model of intentional change. It assumes that individuals do not change behaviours quickly and decisively but a change in behaviour, especially habitual behaviour, occurs continuously through six stages of change. For each stage, different intervention strategies move the individual to the next stage towards maintenance, the ideal stage of behaviour.

Social Learning Theory (SLT)

This is the process by which an individual learns from observing others. Individuals are thought likely to model their behaviour on what they have learned from watching those around them. The best models are those that the individual relates to the most – often their peers or family members. However, some individuals copy the behaviour of media personalities, for example

CONCEPT	SCREENING EDUCATION EXAMPLE	COLON SCREENING OR TESTING
1. Perceived Susceptibility: An individual's perception of the risk of acquiring an illness or disease.	Individual believes they can get colon cancer.	Individual believes they may have colon cancer gene.
2. Perceived Severity: An individual's feelings on the seriousness of contracting an illness or disease or leaving the illness or disease untreated.	Individual believes that the consequences of colon cancer are significant enough to try to avoid.	Individual believes the consequences of having colon cancer without knowledge or treatment are significant enough to try to avoid.
3. Perceived Benefits: An individual's perception of the effectiveness of various actions available to reduce the threat of illness or disease or to cure illness or disease.	Individual believes that the recommended action of using faecal occult test would help to protect them from advanced colon cancer.	Individual believes that the recommended action of getting tested for colon cancer would benefit them by allowing them to get early treatment.
4. Perceived Barriers: An individual's feelings on the obstacles to performing a recommended health action.	Individual identifies their personal barriers to using the faecal occult test (e.g. too embarrassed to talk to their partner about it, feel the test would be messy, worried about the instructions) and explores ways to eliminate or reduce these barriers (e.g. a practice run before using NHS kit).	Individual identifies their personal barriers to getting screening (e.g. embarrassing procedure, will I know the staff, will anyone see me there) and explores ways to eliminate or reduce these barriers.
5. Cues to Action: The stimulus needed to trigger the decision-making process to accept a recommended health action.	Individual receives reminder cues for action in the form of faecal occult test arriving through the post.	Individual receives reminder cues for action in the form of reminder messages from NHS about screening. Sees 'Be clear about cancer' advert on television.
6. Self-Efficacy: The level of an individual's confidence in their ability to successfully perform a certain behaviour.	Individual receives training in using a faecal occult kit correctly from practice nurse.	Individual receives guidance (such as information on where and how to get tested).

▲ **Figure 15.2** An example of using the health belief model (HBM) to show an individual's approach to screening for colon cancer

1. Pre-contemplation

Individuals do not intend to take action within the next 6 months and are often unaware that their current behaviour is problematic or produces negative consequences. They often underestimate the advantages and place too much emphasis on the disadvantages of changing behaviour.

2. Contemplation

Individuals intend to start the healthy behaviour within the next 6 months. They recognise that their current behaviour may be problematic, so consider the pros and cons of changing the behaviour more thoughtfully but they may still feel ambivalent towards changing their behaviour.

3. Preparation (Determination)

Individuals are ready to take action within the next 30 days. They start to take small steps toward the behaviour change, and they believe changing their behaviour can lead to a healthier life.

4. Action

Individuals have changed their behaviour within the last 6 months and intend to keep moving forward with that behaviour change by modifying their problem behaviour or acquiring new healthy behaviours.

5. Maintenance

Individuals have sustained their behaviour change for more than 6 months and intend to maintain it. They work to prevent relapse to earlier stages.

6. Termination

Individuals have no desire to return to their unhealthy behaviours and are sure they will not relapse. Since this is rarely reached, and individuals tend to stay in the maintenance stage, this stage is often not considered in health promotion programmes.

▲ **Figure 15.3** The Stages of Change Model

footballers, pop stars and reality television stars. Learning in a social setting plays a critical role in how individuals gather information and adapt successfully to their environment, but it can also be how they pick up less effective, less healthy habits such as smoking or eating unhealthy foods.

Social Learning Theory (SLT) has been applied to many areas of health education, including the prevention of smoking, substance abuse prevention and violence prevention as well as sexual behaviour. Since SLT aims to change behaviour in the participants, it is a helpful theory to apply to prevention-based programmes.

Theory of Planned Behaviour/Theory of Reasoned Action

The Theory of Planned Behaviour is an extension of the Theory of Reasoned Action. Both theories suggest that an individual's behaviour results from their willingness to carry out the behaviour, which – in the case of smoking, for example – is a result of their:

- attitudes about the outcomes of smoking (or quitting), influenced by how they evaluate these attributes or outcomes
- **subjective** norms (general views) regarding whether other people important to them approve or disapprove of smoking (**normative** beliefs), influenced by how ready they are to comply with these wishes
- perceived behavioural control (how much control they think they have) over smoking when there may or may not be reasons to stop or continue.

In general, the more positive the attitude and the subjective norms are (towards stopping), and the greater the perceived control is, the stronger the individual's intention will be to stop smoking.

> 🔑 **KEY TERMS**
>
> **Subjective** – based on or influenced by personal feelings, tasks or opinions.
>
> **Normative** – relating to, or deriving from, a standard or norm, especially of behaviour.

2.2 Design principles

Information gathering/statistics

Before beginning any health promotion campaign, the Department of Health (DoH) identifies the need for a change of behaviour to reduce ill-health within communities. The National Census, the Office for National Statistics and data from hospitals across the country provide this information so that the focus for new health promotion campaigns is decided.

Consulting with appropriate agencies/organisations/people

People and groups related to the proposed health promotion campaign must be consulted before any action is taken or decisions made. These groups will have up-to-date information around the topic which may help a campaign succeed. For example, if a campaign aims to target older individuals to prevent falls it would make sense to contact Age UK.

Links to national campaigns

A variety of resources is produced for the national campaigns; therefore, it makes sense for local authority health promotion units to run their campaigns on the same dates as the national ones. This will save the local authority the expense of producing their own resources as they will be able to get the resources free from the national campaign. However, the health promotion must be relevant to that local authority.

INDEPENDENT RESEARCH ACTIVITY

(30 minutes)

Visit www.apho.org.uk and examine the health profile for your area. What would be a useful health promotion campaign for your local authority? Compare it to another local authority.

Setting objectives that are specific, measurable, realistic and acknowledge the starting point of the target group/audience

The objectives of the health campaign must be SMART and meet the audience's needs. So a campaign on healthy eating for a group of 10 year olds (Year 5) would be presented differently than to a group of 60-year-olds because of the prior knowledge of the older group.

- **S**pecific – a specific goal has a greater chance of being accomplished than a general goal. For example, educating Year 5 about the value of eating lots of fruit and vegetables is more specific than the general goal of educating them about healthy eating.
- **M**easurable – the Year 5 group's knowledge of fruit and vegetables can be measured with a pre-presentation and post-presentation questionnaire.
- **A**chievable – establish concrete criteria for measuring progress toward reaching each goal. The healthy eating project is achievable as it is not too broad in topic area.
- **R**elevant – identify realistic goals that are most important to the campaign. Eating fruit and

vegetables is realistic and relevant to a healthy eating campaign.
- **T**imed – a goal should be set within a timeframe, for example the presentation could last 20 minutes and take place before October half term.

Ethical issues

A health campaign must be run ethically.

- Rights of individuals – all individuals have the right to refuse to follow health advice. If their GP advises them to cut down on sugary foods and lose weight to prevent diabetes it is still their choice whether they follow the advice or not.
- Rights of others – even though individuals have the right to refuse to change their unhealthy habits, others who work with them, for example GPs, practice nurses etc., still have the right to encourage them to adopt a healthier lifestyle. Health professionals must always act in the best interests of others.
- Not doing harm – although not intentionally, health promotion specialists may do harm by encouraging fear and insecurity. For example, screening has the potential benefit of enabling early diagnosis of disease and successful treatment but it creates worry, anxiety and stress and, sometimes, results in unnecessary treatment.
- Confidentiality – everyone is entitled to confidentiality; for example, those aged under 16 are entitled to confidential sexual health and contraceptive advice and treatment without their parents or guardians being informed.
- Being fair and equitable – incentives to promote behaviour change should be consistent with patient-centred care, where individuals are given all the necessary facts. The health professional should treat the individual fairly and without prejudice, as it may be difficult for that individual to follow the advice however much they wish to do so.

? THINK ABOUT IT

Read the above information on being fair and equitable – what reasons might an individual have that make it difficult for them to follow health advice?

Approaches used

There are several approaches used in health promotion, as shown in Table 15.2:

Table 15.2 Examples of approaches to health promotion

Approach	Aim	Example
Behavioural/ preventative	To change individuals' behaviour through education and persuasion.	Give individuals information about the benefits of eating less processed food and more fruit and vegetables.
Educational	To empower individuals by giving them information and facts so they can make informed decisions.	Give individuals information about reliable, healthy ways of losing weight and they have to decide which is best for them.
Medical	To encourage individuals to use medical science to intervene in health and prevent ill-health; for example, screening.	Encourage individuals to go for screening to pick up early signs of cancer.
User centred	To help an individual who has identified changes they want to make. To help make them, usually on a one-to-one basis with a professional.	Individual wants to give up smoking and GP helps them by discussing the options. A plan is devised that best suits the individual, e.g. GP prescribes nicotine patches as individual thinks this would best for them.
Social	To change the law, for the social and physical environment, to benefit the population's health.	It is illegal to smoke in an enclosed public place or within the workplace.
Fear	To frighten the individual into healthier choices by showing the consequences of an unhealthy lifestyle.	Public Health England campaign featured a decaying roll-up cigarette and the claim that smoking rots the body from within.

Pre-set criteria/outcome measures

Criteria are decided before the health promotion campaign starts. Every campaign has an aim and objectives (see page 269) and its success can be measured by the achieved outcome.

Clear and accurate information communicated appropriately

Information used should be well researched and up to date. Materials for current campaigns can be borrowed from the local health promotion unit. However, the information must be presented in a format that is appropriate for the intended audience. A presentation on healthy eating for 8 year olds would not be suitable for adults as the language and content would be too basic.

Obtaining feedback from participants

The method of obtaining feedback from participants should be decided before the beginning of the campaign. Giving out both pre- and post-campaign questionnaires can indicate how successful the campaign has been. For example, on a healthy eating campaign it can be useful to find out the prior knowledge of the participants by giving them a questionnaire before the campaign and, after the campaign, the same questionnaire can be completed to check what they have learned.

2.3 Government papers/ initiatives/legislation

Saving Lives: Our Healthier Nation (1999)

This presents an action plan to improve the health of everyone, with those at most risk being particularly targeted. It puts forward a comprehensive government plan focused on the main killers: cancer, coronary heart disease and stroke, accidents and mental illness.

Every Child Matters

This was a government initiative, starting in 2003, outlining how different agencies, including care settings, can work together to protect children. There were five key outcomes from Every Child Matters:

1 Be healthy
2 Stay safe
3 Enjoy and achieve
4 Make a positive contribution
5 Achieve economic wellbeing.

The policy was dropped by the government in 2010 but the outcomes continue to be relevant to those working in health, social care and childcare settings.

Choosing Health

Choosing Health: Making Healthy Choices Easier was a 2004 government report that explained its approach to tackling a broad range of public health challenges from smoking, obesity and drinking to mental and sexual health. The key points are listed below.

- Make it easier for people to choose healthy lives.
- Help children and young people to be healthy.
- Help local communities to help people be healthier.
- Make health a way of life.
- Support the National Health Service (NHS) to help people be healthier.
- Help people to be healthier at work.

Smoking ban

It has been illegal to smoke in an enclosed public place and within the workplace since 2006 in Scotland and Wales, and since 2007 in England. This ensured that everyone could catch a train, eat in a restaurant or shop without suffering the negative effects of second-hand smoke. The ban now extends to no smoking in vehicles carrying children in England and Wales.

CLASS DISCUSSION

(20 minutes)

In what ways has the smoking ban had an effect on health? Explain your answer.

Food labelling

Manufacturers are encouraged by the government to have nutritional value labels on foods that can help an individual to choose between products and keep a check on the amount of foods they are eating that are high in fat, salt and added sugars. Some manufacturers use colour-coded nutritional information, which shows if the food has high, medium or low amounts of fat, saturated fat, sugars and salt.

- Red means high.
- Amber means medium.
- Green means low.

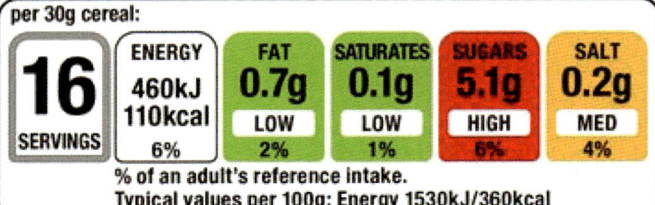

▲ Figure 15.4 Do you find nutritional labelling on food packaging helpful?

Alcohol units

The government now states there is no safe level of alcohol consumption, but the maximum, for healthy adults, is no more than 14 units spread across the week.

INDEPENDENT RESEARCH ACTIVITY

(20 minutes)

Are you aware of how many units of alcohol are in popular drinks?

For example, how many units are in the following?

- One pint of 5 per cent draught lager.
- 500 ml can of 7.5 per cent beer.
- 250 ml glass of 12 per cent wine.
- 275 ml bottle of 4.5 per cent alcopop.
- 25 ml shot of 40 per cent spirit.

Visit enjoyresponsibly.co.uk/unit-calculator to check if you knew the units in the above drinks. Which drink did you think had the most units? Has this changed your perception of alcoholic drinks?

Banning tobacco adverts

Most forms of tobacco advertising and promotion in the UK were banned following the implementation of the Tobacco Advertising and Promotion Act 2002 (TAPA). The law started with a ban on print media and billboard advertising, followed by a ban on tobacco direct marketing and sponsorship within the UK. The ban on tobacco sponsorship of global events – mainly affecting Formula One motor racing – was implemented in July 2005 (source: Ash).

2.4 National campaigns

There have been several recent national campaigns to promote health and wellbeing. Here are some examples.

Physical activity

This Girl Can is a national campaign developed in 2015 by Sport England and a range of partnership organisations. It is designed to get women and girls moving, regardless of shape, size and ability. The idea was to inspire women to challenge cultural assumptions about femininity that prevent them engaging in sport and exercise.

CLASS DISCUSSION

(30 minutes)

Go to www.thisgirlcan.co.uk and watch the video clip for the campaign.

Now go to http://tinyurl.com/lyoknqj

Do you agree with the comments from the *Guardian* that, 'This Girl campaign is all about sex, not sport'?

Diet

The idea of the public health campaign Change4Life, is for individuals to make many small changes to their lifestyle which will add up to a significant change. Eat well, move more and live longer is the catchphrase. Public Health England's One You campaign offers free tools and support to help people to put themselves first and do something about their own health before it's too late.

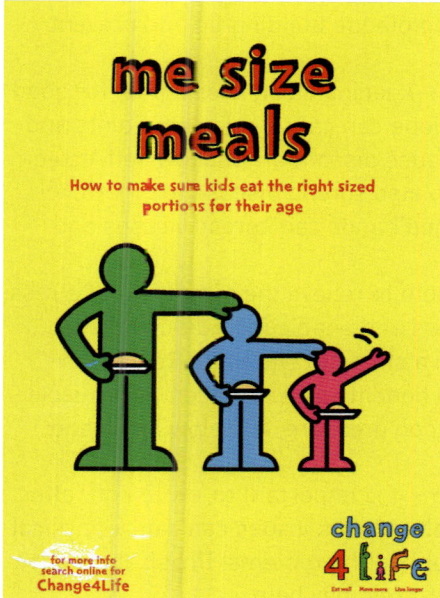

▲ **Figure 15.5** Does Change4Life encourage you to be healthier?

Smoking

One You provides information on ways to quit smoking, such as nicotine replacement therapies, e-cigarettes, free quitting tools and expert support from local NHS stop smoking services, so individuals can choose the best option for their lifestyle.

Heart disease

Cardiovascular (heart and circulatory) disease causes more than a quarter of all deaths in the UK (Source: British Heart Foundation). As a result there have been many different health campaigns linked to heart disease. All healthy eating programmes, exercise regimes, sensible consumption of alcohol and smoking campaigns are related to reducing deaths from heart disease. Change4Life emphasises the dangers of heart disease from obesity.

Diabetes

Change4Life also emphasises that obesity and eating a sugary, empty calorie diet can cause diabetes.

STIs

There have been many different sexual health programmes over the years. Current ones run by the Department of Health (DoH) together with the Department for Education (DfE) and the National Chlamydia Screening Programme (NCSP) include: Sex, Worth Talking About and Chlamydia, Worth Talking About. The NHS has a safe sex campaign – Condom or No Condom.

Mental health

Campaigns on mental health have aimed to take the stigma out of mental health conditions. It is now recognised that 1 in 4 individuals will have a mental health condition in their lifetime. The Mental Health Foundation organises an annual Mental Health Awareness Week to raise awareness of mental health and wellbeing issues. A World Mental Health Day every year also aims to raise awareness of mental health and wellbeing issues.

Alcohol

Alcohol has featured in many health campaigns over the years. The Drinkaware website (www.drinkaware.co.uk) has factual information about all aspects of alcohol such as highlighting the numbers of units in drinks, the dangers of children drinking and an app to reduce alcohol intake. The campaign called 'You wouldn't sober, you shouldn't drunk' aims to stop sexual harassment by people drinking in public places.

> **🔍 INDEPENDENT RESEARCH ACTIVITY**
>
> **Explore the usefulness of a health promotion app**
>
> Download the app from drinkaware.co.uk. Do you think this would be useful for you?
>
> Read the article from http://tinyurl.com/zkukzbx.
>
> Do you agree with the journalist's review of the app? Explain why.

2.5 Targets

In Saving Lives, Our Healthier Nation (1999), the government set the following targets.

- Cancer: to reduce the death rate in people under 75 by at least a fifth.
- Coronary heart disease and stroke: to reduce the death rate in people under 75 by at least two-fifths.
- Accidents: to reduce the death rate by at least a fifth and serious injury by at least a tenth.

- Mental illness: to reduce the death rate from suicide and undetermined injury by at least a fifth.

As a result, health campaigns often focus on these issues.

Local targets come from Public Health England, which collates health statistics for each local authority in England and uses the collected information to produce a profile of each area. The profiles give an overview of health for each local authority in England.

Profiles present a set of health indicators to show how the local area compares to the national average. They help local government and health services make decisions and plans to improve local individuals' health and reduce health inequalities. For example, if an area has a higher teenage pregnancy rate than the national average, reducing the rate will be a target of the local health promotion plan.

2.6 The roles of professionals in promoting health and wellbeing

The following professionals educate and give advice and support to individuals in relation to health.

- School nurses are often the first point of contact for students; easily accessible as they are in school during the day and their priority is to look after students' welfare. Services include providing health and sex education within the school, carrying out developmental screening, undertaking health interviews and administering **immunisation** programmes.
- Midwives are involved in pre- and post-birth care, in counselling, in offering support and education, and helping families prepare for parenthood.
- Dentists educate individuals to care for their mouths and teeth. Dentists will work with patients by preventing and treating dental and oral disease, correcting dental irregularities (particularly in children) and treating dental and facial injuries.
- Dieticians educate individuals about nutrition, enabling them to make informed and practical choices about food and lifestyle in health and disease.

🔑 **KEY TERM**

Immunisation – administering a vaccine to make an individual immune or resistant to an infectious disease.

2.7 Routines to support health and wellbeing

As well as healthy eating and exercise, there are many ways to incorporate healthy routines into everyday life. Here are some examples.

- Brushing teeth twice daily is necessary to keep teeth and gums healthy. If teeth are not brushed properly a film of plaque will form which will cause gum disease and tooth decay. Brushing every surface of the teeth will stop plaque building up and prevent bad breath.
- General hygiene – keeping clean is essential for good health. Poor hygiene can cause skin complaints and infections, and cause discomfort and low self-esteem. Poor hygiene can also spread disease to others, for example unwashed hands can spread viruses and bacteria.
- Relaxation can help to relieve the symptoms of stress, increase calmness and enable individuals to take a step back from a stressful situation. Relaxation has many health benefits as it can decrease muscle tension, lower blood pressure, and slow heart and breath rates.
- Working practice – it is important to 'switch off' after work. Worrying about work issues can cause physical as well as mental health problems. Physical exercise or relaxation exercises may help.

PAIRS ACTIVITY

(10 minutes)

Discuss with your partner how you relax after a stressful day.

KNOW IT

1 Explain two health promotion approaches.
2 Discuss the effects on the health of individuals of the Choosing Health initiative.
3 Discuss why national campaigns such as Change4Life change people's lifestyles
4 Explain how midwives promote health and wellbeing.
5 Explain why confidentiality is important in health promotion.

LO2 Assessment activities

Below are suggested assessment activities that have been directly linked to the pass and merit criteria in LO2 to help with assignment preparation; they include Top Tips on how to achieve best results.

Andrea is the school nurse in a large academy. Concerned about the number of students who binge drink, Andrea decides to have a health campaign on the dangers of drinking too much alcohol.

Activity 1 – pass criteria *P3* *P4*

Describe Andrea's role as a professional promoting health and wellbeing.

Activity 2 – merit criteria *M2*

Analyse the use of routine when promoting health and wellbeing.

Activity 3 – merit criteria *D1*

Do you think Andrea's campaign would be as successful as a national media campaign? Explain why. Evaluate the role of the national media in promoting or influencing health and wellbeing.

TOP TIPS
✔ You might find it useful to talk to health professionals to help complete activities 1 and 2.
✔ Think about the different job roles undertaken by health professionals.

LO3 Understand factors that influence responses to the promotion of health and wellbeing *P5* *M3*

GETTING STARTED
(15 minutes)

Can you think of any barriers that would stop you from following health advice?

Share these with a partner.

3.1 Barriers to following health advice

Location

Where an individual lives can have a huge impact on access to health promotion. For example, gyms may be hard to reach in rural areas because of a poor bus service. The cost of travel could also be unaffordable. Village stores may have fewer healthy food choices than a city supermarket.

Physical disability

It can be difficult for an individual with disabilities to access facilities, for example reaching the top of a flight of stairs with no lift. Adaptations may be insufficient to accommodate a wheelchair. The individual may need assistance to access the equipment and feel awkward asking staff to help. It may be expensive for them to buy their own gym equipment, for example, and they would need enough space to set it up.

Time

Many people take out an expensive gym membership at new year. Often, however, their good intentions soon slip as they do not have the time to continue. Work and family commitments may limit the time available to attend the gym.

Employment

Many people work long hours and are too tired to exercise or cook a nutritious meal so they pick up a high-fat take away on the way home and exercise falls to the bottom of their to-do list. Shift work too can spoil good intentions to keep healthy.

Income

If an individual cannot afford to buy good quality, filling, fresh food they may turn to fast food. Individuals in a low-income family often struggle to pay energy bills, rent and so on so they may have a limited amount of money left for food and exercise classes.

Culture

Culture can affect an individual's views on health promotion. For example, a woman's religion can prevent her from having cervical screening unless a female practitioner is available to carry out the procedure.

Education

Experts think education might help individuals to lead healthier lives (source: Marmot Review: Fair Society,

Healthy Lives (2010), www.instituteofhealthequity.org). Education may enable individuals to make better decisions that affect their long-term health because they are more likely to weigh up evidence presented to them and decide on a course of action.

Socio-economic status

Statistics show that the higher an individual's socio-economic status the more likely they are to live longer and enjoy better health than those with lower socio-economic status. This might be because they have a higher disposable income to spend on healthy food and activities, and better education.

Peer pressure

Younger individuals often change their attitudes and values to conform to their social group's expectations. This may lead them to take risks, such as misuse drugs, drive recklessly or binge drink.

3.2 Possible conflicts

Despite all the evidence for the benefits of healthy lifestyles, some groups benefit, usually financially, from people continuing to live unhealthily. Here are some examples.

Tobacco industry

For many years the tobacco industry refused to admit that smoking damages health, portraying smoking as a social habit for adults who are aware of the risks and choose to smoke for pleasure. It argued that the state should have no role in regulating its activity or its promotion. Obviously the tobacco industry's main aim is to persuade individuals to continue to buy cigarettes so its profit is maintained. The government also collects some of the money from the sale of cigarettes in taxes.

Food manufacturers

The food industry encourages consumers to buy profitable high-fat, high-sugar, low-fibre foods. If consumers are not educated about nutrition they often find it difficult to understand food labelling and how it fits into their dietary needs. The government has encouraged manufacturers to produce healthy versions of bestselling unhealthy foods, with limited success.

Alcohol producers and suppliers

A UK parliamentary group wanted alcoholic drinks to carry a health warning to inform consumers about balanced risk. However, the Portman Group, which was established by the UK's leading alcohol producers to promote responsible drinking, said 80 per cent of people drank 'well within' the government's recommended guidelines and that this proposal was therefore unnecessary. Obviously alcohol producers have an interest in playing down the health risks so that they continue to make profits from the sale of alcohol.

Media sponsorship

Since the implementation of the UK Tobacco Advertising and Promotion Act 2002 (TAPA) and laws prohibiting tobacco advertising in broadcast media, there has been no direct marketing for tobacco. Campaigners are now calling for the phased removal of alcohol sponsorship, for cinema advertising to be restricted to 18-certificate films and a TV watershed. The media are likely to resist this change as it will mean less revenue for them.

Costs of healthy alternatives

Research carried out at the Universities of Cambridge and East Anglia found that healthy food now costs three times as much as junk food. It also reports a sharper rise in the cost of fruit and vegetables from 2002 to 2012 compared to other types of food. Foods classified as healthier (such as fruit and vegetables) were more expensive per calorie than foods high in fat or sugar. Sometimes parents want food that will 'fill up' their children so although they know an apple would be healthier they buy a packet of biscuits for the same price.

3.3 Role of media

The media – newspapers, magazines, TV, YouTube, blogs – constantly present us with images. These may have a positive or negative influence on our attitude towards health.

Advertising and bias

Marketing and advertising are powerful tools to influence behaviour. It is the role of advertisers to sell products by persuading consumers that the item being advertised is desirable, whether they need it or not! A good advertisement can affect individuals' decisions but, when it comes to health, marketing and advertising have traditionally been dominated by industries promoting unhealthy habits and behaviours. In the past the media portrayed smoking and drinking alcohol as glamorous – rich, handsome, successful individuals smoked a certain type of cigarette.

Obviously advertising is biased towards the product it is marketing. Only positive aspects of the product are emphasised, to sell as many as possible, making money for the manufacturer and ensuring continued revenue for the advertiser.

EXTENSION ACTIVITY ➡️

(30 minutes)

Design an effective advertisement for a health campaign of your choice.

Depiction of ideal body form

Some men and women are obsessed by the goal of having an ideal body shape. Many younger people constantly worry about their body not being perfect. Men are often portrayed as needing to be toned and muscled. The media often shows women who are low in weight but curvaceous, which is difficult to achieve. Often the pictures have been changed digitally so not even the original model looked like this.

> **❓ THINK ABOUT IT**
>
> **Case study: Vanda**
>
> Vanda is 17. She did well in her GCSEs and is now in Year 12. She was slightly overweight at a BMI of 25.5 until last year when she started to watch what she ate and took up fanatical exercising. She stopped eating all her favourite foods and now eats only fruit and vegetables. Her BMI is 17 and she is trying reach her favourite model's BMI of 15. Her parents do not realise she is so thin. Her best friend is concerned as she has no energy and is always cold. But Vanda would like to be a size zero.
>
> Why do you think many girls are influenced by their favourite model, pop star or celebrity? Should models' bodies represent the average woman's body?

Promoting health advice

The cost of placing advertisements and using campaigns to promote health must be weighed up against the saving to the NHS if individuals follow the health advice. NICE found that interventions aimed at a whole population, such as mass-media campaigns to promote healthy eating or legislation to reduce young people's access to cigarettes, were the most cost effective.

Reporting initiatives and current advice

The media can be useful in bringing initiatives and current advice to the population. However, media coverage of health issues tends to lack investigative depth. It can also be inaccurate and sensationalist. For example, media reports linking the mumps, measles and rubella (MMR) vaccine to autism and bowel disease meant that many parents did not have their children vaccinated, causing an epidemic of measles. Later, a government-commissioned study found there was no evidence to support this claim.

> **KNOW IT** 💡
> 1 Explain two barriers to following health advice.
> 2 Discuss why the tobacco industry wants people to keep on smoking.
> 3 Discuss why the media are biased towards the products they promote.
> 4 Explain how the media depiction of the ideal body form affects both men and women.

LO3 Assessment activity *P5 M2*

Below is a suggested assessment activity that has been directly linked to the pass and merit criteria in LO3 to help with assignment preparation; it includes Top Tips on how to achieve best results.

Portia wants to lose weight. She decides to go to a slimming club and also joins a gym as she feels extra exercise would speed up her weight loss. She works long hours and sometimes works overtime to earn extra money. Often the bus is late and she does not get home until 9pm and she feels very tired as she left home for work at 7am.

Explain the barriers that may prevent Portia from losing weight.

> **TOP TIPS**
> ✔ Consider factors that might influence individuals' decisions.

LO4 Be able to implement and evaluate a campaign promoting health and wellbeing *P6 P7*

GETTING STARTED 🧍

(15 minutes)

Which health campaign has had the biggest effect on you? Why? What lessons could you learn from it that you could use in your campaign?

If you are planning to carry out a health campaign in your setting, first you need to plan it carefully.

4.1 Aims and objectives

Improving health of individuals and society

A health campaign should aim to improve health by doing the following.

- Providing health-related learning: the overall aim must have a health-related topic with objectives showing how the aim will be achieved. For example, if the aim was to educate children in Year 5 about healthy eating, one of the objectives may be to introduce them to exotic fruits by tasting them. It is a good idea to link into the school's health promotion targets if possible.
- Exploring values and attitudes of the audience. This could be done by carrying out research when handing out the pre-presentation questionnaires. For example, in the above health campaign the children could be asked which fruit they recognise and if they would be willing to try them.
- Providing knowledge and skills for change: continuing with the healthy eating topic, the children could be given flash cards to take away with them identifying the fruits to eat. If the topic linked into the school's health promotion targets, the school kitchen could serve the exotic fruits for lunch.
- Promoting self-esteem and empowerment: the children could build up their self-esteem and empowerment by talking to their parents about their new knowledge of a healthy diet and asking their parents to add the new foods to the family menu.
- Changing beliefs: this could be on a wider scale, for example by asking the school to sell fruit at break time rather than fatty or sugary snacks. Perhaps by encouraging the school to go for a Healthy Schools Award, the whole ethos of the school could be changed.

4.2 Target audience

The audience could be any section of the community. Obviously the topic must suit the audience, for example a sex education talk would not be suitable for older people as many of them would already know the facts. Pregnant mothers would be interested in a talk about diet in pregnancy whereas it would not be applicable for children or older people. For all the groups use simple, easy to understand language and smile while delivering your message. Be engaging and try to have interactive activities so you are not talking all the time. If you are working with children, one way to engage them could be to give out stickers or prizes for their participation. Adolescents and young people may be interested in a health promotion campaign about alcohol especially if you can give them beer goggles to wear which simulate the effects of being drunk.

4.3 Context

Consider carrying out a group talk as this will give you more opportunity to engage with others and to practise your communication skills. There is also more opportunity to analyse anonymous questionnaires where individuals are more likely to be honest about your performance.

4.4 Choice of approach

See LO2.2, page 268.

4.5 Choice of media

These days, many types of media are available to put across information. All have advantages and disadvantages (see Table 15.3).

Table 15.3 Advantages and disadvantages of conveying a health campaign via different types of media

Media	Advantages	Disadvantages
Social media	• Easy to interact with others • Easy to share information • Quick and easy to post content	• Need laptop or mobile phone • Could get inaccurate information
Posters	• Can raise awareness of health issues • Cheap, easy to make • Can give out helplines, addresses etc.	• Impact soon lost • Become ripped and untidy very quickly
Podcasts	• Can reach a lot of individuals • Cost effective	• Need computer, smartphone or tablet • Need to know how to access it • Need to take notes • Cannot ask questions • No camaraderie or engagement

Media	Advantages	Disadvantages
Information booklets	• Cheap to produce • Saves taking notes • Can be read at own pace and referred to later • Easily passed on to others • Can list email addresses, phone numbers etc.	• Have to have literacy skills • Easily destroyed • Not durable
Face-to-face meetings	• Can ask questions • More personal • Nurtures relationships • Reads body language • Clarifies meaning of information	• May be too embarrassed to ask questions • Have to take notes

4.6 Measurable outcomes

What to set

Before beginning the campaign, you must:

- research the needs of your target audience and decide on a topic for your campaign
- set the overall aim
- set the objectives and decide the best way of achieving them.
- identify the resources to be used and their cost
- plan the evaluation methods to be used
- set a timetable for delivery and evaluation.

How to measure

Intended outcomes (what you have achieved) must be measurable so you can evaluate the impact of your campaign. Did you achieve your aims and objectives? Outcomes describe what the recipients should be able to do or demonstrate, in terms of particular knowledge, skills and attitudes, by the end of your health promotion campaign.

Use of pre- and post-campaign questionnaires

Questionnaires can be useful when judging whether a campaign was successful or not. If you give out a pre-campaign questionnaire, you can measure how much prior knowledge the intended audience has and can target your campaign effectively. After the campaign you can check if the audience has gained knowledge by distributing the same questionnaire. The percentages should go up!

Obtaining feedback

The questionnaires will inform you of your success and give some feedback but you could ask the audience what they thought of your campaign at the end of the questionnaire. If your campaign was delivered in a centre, school or care home you could ask the teacher, supervisor or manager for their feedback also.

4.7 Evaluation

Aims and objectives

Reviewing your aims and objectives should help you to decide if your campaign has been successful. For example, if one of your objectives was to educate Year 5 about the value of eating fruit and vegetables, then the pre- and post-campaign questionnaires should help you decide if you met this objective.

Outcome measures/pre-set criteria

This can be judged by what you have achieved (outcome) and whether the aims and the objectives were met.

Strengths and weaknesses

Reflect on all aspects of your work from the beginning of the campaign through to the end. You should evaluate the following.

- Your performance and the performance of your team – what were you pleased with and what needed to be improved?
- Skills used by your team – did you use communication skills effectively? Did you practise the presentation sufficiently? Were you competent with ICT?
- Benefit to your audience – did you engage them? Did they have fun? Was their knowledge extended?
- Quality measures whether it is value for money – was this an expensive campaign? Did it take hours to prepare for little return?

Look for what you did well and what you did not do well.

Aspects to improve

When you examine your strengths and weaknesses you will be able to see how you could improve certain aspects if you were to repeat the campaign.

Likely impact

Considering this is a small health promotion campaign it may have limited impact on the proposed audience. However, even if it changes the behaviour of one person it has had an impact.

LO4 Assessment activity, *P6 P7*

Below is a suggested assessment activity that has been directly linked to the pass criteria in LO4 to help with assignment preparation; it includes Top Tips on how to achieve best results.

- Choose a topic for a small campaign promoting health and wellbeing. Look at national campaigns as you will be able to pick up health promotion materials such as posters and leaflets.

- Choose your target audience, the context and decide on your approach.

- Produce a detailed plan containing aims and objectives, identify your resources and their cost, plan the evaluation methods and set a timetable for the delivery and evaluation. You must also plan your pre- and post-campaign questionnaires.

- Analyse its success.

Read about it

Useful websites

Physical health: www.s-cool.co.uk/a-level-biology/health-and-disease/revise-it/exercise

Management of stress: www.stress.org.uk

Exercise and depression: www.webmd.com

Information on blood pressure and suitable diets: www.bloodpressureuk.org

Advice on pregnancy and fertility: www.babycentre.co.uk

Information on nutrition: www.nutritionist-resource.org.uk

Smoking and the heart: www.bhf.org.uk

All aspects of alcohol: www.drinkaware.co.uk

Public Health Observations – health profiles: www.apho.org.uk

Sexual health and wellbeing: www.ncb.org.uk

Approaches to health promotion: www.educationforum.co.uk

Alcohol units: www.drinkingandyou.com

This Girl Can: www.sportengland.org

Unit 22

Psychology for health and social care

ABOUT THIS UNIT

Psychology is the study of human behaviour and how it is affected by the mind, thoughts and emotions. An understanding of human behaviour is fundamental to those working and interacting with individuals in the health and social care sectors. The focus of this unit is an exploration of various psychological perspectives used to interpret people's behaviour and a consideration of the relevance of these theories for practitioners working in health and social care. Behaviourists and social learning theorists can help to explain how health-related behaviour is learned, while the biological approach considers genetic influence and explains the predisposition that some people may have towards illness. The humanist approach represents a person-centred focus on the individual.

You will learn about a range of psychological theories representing the different perspectives that inspire different approaches to positively influence individuals' health-related behaviours. The link between an individual's physical and mental states is well known and an appreciation of this can only help care practitioners to provide appropriate treatment and interventions. An understanding of health psychology is vital for practitioners to address why individuals ignore symptoms, and how they cope with illness and chronic conditions. By developing knowledge and understanding the differences between individuals' attitudes and behaviours, practitioners can provide person-centred care that meets the needs of the individual.

LEARNING OUTCOMES

The topics, activities and suggested reading in this unit will help you to:

1. Be able to apply psychological theories and approaches to health, social care and child care
2. Understand health psychology
3. Understand the impact of chronic illness and long-term health conditions on individuals
4. Know the psychological impacts of requiring care

How will I be assessed?

You will be assessed through a series of assignments and tasks set and marked by your tutor.

How will I be graded?

You will be graded using the following criteria.

Learning outcome	Pass assessment criteria	Merit assessment criteria	Distinction assessment criteria
You will:	To achieve a **pass** you must demonstrate that you have met all the pass assessment criteria	To achieve a **merit** you must demonstrate that you have met all the pass and merit assessment criteria	To achieve a **distinction** you must demonstrate that you have met all the pass, merit and distinction assessment criteria
1 Be able to apply psychological theories and approaches to health, social care and child care	**P1** Apply psychological perspectives and approaches to health, social care and child care environments, considering how these can support person-centred care	**M1** Evaluate how psychological theory and health psychology contributes to the everyday practice of caring for individuals	
2 Understand health psychology	**P2** Analyse factors that impact on health psychology		**D1** Evaluate the limitations of theories of behaviour change in relation to health psychology
3 Understand the impact of chronic illness and long-term health conditions on individuals	**P3** Explain the psychological impacts of ill-health on individuals	**M2** Assess why individuals may fail to comply with prescribed treatments	**D2** Evaluate the psychological impact when an individual fails to comply with prescribed treatment for a chronic illness or a long-term health condition
4 Know the psychological impacts of requiring care	**P4** Describe the psychological impacts of requiring care		

LO1 Be able to apply psychological theories and approaches to health, social care and child care

P1 M1

GETTING STARTED

Is it nature or nurture? (10 minutes)

Nature refers to an individual's development and behaviour being the result of inherited characteristics and innate drives they are born with.

Nurture refers to an individual's development and behaviour being a result of learning from environmental influences and the people around them.

For each of the following, consider whether you think the main influence on the person's development or behaviour is 'nature' or 'nurture'.

- Michael is an alcoholic. His father was an alcoholic.
- Statistics show that men commit most of the violent crime in the UK.
- Barinder has developed lung cancer.
- Sarah lived to the age of 102.

Share your thoughts with the whole class about what is the major influence in each case – nature or nurture?

Discuss your ideas: is it possible to reach a conclusion – is nature or nurture more influential?

1.1 Psychological perspectives and approaches and 1.2 The application of the theory to practice

An 'approach' or 'perspective' is a viewpoint on something. There are many different psychological perspectives on human behaviour. Each has its own assumptions and beliefs, and each has strengths and weaknesses. A care practitioner's knowledge of the different perspectives will enhance their understanding of human motivation and behaviour, helping them to provide person-centred care that meets individuals' needs.

Biological influences

Theories of biological influence focus on nature. These theories suggest that the influence of inheritance or the body's **physiological** responses are the main factors affecting human behaviour. Thinking, behaviour and emotions are a result of biological factors such as neurochemical levels and brain structures that are influenced by genes.

Influence of genetics

Genetics is the study of heredity – how the characteristics of one generation are passed to the next. All living things contain the genetic material, called **genes**, that makes up **DNA** molecules, and this material is passed on to create the characteristics of the next generation.

Francis Galton is best known for his interest in inheritance. His book *Hereditary Genius* (1869) has been said to have introduced the study of human genetics. Galton also introduced the idea that fingerprints could be used to identify an individual.

His research into the inheritance of certain traits led him to believe that personal characteristics were inborn and not acquired, so they must be biological differences.

Today DNA tests are commonplace and much research is currently being carried out to establish whether certain diseases and conditions are inherited or are caused by defective genes.

Influence of the nervous system and the endocrine system

Hans Selye explored the links between the **nervous system**, the **endocrine system** and illness. He carried out experiments analysing how rats coped with stress and the short- and long-term effects the stress had. This led to Selye developing his 'General Adaption Syndrome' theory where he identified three stages in the stress process. (see Figure 22.1)

A **stressor** is anything that is seen as a challenge or a threat, such as an illness.

At the 'alarm' stage, to prepare the body for action against the stressor, the endocrine system releases hormones such as adrenalin and cortisol to ready the muscles for exertion, then the person attempts to cope with the stress so that the body can return to its normal physiological state.

If the stress continues, or is not managed, the body becomes exhausted and can offer no further resistance. When stress persists over time the person becomes susceptible to disease and illness due to a lowered immune system, or it can lead to conditions such as high blood pressure, heart attacks or mental illness.

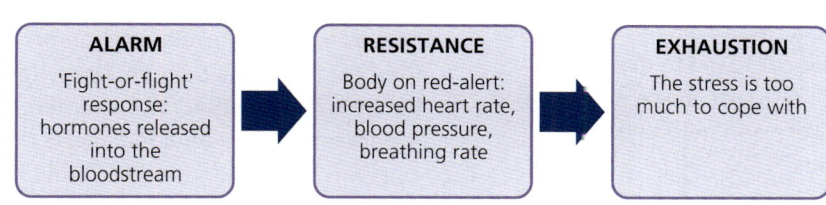

▲ **Figure 22.1** Selye's three stages of reaction to stress

Maturational theory

Arnold Gesell believed that differences among people are inherited rather than resulting from their environment. He identified various developmental milestones that occur at specific ages, forming a pattern of development that can be used as guidelines to track a child's development. From the maturationalist perspective, a child's environment should be adapted to meet their genetically predetermined needs and characteristics.

Biological influences – application of the theory to practice

Genetic predisposition

Developments in biological science research have brought a greater understanding of genetic predisposition to certain illnesses. Individuals can now be tested for their chance of developing some inherited conditions and diseases, like Huntingdon's disease or the BRACA gene for breast cancer. Individuals from families with a known history of certain conditions can have genetic testing and be provided with counselling, enabling them to consider the implications if they are a carrier of a condition that they could pass on to their children.

Stress

The perception of whether something is stressful and whether it can be dealt with varies from person to person. This is an important factor in assessing the impact of an illness or its treatment. Care practitioners, such as social workers or doctors who are deciding on a course of treatment, need to consider how the individual might react to a proposed care plan, or a diagnosis, and whether they will need support to enable them to cope with suddenly requiring carers or treatment.

Constant exposure to stress hormones can affect an individual's health and wellbeing because of its effects on the endocrine and immune systems, as demonstrated by Selye's three stages of stress, so stress needs to be managed. Managing stress means to limit its effects, overcome, or learn to tolerate, the causes of the stress. Table 22.1 lists some examples of ways that care practitioners can help to enable individuals to manage stress.

Table 22.1 Ways of managing stress

Type of support	Examples	How it can help an individual deal with stress
Social	Family, friends, pets, community and faith organisations, third sector support groups	• someone to talk to • reassurance • alleviate fears
Educational	Practitioner to provide information about: illness, tests, side-effects, treatments or services and support available	• knowledge helps understanding of what is happening • helps to feel more in control of the situation
Communication	Practitioners showing empathy, understanding and care to develop trust	• builds self-esteem • feel safe and secure • feel comfortable discussing problems
Physical	Practitioner arranges adaptations to home, mobility aids Community transport provided	• helps maintain independence • reduces isolation
Emotional	Counselling Community support groups	• learn coping strategies • encourages positive thinking • meet people in the same situation

Understanding developmental norms

Every child is unique so the 'norms' of development are just a guideline, indicating generally what a child could be expected to do at a certain stage, rather than age, as the sequence of development is similar for all children. Norms can also be used by health professionals to assess a child's developmental progress, for example their motor skills, speech, language skills and social behaviour, to screen for any differences from normal progression that could indicate a reason for concern.

The Department or Education's 'Early Years Outcomes' document (September 2013) provides a guide to developmental norms for child care practitioners. This can be accessed using the following link: http://tinyurl.com/mxsu2nr.

Behaviourist perspectives

Theories from the behaviourist perspective explain human behaviour as being learned through experience. This relates to the 'nurture' side of the nature–nurture debate. Our experiences mould or shape our personality and behaviour. A key aspect of behaviourism is that it is concerned with how an environmental factor or action (stimulus) can affect an individual's behaviour (response).

Classical conditioning

Ivan Pavlov's investigations into the salivation reflex response in dogs found that the dogs drooled when the lab assistants who fed them appeared, even if they had no food. Pavlov started to ring a bell every time the dogs were fed and eventually just ringing the bell made the dogs salivate. Pavlov called this classical conditioning. So, an unconditioned response can be thought of as completely natural and a conditioned response is something that has been learned. Figure 22.2 shows the process in more detail.

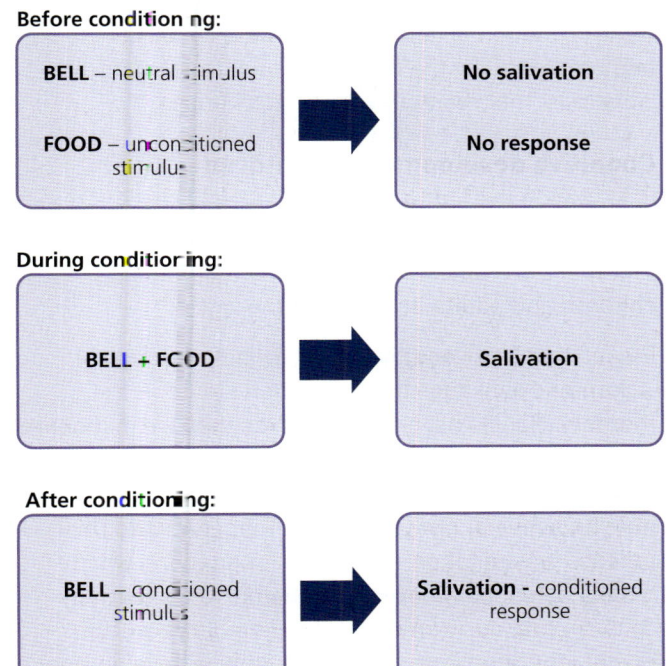

▲ **Figure 22.2** Stages in classical conditioning

Operant conditioning

B.F. Skinner experimented with rats and pigeons using a method called the 'Skinner Box'. He found that they to press a lever that offered them food and to avoid a lever that punished them. Repeating or not repeating behaviour as a result of its consequences is what Skinner called 'operant conditioning'. This is where behaviour that operates on the environment to create pleasant outcomes is likely to strengthen or reinforce that behaviour. So, learning through the consequences of action, or operant conditioning, is where people will repeat actions or behaviour that has previously resulted in them feeling good or better in some way. This is called positive reinforcement.

Behaviourist perspectives – application of the theory to practice

Understanding behaviours and how they can be managed

One way of helping individuals who have an anxiety condition or an irrational phobia is the use of relaxation techniques. Psychologists train the individual to relax using deep breathing and muscle relaxing exercises. Once this skill has been learned, the person conditions the relaxed sensation to a word that they say to themselves, e.g. 'relax'. When they next feel anxiety or panic they say the word 'relax' and their conditioning will induce the relaxed feeling and anxiety will diminish.

Cognitive behavioural therapy has also been found to be very effective in helping individuals overcome anxiety and phobias (see page 286).

Dealing with/changing challenging behaviours

Positive reinforcement is widely used by practitioners in all forms of child care provision to shape children's behaviour. Wanted behaviour is rewarded with praise, smiles, stickers and certificates, whether this is simply putting toys away, sharing or playing nicely with others. The behaviour is rewarded so that it will be repeated and appropriate behaviour patterns established.

In other situations unco-operative or anti-social behaviour needs to be stopped, such as if a child is pulling another child's hair or being aggressive. A way of dealing with this bad behaviour would be 'time out', seating the child well away from others where they will not get any attention. This ensures that they get no 'reinforcement' from others for the inappropriate behaviour and so the inappropriate behaviour diminishes. Behaviourists refer to this as 'extinguishing' unwanted behaviour.

Social learning approaches

People learn from one another in a social context. Behaviours are learned through observation and imitation of role models. Nurture is more influential than nature.

Albert Bandura's social learning theory emphasises the importance of observation and modelling of behaviour, rather than the stimulus and response theory of behaviourists. His research (of which the best known is the bobo doll experiment) shows how an individual will copy behaviour they have observed.

 INDEPENDENT RESEARCH ACTIVITY

Watch a clip of Bandura explaining his bobo doll experiment on YouTube.

Key aspects of his theory are the following.

- Modelling: observing modelled behaviour and imitating or copying it, i.e. learning from other people.
- Intrinsic reward: motivation for the behaviour comes from within the individual – they want to be like the role model. Achieving this is the reward.
- Role models: have more effect on an individual if they are someone with similar values, more powerful, liked and respected, or warm and loving.

Social learning approaches – application of the theory to practice

Practitioners working with children and young people can be very influential and so have a responsibility to provide positive role models. Challenging discriminatory behaviour is an example. Explaining to a child why calling someone a racist name is wrong is important for the child and for others who are observing in developing an understanding of discrimination and equality.

Parents are powerful models for the amount and type of food children eat and the amount of exercise they take part in. Practitioners such as health visitors enable families to be positive role models for their children by promoting healthy eating and exercise. Celebrity and sports role models are used in health promotion campaigns, such as the 'celebrity eats' School Food Trust Campaign. This aims to make eating healthy food and having a sporty

lifestyle appeal to young people by using images of personalities who are generally admired. However, there has also been much debate about extremely thin fashion models, reality TV and soap stars and their link to inspiring eating disorders such as anorexia and bulimia.

Cognitive approaches

This approach looks at innate cognitive abilities, but also recognises that experience shapes these abilities. Knowledge and understanding are developed by experiencing and then adapting to the world around us. Information is taken in from the environment and processed by the brain, forming 'constructs' or 'schemas' that result in behaviour change.

Cognitive development of children

Jean Piaget's theories are about mental processes or cognitive skills and how they develop. He recognised that there is a difference in the way that infants, children and adults understand the world.

Piaget said that cognitive skills develop through 'schemas', packages of information stored in the memory. Babies have basic reflexes that are instinctive, such as sucking and grasping. As time passes more complex schemas (skills) are developed through making sense of new situations. Piaget named this process 'assimilation' and 'accommodation', which means adjusting an existing schema so we learn by constructing our own understanding of the world. Piaget identified four stages of cognitive development, shown in Figure 22.3.

SENSORIMOTOR (0–2 years)

Child learns by doing and deals with the world through its senses, e.g. crying, looking, hearing, touching. At around 8 months, object permanence develops.

↓

PREOPERATIONAL (2–7 years)

Child starts to use one object to represent another, e.g. pretend play. Unable to see a situation from another's point of view. Assumes others see/feel the same as the child does – known as egocentrism.

↓

CONCRETE OPERATIONS (7–11 years)

Can deal with logic but only if it is real (concrete) not abstract, e.g. simple arithmetic.

↓

FORMAL OPERATIONS (11+ years)

Abstract and hypothetical thinking, comparison, reasoning.

▲ **Figure 22.3** Piaget's four stages of cognitive development

Personal constructs

George Kelly felt that individual differences in attitudes and approaches to situations are a result of how we interpret and predict events. He called these interpretations 'personal constructs', meaning that, as an individual gathers information from their experience of the world, they work out, or 'construct', ideas about what or how something should happen.

Our actions reflect how we expect the world to be, based on our interpretations of past events. So our preconceived ideas, based on experience, affect how we interact with other people and new situations. If an individual generally sees people as helpful and pleasant they are likely to engage and interact with others and seek advice. If an individual generally sees others as uncaring or uninterested, they will avoid interaction and interpersonal relationships and just rely on themselves.

Cognitive approaches – application of the theory to practice

Developmental norms

Awareness of stages of cognitive development allows child care practitioners, such as nursery and primary school staff, to provide the optimum learning environment for the child, including those with learning difficulties. Knowledge of developmental norms enables staff to facilitate children's learning, for example knowing whether a child understands object permanence (knows an object exists even though it is not visible) or not enables the practitioner to provide appropriate learning activities for the child and so help them to make maximum progress.

Cognitive behaviour therapy for anxiety and phobias

Figure 22.4 shows the interrelated links between thoughts, behaviour and feelings.

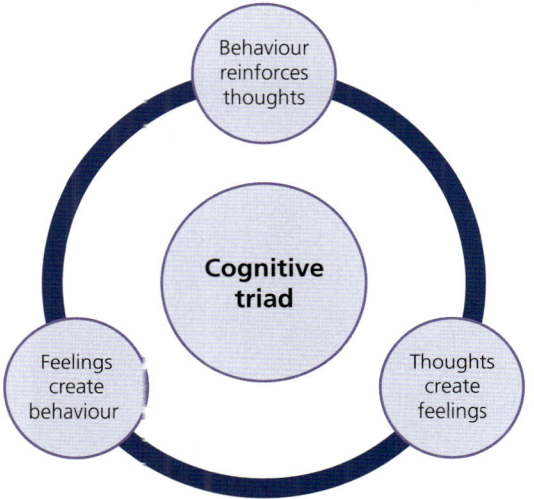

▲ **Figure 22.4** Links between thoughts, behaviour and feelings

- What an individual thinks and believes determines how they feel, e.g. 'I am scared of closed-in spaces'.
- Emotional problems such as anxiety or phobias are the result of distorted thinking, e.g. 'I will suffocate in the enclosed space'.
- Feelings create behaviour, e.g. 'I cannot use a lift'.

Care practitioners aim to change this pattern of negative thinking to help the individual overcome their anxiety or phobia. Cognitive behaviour therapy (CBT) has been found to be an effective method of overcoming phobias. CBT involves a gradual exposure to the fear so the individual becomes less anxious and is desensitised.

For example, someone who is scared of spiders will be asked by a therapist to read about spiders, then to look at pictures of spiders, then visit a zoo to look at real spiders. The final step would be to hold a spider. The therapy works by enabling the individual to gradually take control of their anxious thoughts.

Psychodynamic perspective

The psychodynamic approach incorporates the idea of innate, inborn drives with the influences of social experiences and upbringing during childhood.

The psyche and ego defence mechanisms

Sigmund Freud believed that we are born with biological survival instincts which we have to learn to control to fit in to society and to get on with other people. Freud used an iceberg to represent the 'psyche', which is the conscious and unconscious mind. The 'id' is hidden in the unconscious mind, with the 'ego' and the 'superego' overlapping both the conscious and unconscious parts of the psyche.

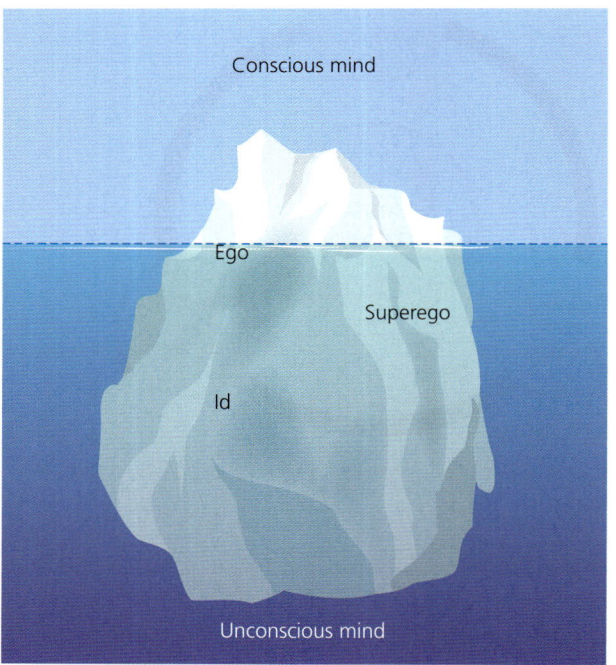

▲ **Figure 22.5** Freud's iceberg model of the conscious and unconscious mind

- The 'id' instincts – the 'I want' demands and desires – exist in the unconscious mind.
- The 'superego' is the moral part of personality. It represents the demands made by society about how to behave in an acceptable way.
- The 'ego' tries to resolve conflicts between the id and the superego.

According to Freudian theory, people are controlled by inner forces that they do not necessarily understand and the way that people cope in life is influenced strongly by early childhood experiences. To deal with problems and conflict, Freud suggested that the mind employs subconscious 'defence mechanisms' to protect the individual from pressure and ward off unpleasant feelings. Some examples of defence mechanisms are shown below.

- Displacement – transferring anger to someone else, e.g. a parent or employer – 'it's their fault'.
- Denial – blocking out reality, removing awareness or acceptance of bad news or information.
- Repression – forcing memories or unpleasant thoughts or situations out of the conscious and into the unconscious mind.
- Rationalisation – reinterpreting memories or events resulting in avoidance of the real reasons for something. Providing ourselves with excuses for something.
- Projection – someone transferring their own, unacceptable thoughts or feelings onto another person.
- Sublimation – changing the way mental energy is directed, satisfying an impulse such as aggression with a socially acceptable substitute, e.g. playing squash.
- Regression – when faced with stress, psychologically the individual moves back in time, e.g. a child regresses to bed wetting.

Attachment theory

John Bowlby considered that children come into the world pre-programmed to make an attachment with one main individual to survive. Attachment is a two-way emotional bond where people depend on each other for their sense of security. Bowlby stated that forming an attachment was an essential part of a child's development, creating a secure base for exploring the world and for forming all future social relationships. If the attachment is broken or disrupted within the first two to three years there will be harmful effects on the child. The effects of this 'deprivation' as Bowlby named it, could result in long-term cognitive, social and emotional difficulties.

Psychodynamic perspectives – application of the theory to practice

Some illnesses or conditions may be a result of an individual's state of mind. Repressed emotions, inadequate attachment and unresolved conflicts can build up and result in anxiety, depression, drug and alcohol abuse or eating disorders.

Psychodynamic therapy is where a patient discusses their condition or problem with a counsellor who uncovers the individual's unconscious motivations and the needs that go beyond the information shared in a normal conversation. For example, defence mechanisms may be causing them to suppress or deny unpleasant experiences, such as childhood abuse, in order to 'cope' with them. A psychodynamic counsellor will try to identify links between past events and how the person thinks and feels now. The aim is to free the individual from the repressed feelings and experiences and enable them to control their life and emotions. Examples of psychodynamic therapy methods are the following.

- Dreams analysis – gives an insight into the workings of the unconscious mind.
- Identifying defences – the counsellor seeks to identify any defence mechanisms.
- Projective techniques – images are used to prompt conversation.
- Free association – an individual says whatever comes into their head and unconscious issues may slip out.
- Interpretation – the therapist will attempt to interpret the real meaning of what the person says.

Art, music and movement therapies also use the psychodynamic ways of working, but aim to encourage alternative forms of self-expression alongside talking. This method can even be used by children and is known as play therapy.

Humanistic approaches

This approach focuses on the social and environmental influences on individuals and how they affect human motivation

Self-concept and self-esteem

According to Carl Rogers' theory, individuals have an 'actualising tendency', an inner strength that enables them to cope and achieve in life. To achieve self-actualisation (when an individual achieves their goals and desires), Rogers thought individuals must have a high level of self-worth, or self-esteem. He believed that feelings of self-worth developed in childhood through interactions with parents and later with others.

Rogers believed that fundamental to developing high self-worth is 'unconditional positive regard'. This is where a person is loved or accepted for what and who they are even if they make a mistake or do something wrong. For example, parents might disagree with something their son has done but still love and support him. The son knows he can make mistakes but will still be valued by the people who matter to him. This contrasts with 'conditional positive regard' where the

individual only receives praise and approval for behaving in ways thought correct. This can lead to people believing they will only be a worthwhile person if they do what others expect of them.

Hierarchy of needs

Abraham Maslow introduced a similar self-actualising theory to that of Rogers. However, Maslow believed that many people do not achieve self-actualisation because their basic needs have not been met. His hierarchy of needs is shown in Figure 22.6.

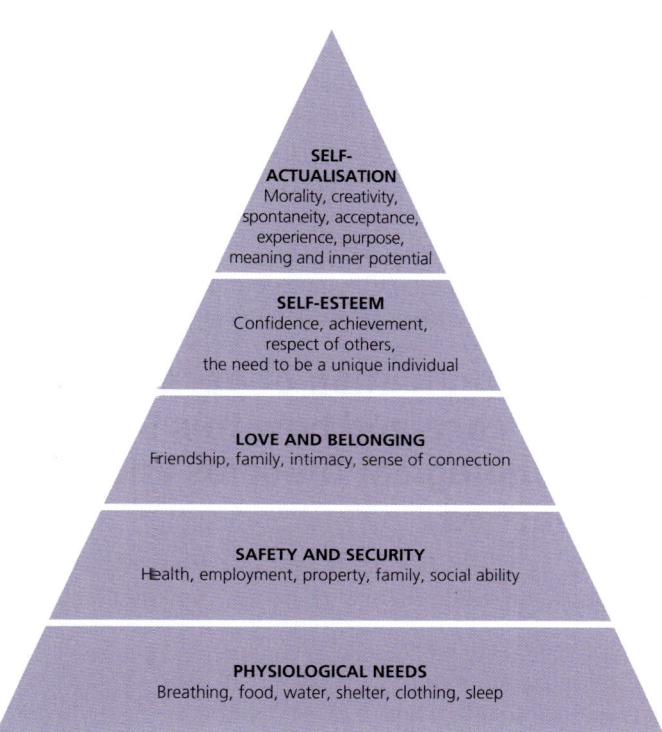

SELF-ACTUALISATION
Morality, creativity, spontaneity, acceptance, experience, purpose, meaning and inner potential

SELF-ESTEEM
Confidence, achievement, respect of others, the need to be a unique individual

LOVE AND BELONGING
Friendship, family, intimacy, sense of connection

SAFETY AND SECURITY
Health, employment, property, family, social ability

PHYSIOLOGICAL NEEDS
Breathing, food, water, shelter, clothing, sleep

▲ **Figure 22.6** Maslow's hierarchy of needs

The basic needs that have to be met for survival are shown at the bottom of the pyramid. Only when those basic physical, and then emotional, needs are met will an individual have the motivation to progress on to trying to meet the higher order needs for personal development and achievement. Only then will a person self-actualise and become the person they want to be

Humanistic approach – application of the theory to practice

The humanistic approach is person-centred, focused on the individual and their needs. For example, a child at school who is tired and hungry will find it difficult to concentrate on learning. This is why some schools provide breakfast clubs. Children also need to feel safe and secure in the classroom, as they will not reach their potential if they are afraid they will be bullied if they ask questions or take part in activities. Teachers have to create a supportive classroom environment where individual students feel valued, respected and safe.

A person-centred approach is essential for an older adult who is moving into residential care, perhaps because they are no longer able to fully care for themselves. They are likely to have mixed feelings and be worried about losing control over their life and losing independence, as well as moving house being stressful. Following Maslow's hierarchy of needs, staff should ensure that the individual's basic needs are met, such as food preferences catered for, and a comfortable room with their own belongings to arrange as they wish gives a sense of control and empowerment. The individual should be welcomed and helped to meet other residents so that a feeling of acceptance and belonging develops. This will make the individual feel respected and valued and more likely to be healthy and comfortable in the new environment as all their needs are being met.

1.3 The application of person-centred care and how this links to psychological theories and approaches

The main principles of person-centred care are that an individual is treated with dignity, compassion and respect.

- Care is personalised.
- Care is co-ordinated.
- Care is enabling.

Health, social care and child care practitioners work collaboratively with individuals who require care or support. Person-centred care enables people to develop the knowledge, skills and confidence they need to effectively manage and make informed decisions because practitioners work with them to ensure they are aware of their options and have all the information they need. This ensures that people are always treated with dignity, compassion and respect, and are supported to recognise their own strengths and abilities to enable them to live an independent and fulfilling life. For more on person-centred care, see Unit 6 (page 123).

An understanding of psychological theories helps practitioners to use a whole person approach. Just focusing, for example, on treating the physical symptoms of illness may be misleading as they could be a result of stress, the causes of which need to be

established and addressed, or the effect of a deep-seated emotional issue that requires therapy to resolve.

Each psychological theory or approach has its strengths and weaknesses; however, if used appropriately, it can make a valuable contribution to providing care that meets an individual's needs.

LO1 Assessment activities

Below are suggested assessment activities that have been directly linked to the pass and merit criteria in LO1 to help with assignment preparation; they include Top Tips on how to achieve the best results.

Scenario: your application for a work placement at a national charity providing care and support for older adults has been successful. Before you start the placement, the charity has asked you to carry out some research into psychological theories and approaches relevant to health and social care.

Activity 1 – pass criteria P1

Produce information for your placement portfolio that explains how to apply psychological perspectives and approaches to health, social care and child care environments and how these can support person-centred care.

Activity 2 – merit criteria M1

After your first few sessions working at the charity, write up an evaluation, based on your observations and research, about how psychological theory and health psychology contribute to caring practice.

Evaluate how psychological theory and health psychology contribute to the everyday practice of caring for individuals.

LO2 Understand health psychology
P2 D1

GETTING STARTED

Why was I ill? (10 minutes)

Think about the last time you were ill, for example with a cold, headache, nausea, flu, aches and pains. Consider to what extent factors, other than biological ones, may have contributed towards you being ill.

2.1 The role of health psychology

Health psychology has two main roles, first to promote general wellbeing and healthier lifestyles and second to develop understanding of the impact of psychology on physical illnesses.

Promote general wellbeing and healthier lifestyles

- Identifying behaviours that may be damaging to an individual's health, for example smoking, poor diet, alcohol intake, drug abuse.
- Encouraging positive health behaviours, such as healthy eating, exercise, health checks, self-examination, and preventative medical screenings such as cervical smear tests and mammograms.
- Using psychological theories and interventions to support prevention and health related behaviour change.

Understand physical illnesses and the impact of psychology on these

- Investigates an individual's cognitive behaviour to determine their health and illness behaviours.
- Uses a range of models and frameworks to develop interventions, for example to change health beliefs, to increase an individual's internal control or self-belief.

- Investigates the nature and effects of communication between health professionals and patients, with a view to improving communication and mutual understanding.
- Looks at the psychological impact of illness – the mental and emotional reactions to illness, not only of individuals but also their families and carers.

The theories covered in LO1 show that psychological factors can play a significant role in health, wellbeing and illness. The mind can affect the cause, effects, treatment and an individual's response to illness. The government document The Health of the Nation (1992) identified five areas for improving the nation's health, all of which required people to change their behaviour rather than to have any medical treatments or interventions. An example Health of the Nation target is reducing the number of deaths from coronary heart disease. This can be achieved if individuals stop smoking, eat a healthy diet and exercise regularly – that is, behaviour change rather than medical treatment. So it can be seen that the role of health psychology is to promote general wellbeing and healthier lifestyles through behaviour change.

INDEPENDENT RESEARCH ACTIVITY

What is a health psychologist? (30 minutes)

Using the link below, and any other sources of information available to you, research the job role of an NHS health psychologist.

http://tinyurl.com/hkx3et2

2.2 Factors that impact health psychology

The overall health of the population has improved due to the availability of health care, better work and living conditions and more health awareness, such as the dangers of smoking, alcohol and a diet high in fat and sugar. However, a range of factors still influence health inequalities in society. Some poorer members of society live in deprived areas, experience unemployment and suffer from more illnesses than individuals who live in more affluent areas that provide a better environment. Age, gender and level of education also have an impact on health and wellbeing. The statistical information shown in Table 22.2 demonstrates the impact these factors have on individuals' health behaviour and their general wellbeing.

Table 22.2 Factors that influence health (Source: the Office for National Statistics and the NHS)

Factors	Impact
Cultural	• Cultural differences in eating habits may mean that different health issues arise within different cultural groups, for example: people from African Caribbean communities are more likely to develop Type II diabetes than the rest of the population. This is linked to diet, genetic differences in processing and storing fat, and unequal access to health services.
Ethnicity	• The 2011 census showed that 10 per cent more Pakistani and Bangladeshi women reported being limited in their choice of activities due to a health problem or disability than white British women. • Black and south Asian people are three to five times more likely to have kidney failure than white people.
Age	• People aged 65 and over are most likely to drink alcohol at least five days a week. • 16–24 year olds were most likely to have drunk very heavily at least once in the last week.
Gender	• A higher proportion of women (21 per cent), than men (16 per cent) suffer from anxiety or depression. • Women live longer in good health than men.
Education	• Someone whose highest qualification is a GCSE grade D–G is four times more likely to be a smoker than someone with a degree.
Socio-economic	• Smoking rates are higher in areas of social deprivation – people in the least deprived areas are most likely to have given up smoking. • Smokers were more than twice as likely as non-smokers to have drunk very heavily at least once in the last week. • Alcohol-related death rates for those in routine occupations (e.g. bar staff, cleaners and labourers) were four times greater for men and two times greater for women, than those in professional occupations (e.g. doctors, IT strategy and planning professionals and lawyers).
Environmental	• The more deprived the neighbourhood, the more likely it is to have environmental characteristics presenting risks to health. These include poor housing, high crime rates, poorer air quality, lack of green spaces and places for children to play, traffic risks. (The Marmot Review – Fair Society, Healthy Lives. 2010, p. 78) • In England, people living in the poorest neighbourhoods will, on average, die seven years earlier than people living in the richest neighbourhoods. (Marmot Review, p. 11)

2.3 Theories of behaviour change

Learning theories

Learning theories help to explain the ways that individuals change, or do not change, their behaviour. The theories are useful for health and social care practitioners because they provide a basis for practice. For example, theories can help to explain how health behaviours are acquired through classical and operant conditioning; a behaviourist approach (see LO1 page 283) could be where positive reinforcement is given for example when someone makes healthy eating choices. Social learning (see LO1 page 284) is when, for example, a parent exercises regularly and involves their children, so modelling healthy behaviour.

Social cognitive theory

This focuses on the movement between stages as an individual makes changes to their behaviour. It suggests that behaviour results from weighing up the pros and cons, or the value to the individual, of any suggested action. It is based on Badura's social learning theory (see LO1 page 285). Table 22.3 shows how it works for someone considering starting to take part in exercise.

Theory of reasoned action (TRA) and theory of planned behaviour (TPB)

These are similar approaches and both involve behavioural intentions and planning as an important feature to successfully achieve behaviour change. The belief is that if we plan we are more likely to do it and more likely to achieve the intended outcome. Figure 22.7 demonstrates the approach.

Table 22.3 An example of applying social cognitive theory

Expectancies	Situation expectancies – lack of exercise can lead to obesity and heart disease. Outcome expectancies – behaviour can reduce harm – exercising will reduce the chances of obesity and heart disease. Self-efficacy expectancies – I am capable of doing this if I want to.
Incentives	Rewards/benefits – I will be healthier, I will live longer; others will admire my behaviour/weight loss; I will feel better about myself.
Social cognitions	Health belief: Susceptibility to illness – my chances of getting heart disease are high. Severity – heart disease is a serious illness. Costs – exercise will make me tired; exercise takes up a lot of time. Cues to action – Internal: symptoms, e.g. breathlessness, weight gain. External: information from, for example, GP or health education leaflets.

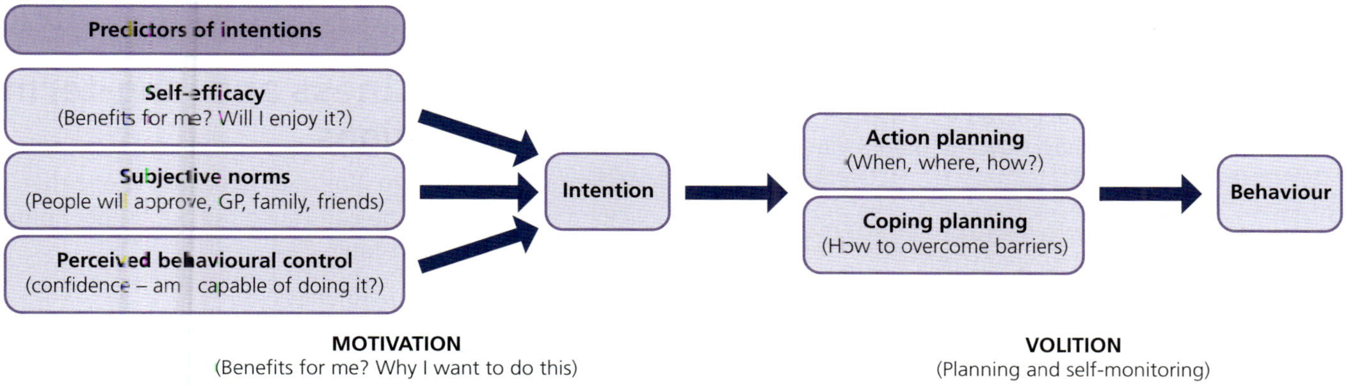

▲ **Figure 22.7** Theory of planned behaviour

INDEPENDENT RESEARCH ACTIVITY

Search on YouTube for a clip called 'Introduction to the Theory of Planned Behaviour' which gives a useful description of the theory of planned behaviour in action related to exercising. The clip is presented by Nathan Smith, from the University of Birmingham, School of Sports Science.

For more details about the health action process approach (HAPA), search for a video called 'hapa2014' on YouTube.

The trans-theoretical model identifies five stages of behaviour change, described in Figure 22.8.

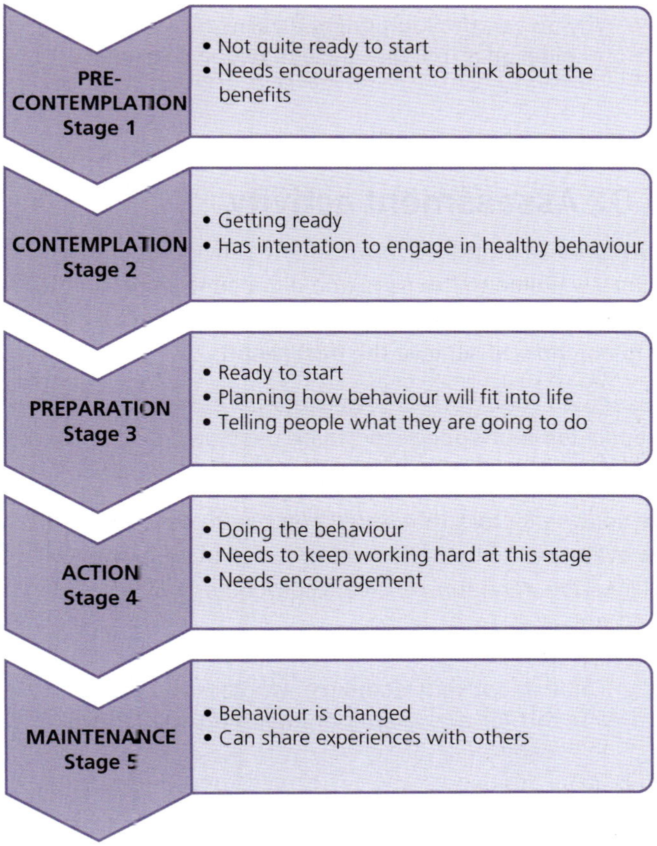

▲ **Figure 22.8** The five stages of the trans-theoretical model of behaviour change

Further details of the trans-theoretical theory are given in the YouTube clip presented by Nathan Smith, from the University of Birmingham, School of Sports Science. Search for 'Trans-Theoretical Model of Behaviour Change'.

GROUP ACTIVITY

(40 minutes)

Use the link below to access Brendan and Debbie's story.

http://www.nhs.uk/Conditions/Obesity/Pages/Realstories.aspx

In small groups consider Brendan and Debbie's journey to overcome their obesity.

● Reflecting on the theories of behaviour change that you have studied, which relates best to the way Brendan and Debbie achieved their weight loss?
● Draw a diagram to show how the theory was followed.

KNOW IT

1 What is 'health psychology'?
2 Describe four factors that could impact on health psychology.
3 Explain three key features of social cognition theory.
4 Why do you think planning and incentives are considered important for behaviour change?

LO2 Assessment activity *P2 D1*

Below is a suggested assessment activity that has been directly linked to the pass and distinction criteria in LO2 to help with assignment preparation; it includes Top Tips on how to achieve the best results.

Based on your work experience and research, write a report for your supervisor, to be used as a discussion document at a staff meeting. Your report should:

● analyse factors that impact on health psychology. *P2*
● evaluate the limitations of theories of behaviour change in relation to health psychology. *D1*

TOP TIPS ☑

✔ Think about your audience: who are you producing a report for and what language/information will they expect?
✔ Make sure your report is professionally produced. Check for typos and grammatical errors.

LO3 Understand the impact of chronic illness and long-term health conditions on individuals *P3 M2 D2*

GETTING STARTED

What is a 'chronic' illness? (10 minutes)

Discuss illnesses that you know about that last for a long time.

Do you know anyone who has a chronic or long-term illness? How does it affect them?

Write a group definition of 'chronic illness'.

3.1 Chronic illness and long-term health conditions

A chronic or long-term illness or condition is one that is long lasting: it can be controlled but not cured. Some examples are given in Table 22.4.

Table 22.4 Types of chronic illness

Illness or condition	Description
Arthritis	A painful degenerative disease that causes inflammation in the joints.
Dementia, Alzheimer's	Alzheimer's is the most common form of dementia. It involves a gradual loss of mental ability associated with the death of brain cells. It causes a range of problems including memory loss, confusion and personality changes.
Chronic obstructive pulmonary disease (COPD)	This is the name for a collection of lung diseases including chronic bronchitis, emphysema and chronic obstructive airways disease. People with COPD have breathing difficulties due to the narrowing of their airways.
Heart disease	Angina, heart attacks and heart failure are examples of heart disease. Walls of the arteries become blocked with fatty deposits, a process called atherosclerosis.
HIV/AIDS	The virus causes progressive damage to the immune system. AIDS is the final stage of HIV infection, when the body can no longer fight life-threatening infections; early diagnosis and treatment can prevent or control the deterioration.
Back pain	Long-term back pain has various causes: through injury, a slipped disc, sciatica, or a disease such ankylosing spondylitis which is a long-term condition that causes pain and stiffness where the spine meets the pelvis.

3.2 Psychological impacts of ill-health

Table 22.5 Examples of the psychological impacts of ill-health

Psychological impact	Explanation
Negative attitude	Always expecting the worst. Can lead to anxiety, depression or disengagement. Research has indicated that people with more positive attitudes have been generally found to cope more successfully with illness.
Depression	This could be an individual's reactive response to their life circumstances. They may feel unable to cope with their illness and so feel unable to cope with day-to-day life. This can lead to suicidal thoughts.
Denial	Ignoring or pretending that something is not happening. Hoping that if it is ignored it will go away. For example, an individual may ignore symptoms because if acknowledged it would mean admitting there is something wrong or that they need help.
Disengagement	Lack of interest in others and in activities. Can result in social exclusion and a lack of connection and social interaction with others.
Anxiety	It is normal to feel slightly nervous and worried at times, but if these feelings become more severe and result in panic attacks, fainting, vomiting, or fear that stops an individual living a normal life, therapy or treatment will be required to develop coping strategies.

3.3 Prescribed treatments

Table 22.6 Examples of treatments for chronic and long-term conditions

Prescribed treatments	Description
Medications	Used to treat symptoms or combat the effects of an illness such as pain or to delay the progress of a condition. Medication can take many different forms such as tablets, medicine, inhalers, creams and lotions. Injections are also used, such as insulin for Type I diabetes.
Dietary	Advice on a healthy diet may be appropriate for some conditions where weight loss is beneficial, such as arthritic knee joints, e.g. less fat, less sugar, less alcohol. Other diseases may require vitamin or mineral supplements. A healthy diet can reduce the risks of some cancers and heart disease.
Relaxation techniques	These techniques can be used to relieve stress, anxiety or depression, for example, or to help with sleep problems, pain and headaches. All relaxation techniques combine breathing more deeply with relaxing the muscles. Yoga or tai chi are sometimes recommended.
Counselling	Talking therapy allows an individual to talk about their problems and feelings in a safe and supportive environment. The counsellor will listen with empathy and will help an individual to deal with negative thoughts and feelings. (See also CBT and psychotherapy in LO1.)
Complementary therapies	Sometimes referred to as CAMs (complementary and alternative medicines). Covers a range of treatments and medicines such as acupuncture, homeopathy, chiropractic, herbalism, meditation, colonic irrigation and aromatherapy. The NHS has recommended the use of the Alexander Technique for Parkinson's disease, acupuncture and massage for persistent low back pain and ginger and acupressure for reducing morning sickness.
Exercise	Helps by strengthening muscles and the cardiovascular system and so helps prevent heart disease, diabetes, obesity. It also induces feelings of wellbeing, which can help mental health.

3.4 Impacts of treatment

Treatment of a health condition can be both a positive, and a negative, experience. The treatment may improve, or remove, any symptoms, which is a positive impact. Having treatment that works makes the person feel better and more in control of their life because taking, or having, the treatment makes them feel they can do something about their illness.

However, many treatments have negative side effects, such as hair loss, constant nausea or weight gain, or the treatment could be painful and tiring to endure, such as physiotherapy or chemotherapy sessions. Treatment can sometimes be for a short time or may be longer term or for the rest of an individual's life. Having to endure complex treatment in the long term can cause feelings of stress or depression especially if there are unpleasant side effects. Individuals may feel more ill by having the necessary treatment but fear the consequences if they do not endure it.

PAIRS ACTIVITY

(30 minutes)

Read 'Chronic obstructive pulmonary disease – Lynn's Story' which can be accessed by the following link:

http://tinyurl.com/gsbh6kj

Work in pairs to discuss how Lynn has coped with the impact of the treatment of her COPD.

Failure to comply with prescribed treatments

There is a wide range of reasons why individuals may not comply with treatments they have been prescribed. Table 22.7 gives some examples of the causes of non-compliance.

The use of health psychology theories such as those covered in LO2 can help and support individuals to comply with prescribed treatments. For further reading

Table 22.7 Why individuals fail to comply with prescribed treatments

Reason	Explanation
Side effects	Undesirable side effects of medication such as weight gain, nausea, impotence, depression can cause individuals to stop the treatment.
Time and complexity of treatment	Research has shown that short-term treatment is more likely to be successfully completed than longer-term treatments (Russell 2004: pp. 143–44). Long-term and chronic conditions are much more demanding to manage, often requiring not just medication but significant lifestyle changes such as in diet, or exercise.
Not using a person-centred approach	Prescribed treatment should involve a 'two-way' dialogue so that patients are fully informed and involved in all decision making from the start. Not using this approach reduces patient compliance as they feel treatment is imposed on them and they feel a lack of control.
Fear	Patients may have doubts or concerns about taking the medication but not feel able to discuss these with the health professional, or may lack confidence to question the 'expert'.
Lack of knowledge or information	The individual may not have been given enough information about their need for the prescribed treatment; they may not understand information they have been provided with.
Poor patient–practitioner communication	If a practitioner uses an authoritarian approach that focuses on medication and treatment it can lack patient focus. A patient may be very concerned about a particular symptom that is in fact medically not important, and so it is ignored as irrelevant by the practitioner. However the patient needs to have that symptom addressed by the practitioner to feel secure and confident in the treatment prescribed.
Lack of social support	Learning and behaviour change theories covered in LO2 demonstrate the need for support from others such as family and friends to enable treatment and lifestyle changes to be achieved.

on this topic, Russell (2014: Chapter 6 – Adherance to treatment) provides useful insights into patient non-adherance to prescribed treatments.

LO3 Assessment activity P3 M2 D2

Below is a suggested assessment activity that has been directly linked to the pass, merit and distinction criteria in LO3 to help with assignment preparation; it includes Top Tips on how to achieve the best results.

Find two real life case studies of individuals with different chronic or long-term health conditions. Use an authoritative source such as a charity's website.

Create two handouts for the charity to use when training new volunteers. The handouts should do the following.

- Explain the psychological impacts of ill-health on individuals. **P3**
- Assess why individuals may fail to comply with prescribed treatments. **M2**
- Evaluate the psychological impact when an individual fails to comply with prescribed treatment for a chronic illness or a long-term health condition. **D2**

TOP TIPS

- ✔ Make sure that you choose case studies from official charity websites.
- ✔ Think about what work the charity does and what information new volunteers would need.
- ✔ Make sure that you include all the relevant information the criteria ask for.

LO4 Know the psychological impacts of requiring care P4

GETTING STARTED

(10 minutes)

George is 89 years old and is thinking of going to live in a care home because his mobility is not what it was. He finds it difficult to manage the stairs in his house and struggles with food shopping because he cannot walk very far. His daughter works full time and lives too far away to help him.

What impact would this move have on George's quality of life? Write a list of positive effects and a list of negative effects.

Discuss your lists with the rest of the class.

4.1 Positive and negative psychological impacts of requiring care

Learned helplessness is when an individual believes that they cannot do things by themselves and need to rely on others. This can happen when an older person goes to live in retirement home – for instance, because they are 'in care' they says they cannot look after themselves any more, when in reality they are capable of continuing to perform daily tasks. Staff who make choices for them, about meals and what to wear, for example, contribute to the development of learned helplessness. Health and social care practitioners can limit learned helplessness through using a person-centred approach that focuses on the individual's capabilities.

Empowerment due to receiving care is a positive outcome, for example an individual with arthritis who has been struggling to cook meals, get dressed and have a shower may feel empowered if they are helped by care assistants visiting their home every day. This results in an improved outlook on life and reduces the risk of developing learned helplessness because they are being enabled to be as independent as possible. As long as an individual feels that they have maintained control over their life, and feel safe and secure, receiving care will have a positive impact on self-esteem.

Opportunities for activities and social contact let an individual maintain a sense of belonging and wellbeing. Encouraging individuals to attend a day centre or lunch club would help to provide social stimulation for someone who is usually alone at home due to having a chronic health condition. Providing transport would enable the individuals to take part in activities, which may enhance their quality of life and prevent them from becoming socially isolated.

Changes to independence and financial situation, or chronic illness that results in an individual requiring care, can lead to dependence on others for transport, food shopping and daily living tasks such as bathing. This can cause an individual to feel depressed and have low self-esteem, as they may struggle to accept the fact that they are now dependent on others. Some individuals may feel that they are a burden to their family and carers and so not ask for help that they need. They may become disengaged from society, feeling they are no longer valued and spend long periods of time alone.

Financially, chronic illness may have a significant impact on income. If the individual can no longer work, or has to work part time, income may be reduced or lost so they have to rely on state benefits. This can drastically affect quality of life by restricting what they can spend on leisure, food, heating and housing costs and, again, also affects their ability to be independent and self-sufficient.

If well managed by practitioners using a person-centred approach, receiving care can have positive results. If an individual is involved in decision making regarding their individual care plan and the principles of person-centred care are adhered to then their needs will be met, as demonstrated by the humanistic approach described by Maslow's hierarchy of needs and actualising tendency (see LO1 page 288).

THINK ABOUT IT

Case study

Choose one of the real life case studies which can be accessed by the following links.

Coronary heart disease:

http://tinyurl.com/h296dcq

Deep brain stimulation treatment for Parkinson's:

http://tinyurl.com/j576rsp

Arthritis:

http://tinyurl.com/hvbn6dg

1 Describe the illness or condition.
2 What are the psychological impacts on the person, and their family and friends, of the illness or condition?
3 Why might the person fail to comply with prescribed treatments?
4 Describe the psychological impacts of requiring care for the condition.

KNOW IT

1 Give four examples of chronic or long-term illnesses.
2 Name three types of prescribed treatments and give examples of why they would be prescribed.
3 Explain one positive and one negative impact of receiving treatment for a long-term illness.
4 What is the meaning of the term 'learned helplessness'?
5 How could staff at a nursing home empower the residents?

LO4 Assessment activity *P2*

Below is a suggested assessment activity that has been directly linked to the pass criteria in LO4 to help with assignment preparation; it includes Top Tips on how to achieve the best results.

Write a diary for a week from the perspective of an individual with a chronic illness. The diary will be used to help give new volunteers an insight into the experience of an individual living with a chronic illness.

The diary should describe the psychological impacts of requiring care.

TOP TIPS

✔ Think about how you would feel if you had a chronic illness – what frustrations do you think you would experience?
✔ Think about the range of physical and psychological limitations an individual might encounter.

Read about it

Cardwell, M. (2010) A-Z Psychology Handbook, 4th edition, Philip Allen.

Fisher, A. et al. (2012) Applied A2 Health & Social Care for OCR, revised edition, Oxford.

Moonie, N. et al. (2007) Core Themes – Health and Social Care, Heinemann.

Russell, J. and Roberts, C. (2014) Introduction to Psychology for Health Carers, CENGAGE Learning.

Unit 23

Sociology for health and social care

ABOUT THIS UNIT

Sociologists provide us with different perspectives that can be used to examine and analyse health and illness. By studying this unit you will be able to use a sociological approach when considering questions such as whether health is a matter of personal choice or instead determined by other factors such as genes, economic status, access to information and health care.

What determines ill-health? Is it a person's own opinion that they feel ill, or does it have to be an officially recognised and named disease in order to be classed as illness? Applying sociological theories to the ways society functions and to an individual's beliefs, values and practices, will enable you to develop your understanding of contemporary issues in the health and social care sectors.

LEARNING OUTCOMES

The topics, activities and suggested reading in this unit will help you to:

1 Understand sociological perspectives
2 Understand sociological perspectives about health and social care
3 Understand patterns and trends in health and illness among different social groups
4 Understand sociological perspectives about the organisation and management of health and social care

How will I be assessed?

You will be assessed through a series of assignments and tasks set and marked by your tutor.

How will I be graded?

You will be graded using the following criteria.

Learning outcome	Pass assessment criteria	Merit assessment criteria	Distinction assessment criteria
You will:	To achieve a **pass** you must demonstrate that you have met all the pass assessment criteria	To achieve a **merit** you must demonstrate that you have met all the pass and merit assessment criteria	To achieve a **distinction** you must demonstrate that you have met all the pass, merit and distinction assessment criteria
1 Understand sociological perspectives	**P1** Describe sociological perspectives **P2** Explain the purposes of sociological research and the methods used	**M1** Use sociological theory to compare medical and social models of illness	
2 Understand sociological perspectives about health and social care	**P3** Explain how sociological perspectives relate to issues in health and social care		
3 Understand patterns and trends in health and illness among different social groups	**P4** Explain patterns and trends in health and illness among different social groups	**M2** Analyse data on health outcomes and comment on the distribution using sociological theory	**D1** Evaluate patterns and trends in health and illness among different social groups
4 Understand sociological perspectives about the organisation and management of health and social care	**P5** Describe who is responsible for promoting good health **P6** Explain how sociological perspectives relate to the organisation of health and social care		

LO1 Understand sociological perspectives *P1 P2*

GETTING STARTED

What is 'sociology'? (10 minutes)

In small groups discuss what you think 'sociology' is about – use a textbook, the internet or a dictionary for information. Agree on one sentence that you think describes it. Each small group can then feed back to the whole group and decide on a whole group definition.

1.1 Sociological theory

Society is complex and constantly changing; using sociological theory can help us to understand, explain and question our social world. The different theoretical perspectives provide viewpoints that are used to explain society and how it functions.

Sociologists develop theory that helps to explain the social world. They carry out research on people and groups within society to help develop their theories. The social world is complex and so a number of different theoretical perspectives try to explain it; sometimes these perspectives agree and sometimes they conflict. LO1 considers some of the main sociological theories.

Grand theory

Karl Marx (1818–1883), Émile Durkheim (1820–1903) and Max Weber (1864–1920) have been called the founders of sociology. Their theories developed in response to the evolution of modern society which, due to the Industrial Revolution, moved from being rural, agriculturally and family based to being highly industrialised, scientific and mostly functioning in an urban environment. The culture of social groups, in general, moved from tradition, family and religion to being influenced by technological, scientific and rational thinking.

Marx

Marx based his theory on the economic structure of society, where he saw conflict between the different groups within the population. Marx believed that the wealthy industrialists and business owners, or 'capitalists', had all the power and influence over society.

Marx argued that the economic system defined society and people's place within it. He said that the workers, or 'proletariat', were exploited by the land-owning capitalists because they only had their labour to sell. This small, but powerful, capitalist elite benefited from their workers' labours and became very wealthy, while the workers, who were the majority of the population, lived in relative poverty. This unequal relationship between the capitalists and the proletariat resulted in conflict which he hoped would lead to a revolution where the proletariat would take over all the factories and institutions and put them into public ownership so that the wealth created would benefit everyone, not just a select few.

Marx believed that the capitalists' power as the ruling class enabled them to influence the whole of society through the **socialisation** process where their ideas, values and attitudes were passed on. Marx felt that this was so successful because the proletariat did not realise that they were being exploited and were being used to serve the interests of the upper classes.

Conflict sociologists, such as Marx, view the relationship between groups in society as one of domination and subordination, in which the dominant group act as oppressors.

Durkheim

Durkheim's theory is **structuralist**, as it focuses on the view that society is made up of social structures, groups and institutions, e.g. the family, religious groups, health and social care services, the education system, the judicial and political systems. People are held together in society through work, family and community.

Durkheim argued that 'social facts', such as beliefs, values, morals and cultural norms, go beyond the individual and, through shared membership of institutions such as families, they provide social restraint by guiding and controlling behaviour as they have become internalised through socialisation.

Durkheim investigated how different **social institutions** produce differences in individuals' behaviour. For example, he suggested that suicide is caused by a lack of social integration. He argued that the stronger social support found among Catholics would result in lower suicide rates, because they are a more closely integrated and more distinct social group than Protestants. He compared the suicide rates of Catholics and Protestants who were similar in other social characteristics – marital status, where they lived, age etc. He found that the official statistics on suicide showed that Catholics did have a lower suicide rate than Protestants. He also found that suicide rates were higher among men than women, for single people, for people without children, among soldiers than civilians, and in times of peace rather than in times of war.

Durkheim's research supported his theory that social factors are more influential than a person's psychology or biology, and enabled him to argue that causes of suicide were to be found in social factors and not individual personalities.

🔑 **KEY TERMS**

Capitalist – the Marxist term for industrialists, factory and business owners who provide employment for others.

Proletariat – the Marxist term for workers who sell their labour to earn an income.

Socialisation – the process where people learn the values, attitudes and norms of their society.

Structuralist – a sociological perspective that is concerned with the overall organisation or 'structure' of society.

Social institutions or structures – the elements that make up society, e.g. family, school, workplace, judicial system, health and social care services.

Weber

Weber used social action theory, also known as the **interpretivist** approach. Action is 'social' because actions are viewed as 'appropriate' or not, depending on the social circumstances and accepted ways of thinking. Weber focused on the meanings and motives behind actions. Using this approach, a researcher observes society from the point of view of the individual in order to interpret what is happening and why from their perspective.

Weber identified four types of social action in order to understand motivation.

1 *Emotional actions* are motivated by feelings, for example losing your temper and shouting.
2 *Traditional actions* are motivated by customs or habits, for example giving presents at Christmas.
3 *Value-rational actions* are motivated by commitment to a particular value, such as patriotism or loyalty.
4 *Instrumental-rational actions* are based on a strategic cost–benefit analysis. Working for wages for example or a 'what's in it for me' approach.

Weber recognised that many actions fall into more than one of these categories.

Weber also used the term '*verstehen*', which is a German word for interpretive understanding of social actions. He described two types of understanding.

1 '*Aktuelles verstehen*' – understanding derived from direct observation.
2 '*Erklärendes verstehen*' – where the sociologist must put themselves in the mind of the individual whose behaviour they are trying to explain, in order to try to understand their motives.

The social action perspective examines smaller groups and individuals and sees society as a product of human activity; unlike structuralism, which sees society as being shaped by its structures and institutions.

In 1905 Weber published *The Protestant Ethic and the Spirit of Capitalism*. In this he emphasised the hard work and frugality that led to prosperity, known as the Protestant work ethic. He stated that societies that are more Protestant tended to be more bureaucratic. To him this was a good thing, as workers are more likely to take pride in their work and are less alienated than in the Marxist worldview where power is in the hands of the elite.

Applying theory to sociological questions

Sociology considers questions about how and why society works as it does. Sociologists examine why society changes – as a whole, but also at group and individual level. It looks at problems and issues within society. An example is increasing obesity levels in the population, despite the availability of good quality food and health advice. What social and economic forces make this happen?

Sociologists will look for the dominant views of society and how these shape the lives of the population. Understanding changes in the cultural values and norms of society, such as marriage, the family and an ageing population, all involve, and are affected by, constantly changing and developing social expectations.

Using theory to analyse situations, events or developments in society, a sociologist will have a hypothesis, or idea, about why something is happening and will then gather facts and evidence that will either confirm or disprove the hypothesis. Gathering and analysing the 'social facts', as Durkheim would say, can help to provide reasons and explanations.

1.2 Macro perspectives

Macro sociological analysis involves studying the large-scale structures or aspects of society. Looking at the 'big picture' includes historical change over time, and the rise and fall of political systems or class hierarchies. Grand theories such as Marxism and functionalism use this approach, looking at how society works as a system made up of interdependent parts.

Social systems

Socio-economic status

An individual's socio-economic status is based on the concept of '**social class**', introduced by Marx. Social class is determined by economic factors such as level of income, type of housing and occupation. Socio-economic status combines factors such as income and occupation with other factors such as education.

> 🔑 **KEY TERM**
>
> **Interpretivist** – a sociological perspective that focuses on understanding the motivation and meaning of individual behaviour.
>
> **Social class** – the classification of people according to their occupation and income to be working class, middle class or upper class.

The Office for National Statistics provides a broad classification of occupations into social classes, shown in Table 23.1. The government uses this classification to analyse trends in the population such as mortality rates.

Table 23.1 UK National Statistics Socio-economic Classification (NS-SEC class) (source: www.ons.gov.uk)

NS-SEC class	Occupation	Type of job
1	Higher managerial and professional occupations	Doctors, lawyers, dentists, vets, general managers, accountants, clinical psychologists, scientists, chaplains
2	Lower managerial and professional occupations	Teachers, nurses, midwives, physiotherapists, occupational therapists, social workers, radiographers, chiropodists, librarians, laboratory technicians, careers advisors
3	Intermediate occupations	Secretaries, fire fighters, police constables, hospital-based nursing assistants, ambulance staff, nursery nurses
4	Small employers and own-account workers	Builders, car sellers, shop owners, roofers, painters & decorators, joiners, taxi drivers, beauticians
5	Lower supervisory and technical occupations	Computer maintainers & installers, electricians, plumbers, gardeners, television engineers
6	Semi-routine occupations	Dental nurses, shop assistants, postal workers, security guards, receptionists, traffic wardens, hospital porters
7	Routine occupations	Bus drivers, waiters & waitresses, cleaners, bar staff, car park attendants, flight attendants, hairdressers
8	Never worked and long-term unemployed	Students, people not classifiable, unemployed

Family

The family is a fundamental structure of society. It has undergone many changes over the last century and there are now many different types of family.

Everyone is affected by their family, positively or negatively; a family gives its members a place in society and it is the main unit of socialisation and preparation for adulthood. Sociologists such as Durkheim argue that because of this the family is a positive institution that is beneficial for individuals and society as a whole. However, Marxists would argue that it is damaging as it perpetuates gender and economic inequalities in society.

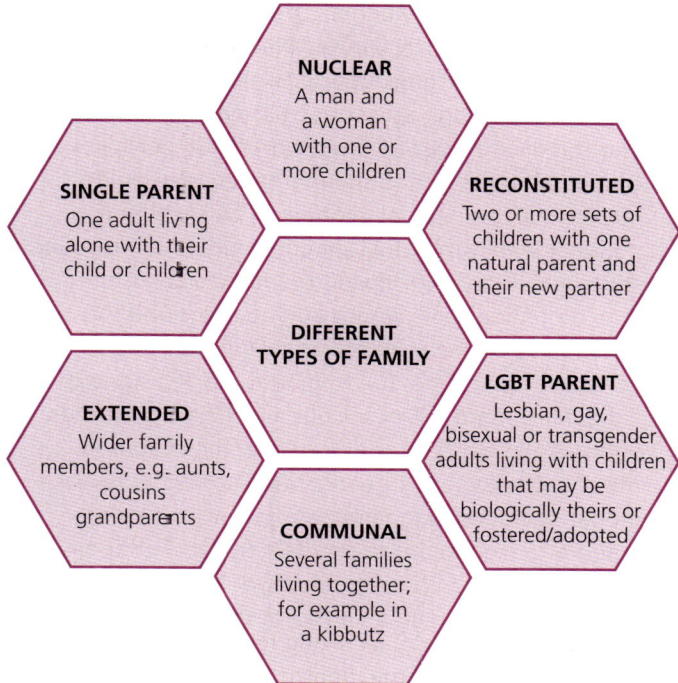

▲ **Figure 23.1** Different types of family structure

Gender

In sociological terms there is a distinct difference between 'sex' and 'gender'. Sex refers to the specific biological and physiological differences between males and females. Sociologists say that the gender differences between men and women are socially constructed – that is, they are created by society. For example, different gender roles have different expectations. Gender socialisation is the way that the behavioural expectations of society for men and women are transmitted. Generally, women are expected to be nurturing, caring and passive whereas men are seen as active, aggressive, dominant and unemotional. Sociologists say that gender expectations affect how an individual experiences their life and who they become.

Structures

Structuralism is a top-down perspective that examines the way in which society as a whole fits together. Functionalism and Marxism are both structuralist perspectives – they perceive human activity as the result of social structure.

● Political structures – in the UK examples include political parties (Labour, Conservative etc.), the House of Lords and House of Commons, trade unions.
● Social structures – the family, church-based organisations and voluntary organisations, school, workplace, judicial system, health and social care services.

- Global structures – such as the World Health Organization, the UN (United Nations), NATO (North Atlantic Treaty Organization), Greenpeace. These organisations look at issues such as health, security and the environment from a worldwide perspective. Globalisation refers to the increased worldwide interconnectedness of economic, cultural and political structures. Instant communication through the internet and worldwide media has resulted in a 'global culture' where societies around the world have become increasingly similar, sharing consumer products due to global marketing, e.g. Nike, McDonald's, Coca-Cola and TV programmes such as Big Brother and The X Factor. A shared mass culture means people have access to diverse global social media, religions, music and food, leading to significant social and cultural changes. Globalisation can provide material improvements but can also be seen as a threat to cultures and identities in society.

1.3 Micro perspectives: interconnections between personal experience and social circumstances

Micro perspectives involve studying how society works at a person-to-person level. A micro perspective looks at one-to-one interactions between individuals, such as how people deal with social situations like job interviews or personal confrontations. It examines how people make decisions about their lives. Sometimes these decisions make sense (e.g. taking a job for money to buy food to live), and sometimes they do not seem to make sense at all (e.g. spending money on smoking, which will affect health).

Structural changes in the family (see Figure 23.1) have been significant and the impact on relationships is of interest to sociologists to determine whether, for example, there is now more equality between men and women in their relationships. To investigate how the changes in family structure have impacted on family roles and relationships, sociologists carry out research to look at who carries out the household chores and, if they are shared, who takes responsibility for child care, managing finances and decision making.

1.4 Purposes of sociological research

Sociologists are concerned with the study of society, social institutions and social groups. Sociology does not attempt to analyse and explain an individual's behaviour; it examines the **social groupings** in society and uses these to answer questions. For example, to increase knowledge and understanding it will look at social class or age group as a basis for investigating patterns in health and illness. Research could also be carried out to monitor or review policies, practices or specific services, to test out new treatments and establish the benefits for particular groups of people or to identify the needs of specific population groups.

> 🔑 **KEY TERM**
>
> **Social groupings** – the classification of people by, for example, their gender, social class, ethnicity, age, locality.

1.5 Methods of investigation in sociology

Sociologists will choose different methods to carry out their investigations depending on what they are researching and what type of information they hope to obtain.

Scientific methods versus interpretive approaches

In theory, the most reliable research method is the laboratory-based scientific experiment. The results are measurable because it is carried out in controlled conditions. This means it can be carried out in exactly the same way by someone else who will get the same results. However, this method is not always ideal for sociological research because it involves situations set up by the researcher and so the findings may not apply to real life. Some sociologists believe that scientific experimental approaches cannot adequately explain the social world because people and society are complex and not easily predictable or measurable.

'Field experiments' can be more suitable as they are based in the real world, such as in a hospital or school, and it is possible to learn more about social groups and how people behave. Research methods such as tick-box questionnaires, **structured interviews**, **closed questions** and observational checklists allow facts to be obtained in pre-planned and controlled way. There is, however, less control in a field experiment compared with a laboratory experiment.

An interpretive approach to research related to health and social care uses methods such as semi-structured or **unstructured interviews** and observation of naturally occurring action. The aim is to obtain information about the experiences of individuals or groups from their own perspective an 'insider's' view. It could, for example, involve finding out how people define their own state of health or how they view their interactions with health professionals. This kind of research could then lead to identifying patterns that could be linked back to structures such as family or social class.

KEY TERMS

Structured interview – an interview where the interviewer asks pre-prepared questions and records the answers.

Closed question – a question with a limited number of answers to choose from.

Informal or unstructured interview – an interview where the interviewer does not keep to a prepared list of questions.

Quantitative versus qualitative approaches

Data collected for sociological research studies will either be quantitative or qualitative.

Quantitative data uses numbers and statistics and is often presented in a graph or table. Health and social care data gathered by the Office for National Statistics (ONS) is an example of a quantitative approach. The ONS is responsible for collecting and publishing official statistics related to the economy, population and society at national, regional and local levels. It also conducts the census in England and Wales every ten years. The government obtains a lot of information from the ONS that is then used to inform decisions about policy.

Qualitative data is presented in words rather than in numbers, is descriptive and may involve attitudes and viewpoints. It is used for exploratory research to gain an understanding of underlying reasons, opinions and motivations; it can provide insights into problems and issues through analysis of the experiences and views of individuals.

INDEPENDENT RESEARCH ACTIVITY
(30 minutes)

Using the internet or any other source of information available to you, such as newspaper articles or textbooks, find an example of health-related research.

Reflect on the piece of research to answer the following questions.

- Which method(s) has the researcher used?
- Is the information and data obtained qualitative or quantitative?
- Why do you think the researcher has used the methods they did?

KNOW IT

1 Why is Marx called a 'conflict structuralist'?
2 What did Durkheim mean by the phrase 'social facts'?
3 What is 'social action theory'?
4 Explain the difference between 'micro' and 'macro' sociology.
5 Explain the difference between qualitative and quantitative research methods.

L01 Assessment activity *P1 P2*

Below is a suggested assessment activity that has been directly linked to the pass criteria in LO1 to help with assignment preparation; it includes Top Tips on how to achieve the best results.

Staff at your local health centre want to know more about sociological approaches to health and social care to inform their work. Because you are studying Level 3 Health and Social Care, you have been asked to provide information for them.

- Prepare a presentation, with presenter's notes, that describes sociological perspectives.
- Produce an information booklet that explains the purposes of sociological research and the methods used.

TOP TIPS

✔ Think about the difference between a presentation and an information booklet – how would this have an impact on the way you present your information?
✔ Think about the difference between describing and explaining something.

LO2 Understand sociological perspectives about health and social care *P3 M1*

2.1 Medical and social models of illness

Sociological perspectives about health, social care and illness have challenged the traditional view that health and illness have purely biological causes and medical treatments. It is now recognised that health and illness has a social element. However, different perspectives explain why some individuals, or groups of people, suffer illness and have shorter lives than others. Structuralist perspectives explain health as being affected by the economic and political structures of society. Durkheim would state that 'social facts' and influences are more important and Weber would stress the motivation behind individual lifestyle choices.

Causes and origins of illness

The role of scientific investigation in understanding illnesses

The medical model of health and illness focuses on the biological aspects of disease and illness and is practised by doctors and other health professionals. It is associated with the diagnosis, treatment and cure of the disease or illness. Health is seen as an absence of disease or illness.

A health service provider may be more likely to use a medical model of health because, historically, the NHS has diagnosed and treated ill-health. Tax payers want to see value for the money spent on the NHS. For example, the children's immunisation programme protects children from diseases that can be fatal or seriously damage future health and quality of life. This provides quantitative data about how infection rates decrease as a direct result of the vaccination programme.

The limitations of science in establishing causes

The medical model encourages service users to give control of their care to health care experts and passively expect to be treated. They become dependent on this perspective, not challenging it, just accepting what they are told and taking the care pathway they are instructed to. It can be appropriate for acute, short illnesses which require specific treatment (such as a broken arm), but is generally less appropriate for long-term or chronic illnesses or incurable disabilities. Often personal and social circumstances play a part in both physical and

mental illnesses, and may, in some cases, be the trigger for the condition rather than a biological cause.

Scientific rationality and health and social care

Scientific rationality is based on logic, facts and sound judgement which should underpin any scientific or medical investigation, treatment or action. Many advances in medical knowledge are due to research taking this approach, for example the development of treatments for cancer. The following sections outline some theories that influence decision making in health and social care.

Judging actions: consequentialist perspectives

Consequentialist theory states that right or wrong depends on the consequences of an action. The better the consequences, or results, the better the action is that has been taken. Jeremy Bentham was a philosopher and social reformer. He said:

'That action is best, which procures the greatest happiness for the greatest numbers.'

(Source: http://plato.stanford.edu/entries/ utilitarianism-history)

This approach is used in the UK by the National Institute for Health and Care Excellence (NICE). Part of the work carried out by NICE involves deciding what drugs, treatments and procedures can be provided by the NHS. NICE weighs up the costs and benefits of a drug or treatment to inform the decision about whether it is effective enough to be funded by the NHS. NICE has to look for the greatest benefit for the greatest number of people. This sometimes results in treatments being withheld, not because they are ineffective, but because the expense outweighs the number of people who would benefit.

Judging actions: deontological perspectives

Deontological ethics or moral principles are used to judge whether an action is right or wrong based on how well the action adheres to a rule or set of rules. It is sometimes called 'duty' or 'obligation'. For example, the Hippocratic Oath, written by Hippocrates in Ancient Greece, is still taken by new doctors and is used as a guide to their conduct. The Oath requires physicians to treat the ill to the best of their ability, to preserve a patient's privacy, to teach knowledge of medicine to the next generation and to do no harm.

Instrumental rationality

This is an approach to decision making that balances options against one another and the decision is made by making a strategic judgement. The costs are considered, that is what will it take to achieve – for example, time, effort, staffing, training or money. Then the benefits will be weighed against the costs and a decision made.

Value questions

Sociologists carrying out research and health and social care professionals working with individuals must always be impartial and objective. Their own personal values, beliefs or moral judgements must not be taken into account as this would lead to bias and possibly unfair treatment. Weber stated that 'value neutrality' should be the aim of sociologists, who should be aware of their own values and not carry them into their work. For example personal opinions about people's lifestyle choices or views on sexuality, race or religion should be put to one side and the diverse nature of individuals respected.

Diagnosis

Personal and social impact and illness as deviation from normality

Talcott Parsons (1902–1979), an American sociologist, felt that, for society to function properly and efficiently, its members need to be healthy. He called illness 'deviance' from the norm and said that members of society who were ill were performing 'the sick role'. This was his way of explaining how the cultural expectations about being ill affect how ill people behave. In his book *The Social System* (1951), Parsons identified four aspects of 'the sick role', shown in Figure 23.2.

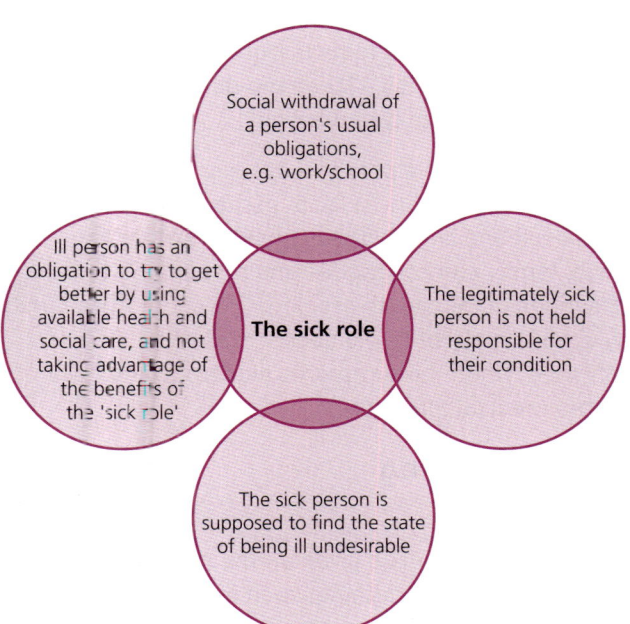

▲ **Figure 23.2** Talcott Parsons' 'sick role'

However, Parsons' theory is not supported by all sociologists. Some feel that, while it is useful in helping to analyse how society assigns roles, and has expectations of how ill people should behave, it does not take account of situations where the individual does not want to acknowledge that they are ill.

An individual may not want an employer or family members to know about their illness, or they may be in denial that they are ill at all. They may be diagnosed with a mental illness or a particular infectious disease and want to avoid talking about it because of the social stigma attached to that condition. There are also situations, such as one parent families, where the parent simply cannot withdraw into the 'sick role' because they need to work and support their family. Other individuals may feel that being ill is a weakness and so refuse to adopt the 'sick role', instead hoping that the effects of illness will go away. Sociological research has found that there are also common attitudes regarding what is seen as 'normal' illness, such as headaches, aches and pains associated with the ageing process and feeling 'run down' – these are seen as an inevitable, normal part of life. This is in contrast to 'real' illness that demands a visit to a health professional.

Relationship between psychological and physical factors in illness

The research of psychologist Sigmund Freud suggested that some illnesses or conditions may be a result of an individual's state of mind, where repressed experiences and feelings may appear as a physical or emotional problem which in fact has its roots in the mind. Repressed emotions, inadequate attachment and unresolved conflicts can build up and result in anxiety, depression, drug and alcohol abuse or eating disorders.

Psychodynamic therapy is where a patient discusses their condition or problem with a psychodynamic counsellor, who may use a variety of ways to uncover the individual's unconscious motivations and the needs. A psychodynamic counsellor will try to identify links between past events and how the person thinks and feels now. The aim is to enable the individual to be free from the repressed feelings and experiences in their unconscious mind and more able to control their life and emotions.

Behavioural psychologists believe that behaviour is learned by being rewarded through positive or negative reinforcement. So, for example, treating an individual with an alcohol or drug dependency may use aversion therapy, which produces an adverse reaction if they attempt to take drugs or have an alcoholic drink.

Social definitions of illness

Also known as the 'social model of health', this focuses on the social, environmental and economic factors that can impact negatively on health rather than perceiving illness to have its origins within the individual. During the nineteenth century, improving water supplies, providing sewerage systems, better housing and health education programmes and policies attempted to prevent illness in the first place. This is known as the 'public health approach' and helped to reduce ill-health and premature death by the beginning of the twentieth century.

The idea is that social change is required to prevent illness. Issues wider than just biological illness and medical treatment need to be considered, such as reducing social inequalities, providing access to health care, improving the physical environment, and empowering individuals with the knowledge and confidence to make positive decisions about their own health and participate in healthy behaviours. Providing access to health care for all does not just involve having hospitals and GP surgeries in all areas, but overcoming cultural, educational and language barriers that prevent individuals from being proactive about their health.

Advantages of the social model are that it helps to prevent illness. This can be cost effective, which helps the economy and the NHS, and it improves individuals' quality of life. The difficulties are that many people do not receive or understand the health promotion messages and information. Some ignore the messages and are not motivated to change because they enjoy things like getting a suntan or smoking, and changing lifestyles is hard work. Also, of course, not all diseases can be prevented.

> ### ❓ THINK ABOUT IT
>
> #### Case study: Josh
>
> Josh is 7 years old and has asthma. He lives with his mum and younger brother in a house next to a busy main road. The house is damp and run down. Josh's mum enjoys smoking; it is her only luxury and she spends all the rest of her money on the house and her children.
>
> 1 What could be a trigger for Josh's asthma?
> 2 The family is visited by a health professional who uses the medical perspective. What type of treatment would be offered to Josh for his asthma?
> 3 What would a health visitor who uses the social model of illness recommend to help with Josh's asthma?
> 4 What are the strengths and weaknesses of each approach?

Role and responsibility of professionals

Professional judgement and expert knowledge

There is a high level of trust involved in the doctor–patient relationship, and the patient's interests must be protected. Functionalists suggest the following features of professionalism apply to the medical profession.

- Doctors have gained specialised, expert medical knowledge through their training.
- Doctors should work altruistically, that is motivated by an unselfish concern for the welfare of others.
- All patients should be treated fairly and equally based on their needs, regardless of social class, sexuality, gender or ethnicity.
- Only qualified individuals may practise medicine.
- Professional should be controlled by a code of professional and medical ethics.

These features could equally apply to any health and social care practitioner.

Personal experience and knowing whose knowledge counts

Irving Zola (1935–1994) was a medical sociologist and supporter of disability rights. In his book, *The Patient's Perception of the Illness* (1973), he identified five 'social triggers' that influence the judgement that the symptoms need professional health care.

1 Perceived interference with work-related activity.
2 Perceived interference with social or personal relations.
3 Perceived interference with social relationships.
4 A monitoring of symptoms (setting a deadline – if I'm not better by Monday, I'll see the doctor).
5 Pressure from family and friends.

Zola's theory is that a person's decision to seek professional medical help for a 'perceived' illness is in fact a social one and involves consulting others such as friends, family and colleagues and responding to their perceptions of the health problem. Pressure from family may speed up a visit to the doctor to have the illness 'confirmed' when the symptoms alone may not have required medical attention.

Decision making

Informed choice

This is when someone is given all the facts and information about something, such as a course of medication and alternative options, so they can consider whether to agree to the treatment or not.

Shared decision making

Any treatment, procedure or action in health and social care should always be discussed fully with the individuals involved and only carried out if agreement is reached and consent given. The Health and Social Care Act (2012) introduced the principle of 'No decision about me without me', which now guides all practice. Patients are free to choose their GP, consultant, treatment and hospital or other local health service.

Professional choice

Some health care providers have suggested, for example, that there should be restrictions on treatment for cardiovascular disease for smokers. In practice, some health services are already restricted because of an individual's lifestyle. For example, patients with alcoholism who do not give up drinking are not candidates for liver transplants. In some areas, individuals who are obese have to lose weight before they are offered bariatric surgery such as a gastric band.

Paternalism and trust

Feminist writers feel that paternalism (power of men over women) exists, for example through male doctors' control over women through the medicalisation of pregnancy and birth. The male doctors hold the power and women are dependent on them and so have to trust them to work in the mother's best interests. However, many doctors are now women so paternalism may not be as common as it once was.

Today a patient can be considered to be a 'consumer' of health and social care services. This is due in part to initiatives such as the 2012 Health and Social Care Act, but also to individuals becoming less accepting of the traditional 'expert' view. Increased 'consumer' knowledge leads to patients asking questions and challenging the views of professionals. Some question the reliance on the scientific approach of the medical model and look to complementary or alternative therapies instead. This raises the question of who is responsible for good health – the government? The doctor? The individual?

PAIRS ACTIVITY

(40 minutes)

Jonathan is 25 years old and is severely obese.

- In pairs, discuss who is responsible for Jonathan's health and wellbeing.
- Consider how a 'shared decision-making approach' could benefit Jonathan.
- Share your thoughts with the rest of the group.

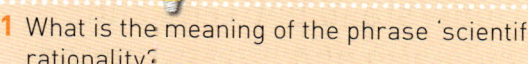

KNOW IT

1 What is the meaning of the phrase 'scientific rationality'?
2 Give examples of what is meant by 'value questions'.
3 Describe Parsons' theory of the 'sick role'.
4 Explain what Freud thought was the basis of illness.
5 Give a definition of the medical model of illness.
6 Give a definition of the social model of illness.

LO2 Assessment activities

Below are suggested assessment activities that have been directly linked to the pass and merit criteria in LO2 to help with assignment preparation; they include Top Tips on how to achieve best results.

Your work for this activity should relate to two particular issues of your choice. Examples could include: childhood obesity, social care provision for an ageing population, smoking, binge drinking.

Activity 1 – pass criteria *P3*

Write an additional section to the information booklet you started in LO1. This section should explain how sociological perspectives relate to issues in health and social care

Activity 2 – merit criteria *M1*

Produce a display for the staff notice board at the health centre. The content of the display should use sociological theory to provide a comparison of the medical and social models of health.

TOP TIPS

- ✔ Choose two issues that you find particularly interesting and research them thoroughly.
- ✔ Think about how you could display your information – what could you do to make your work eye-catching?

LO3 Understand patterns and trends in health and illness among different social groups *P4 M2 D1*

Statistical trends in the levels of health, illness and wellbeing are available from three main sources. Government statistics are available from the ONS website where there is up to date data on many aspects of health and social care related issues, as well as 'Social Trends' which detail population patterns. Third sector organisations such as Mind and the British Heart Foundation also collect and publish data. Authors and academic researchers produce articles and textbooks analysing social trends.

3.1 Health inequalities between different groups

Socio-economic

Social class is no longer considered by sociologists to be as important as it used to be to individuals as a definition of themselves and their place in society. However, there is still a socio-economic hierarchy in the UK that does affect individuals' life chances. Government statistics show those with a lower income suffer higher levels of illness and premature death, while those with higher incomes have better health and longer lives. This is demonstrated in Table 23.2, which is adapted from an ONS bulletin released in October 2015 showing the trend in life expectancy at birth by socio-economic position, for England and Wales.

Table 23.2 ONS Life expectancy at birth by socio-economic position

NS-SEC Class	Class Label	Life expectancy	
		Male	Female
1	Higher managerial and professional	82.5	85.2
2	Lower managerial and professional	80.8	84.5
3	Intermediate	80.4	83.9
4	Small employers own account workers	80.0	83.5
5	Lower supervisory and technical	78.9	81.9
6	Semi-routine	77.9	81.7
7	Routine	76.6	80.8
8	Unclassified	74.0	78.5

(Source: http://tinyurl.com/hkoys6l)

Theories relating to health trends

Ulrich Beck stated that we live in a 'risky' society where tradition has less influence and people have more choice. Individuals calculate the risks and rewards of actions and decisions. In previous generations, everyone was expected to marry then have children. Women looked after the house and men were the wage earners and decision makers. Two trends have undermined this traditional patriarchal family – gender equality and greater individualism where actions are based on self-interest rather than a sense of obligation to others.

Beck stated that this has resulted in the 'negotiated family' that does not conform to any traditional or standard norm. The members decide what is best for themselves by negotiation, and enter the relationship on an equal basis. It is seen as a less stable type of family since a member can easily leave if they feel their needs are not being fulfilled.

Peter Townsend defined relative poverty in the late 1970s by using a list of 12 items as indicators of poverty and deprivation. The items are Townsend's decisions about what most people wanted and expected at the time.

1 No holiday away from home in the last 12 months.
2 Has not had a relative or friend to visit for a meal or snack in the last four weeks (adults).
3 Has not been to a relative or friend for a meal or snack in the last four weeks (adults).
4 Has not had a friend to play or for tea in the last four weeks (under 15 years).
5 Did not have a party on last birthday (children).
6 Has not had an afternoon or evening out for entertainment in last two weeks.
7 Does not have fresh meat (including meals out) as often as four times a week.
8 Has had one or more days in last two weeks without a hot meal.
9 Has not had a cooked breakfast most days of the week.
10 Household does not have a fridge.
11 Household does not usually have a Sunday joint.
12 Household does not have sole use of a toilet, a sink or wash basin with running water, a fixed bath or shower and a cooker.

(Source: Townsend (1979) Poverty in the United Kingdom, p. 250)

Richard Wilkinson wrote about the 'Socioeconomic determinants of health' (*British Medical Journal* February 1997, pp. 591–594). He discussed whether the health disadvantages of the least well-off reflect the direct effects of bad housing, poor diets, inadequate heating and air pollution, or if it is more a matter of the effects of differences associated with social position – of where you stand in relation to others. The indirect effects of social circumstances include increased exposure to behavioural risks, including smoking, drinking and eating 'for comfort'; most of the direct effects are likely to centre on the physiological effects of chronic mental and emotional stress.

Gender

Statistics show that women live longer in good health than men (see Table 23.2); however, a higher proportion of women (21 per cent), than men (16 per cent), suffer from anxiety or depression. This could be due to gender social differences, as women are socialised to express their feelings and talk about their problems, which could account for more women being diagnosed with mental illness because they are more likely to go to their GP to talk about their symptoms. They are also more likely to have a consultation with a GP as they generally take responsibility for child care, including the child's health, so they are more likely to discuss their own health and wellbeing at the same appointment.

Men can suffer from gender expectations that they should be tough and not make a fuss. A cultural expectation is that men do not talk about mental health and they don't behave proactively regarding their health in general. Young men are subject to peer pressure to indulge in risky behaviours, such as unprotected sex, binge drinking and extreme sports, in order to demonstrate their masculinity.

Ethnicity

Members of certain ethnic groups tend to live in deprived areas, experience unemployment and suffer from more illnesses than those who live in more affluent areas that provide a better environment. They also experience greater stress and hostility through racism.

The statistical information shown in Table 23.3 demonstrates the impact of these factors on individuals' health behaviour and their general wellbeing.

Table 23.3 Differences in health outcomes due to ethnicity

Factors	Impact
Cultural	- Cultural differences in eating habits may mean that different health issues arise within different cultural groups, for example: people from African Caribbean communities, are more likely to develop Type II diabetes than the rest of the population. This is linked to diet, genetic differences in processing and storing fat, and unequal access to health services.
Ethnicity	- The 2011 Census showed that Pakistani and Bangladeshi women reported rates of activity limitation due to a health problem or disability 10 per cent higher than for white British women. - Black and south Asian people are three to five times more likely to have kidney failure than white people. - Sickle cell anaemia is a serious inherited blood disorder where the red blood cells, which carry oxygen around the body, develop abnormally. The disorder mainly affects people of African, Caribbean, Middle Eastern, eastern Mediterranean and Asian origin. In the UK, sickle cell disorders are most commonly seen in African and Caribbean people.
Environmental	- The more deprived the neighbourhood, the more likely it is to present risks to health because of poor housing, high crime rates, poorer air quality, lack of green spaces and places for children to play, traffic risks. (The Marmot Review – Fair Society, Healthy Lives 2010, p. 78.) - In England, people living in the poorest neighbourhoods, will, on average, die seven years earlier than people living in the richest neighbourhoods (Marmot Review, p. 11).

(Source: ONS (www.ons.gov.uk/ons) and NHS (www.nhs.uk))

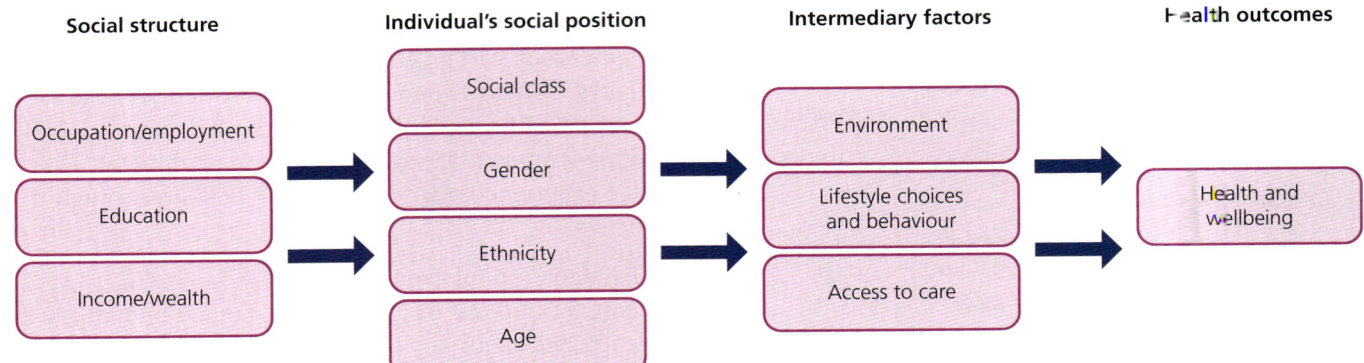

Social structure	Individual's social position	Intermediary factors	Health outcomes

Social structure: Occupation/employment, Education, Income/wealth

Individual's social position: Social class, Gender, Ethnicity, Age

Intermediary factors: Environment, Lifestyle choices and behaviour, Access to care

Health outcomes: Health and wellbeing

(Source: Adapted from Graham and Kelly (2004) NHS Briefing paper Health Inequalities: Concepts, Frameworks and Policy (www.nice.org.uk))

▲ **Figure 23.3** Causes of differences in health outcomes

3.2 Causes of differences in health outcomes

Factors affecting health outcomes are summarised in Figure 23.3. This shows how social position can be considered fundamental to heath as it is the pivotal link between the determinants that influence people's health. It shows where education and employment or unemployment, which are societal level factors, connect with other determinants influencing the extent to which they are exposed to risk factors that directly affect their health. These include:

- material factors, such as physical environment, poor quality housing, level of income, workplace hazards
- behavioural factors, such as smoking, exercise, diet, alcohol consumption, exercise
- psychosocial factors, such as stress, risk-taking behaviour, perceived inequality
- regulating human behaviour, such as Durkheim's 'social facts' – beliefs, values, morals and cultural norms (see LO1).

3.3 Role of social networks in promoting good health

Work/life balance and social capital

Robert Putnam defines social capital as:

'features of social life – networks, norms and trust – that enable participants to act together more effectively to pursue shared objectives ... To the extent that the norms, networks and trust link substantial sectors of the community and span underlying cleavages ... those who have wider and more closely integrated networks ... feel a sense of wellbeing'.

(Source: Putnam, 2001)

Putnam found a strong correlation between income equality and the strength of local community and social cohesion. He states that equality is an essential feature of civic community life, and that a better integration into a social network, friendship groups and having a good work/life balance benefits health. The right balance may vary over time as circumstances change, but a good work/life balance improves an individual's quality of life.

KNOW IT

1 Explain, with examples, what is meant by 'socio-economic' factors.
2 Give examples of different groups in society affected by health inequalities.
3 Name three causes of differences in health outcomes.
4 Describe Beck's theory of a 'negotiated family'.

LO3 Assessment activity *P4 M2 D1*

Below is a suggested assessment activity that has been directly linked to the pass, merit and distinction criteria in LO3 to help with assignment preparation; it includes Top Tips on how to achieve the best results.

This activity must be based on information from authoritative sources, using relevant case studies, for example, from the NHS Choices website or information from the ONS social trends website.

- Produce a report that explains patterns and trends in health and illness among different social groups.
- Analyse the data on health outcomes and comment on the distribution using sociological theory.
- Evaluate patterns and trends in health and illness among different social groups.

LO4 Understand sociological perspectives about the organisation and management of health and social care *P5 P6*

GETTING STARTED

The future of healthcare? (20 minutes)

Read the following article, from the *Health Service Journal* website, about a roundtable discussion by a panel of expert healthcare commissioners and strategists. They considered 'How can patients use technology to monitor and care for themselves?'

http://tinyurl.com/j2sss84

● Do you think it is a good idea to use your smartphone to monitor your health? Why?
● Do you think there are benefits for the GPs and hospitals and the NHS as a whole?
● Are there any barriers for patients in using technology to manage their health care?

4.1 Rights and responsibilities for promoting good health

The professional

The growth of preventative and promotional health care has resulted in increasing numbers of health professionals monitoring apparently healthy people for evidence of risk factors in their bodies, their behaviour or their social environments. This has been described as 'surveillance medicine' and demonstrates the move from sickness to health. However, it is not the role of health professionals to make value judgements on the way others choose to live, particularly if their behaviour does not cause harm to others, and they should not create health panics and unnecessary worry. The idea behind surveillance medicine is that prevention is better than cure.

The individual

People are now faced with a mass of evidence that health is to a large extent dependent on what they do for themselves. Many of the diseases of modern society are linked to behavioural factors such as sedentary lifestyle, poor diet, and use of drugs, alcohol and smoking.

The state

The government has the responsibility for attempting to reduce health inequalities by using social policies to address the issues. A government report, Our Healthier Nation (1999), introduced initiatives to reduce deaths from heart disease and cancer, introduced smoking cessation clinics and established health action zones. This formed the basis of health promotion strategies in the UK. Other national health promotion campaigns include Smokefree, Change4Life and Drinkaware. These all have their own websites and contact details for health practitioner support, along with resources such as leaflets, video clips, apps and many other forms of help, including local clinics.

GROUP ACTIVITY

Health promotion (40 minutes)

In small groups, use the internet to find out about a government health promotion campaign.

● What resources are available?
● How useful are they?
● Do you think it will motivate individuals?
● Are there any links to the sociological perspectives you have studied?

4.2 Division between health and social care

Current policy directions in health and social care

Following the Francis Report into poor quality treatment and the high number of unnecessary deaths at the Mid-Staffordshire NHS Trust, the NHS addressed the importance of good quality patient–practitioner interaction to support patient recovery. The introduction of the Care Certificate for health and social care assistants is aimed at enabling care workers to provide the highest standard of care that supports service users' dignity, health and safety, and privacy. Revalidation of nurses and midwives every few years is another initiative introduced with the aim of improving standards of care.

The Health and Social Care Act 2012 is underpinned by two main principles: first enabling patients to have more control over the care they receive; and second that those responsible for patient care – the doctors, nurses and others – have the freedom and power to commission care that meets local needs. Key aspects include GP-led Clinical Commissioning Groups, health and wellbeing boards to tackle inequalities in people's health and wellbeing, and an increased focus on prevention, with local councils taking over responsibility for health improvement, for example, obesity, anti-smoking, screening, vaccinations. Full details of the Act can be found in Unit 2, page 32.

Decline in NHS provision of long-term care

The Barker Report (2014) on health and social care recommended that care should be built around patient needs, merging health care and social care. The report stated that the cost of providing free social care could come from a mix of new taxes, cuts to benefits and prescription exemptions. The report compared the care given to cancer patients, who get their treatment free, with the support needed to help people with dementia, which often falls into the means-tested social care system. Dame Kate Barker, who produced the report, said the country was facing 'difficult questions' but added the current system was simply 'not fit to provide the kind of care we need and want'.

4.3 Efficiency and effectiveness

Scientific rationality and utilitarianism (e.g. greatest good for the greatest number) and calculating costs and benefits and values (e.g. who takes priority) are covered in LO2.1

Role of performance targets in health and social care

Targets are set for GPs to increase the uptake of health screening and vaccinations. Accident and emergency departments have targets for waiting times and

ambulances have to meet response time targets. These are all in place to provide a high-quality service and also to make efficient, cost-effective, use of NHS resources.

Health improvement programmes identify the most important health need of the local population and then strategies are developed to meet these local needs. This aims to improve the health of local residents, but also aims to save the NHS money in the long term, as illness is either avoided or picked up earlier when it is easier, and cheaper, to treat.

Calculating costs and benefits

NICE (the National Institute for Health and Care Excellence) helps to improve outcomes for individuals using the NHS and other public health and social care services. NICE considers whether a treatment benefits patients, will help the NHS meet its targets – for example by improving cancer survival rates – and whether the treatment is value for money or cost effective. It also provides evidence-based guidelines on how particular conditions should be treated, provides guidelines on how public health and social care services can best support people and provides information services for those managing and providing health and social care.

The CQC (Care Quality Commission) registers, monitors and inspects a range of services, including hospitals, GP practices, walk-in centres, out-of-hours services and care homes. The CQC sets out the standards of care required and checks that services meet the required standards of quality and safety and then publishes inspection reports. It awards ratings that service providers have to display by law. To improve standards, the CQC can issue 'requirement notices' or 'warning notices' to set out what improvements the care provider must make and by when or placing a provider in 'special measures' to closely supervise the quality of care to help them improve within set timescales. Alternatively, the care provider can be held to account for their failings by being issued with a caution, a fine or can be prosecuted in cases where people are harmed or placed in danger.

LO4 Assessment activity *P5 P6*

Below is a suggested assessment activity that has been directly linked to the pass criteria in LO4 to help with assignment preparation; it includes Top Tips on how to achieve the best results.

You have been asked to provide a second session for the health centre staff. Produce a presentation with presenters' notes that describes who is responsible for promoting good health. For example, your presentation could be based on the roles of the government, the professional and the individual in smoking cessation (or any other relevant health issue).

- Include who is responsible for promoting good health. **P5**
- Produce an additional document that explains how sociological perspectives relate to the organisation of health and social care. **P6**

TOP TIPS
- ✔ Think about your audience and the language you should use for them.
- ✔ Make sure that your notes include lots of relevant information.

Read about it

Aggleton, P. (1990) *Health (Society Now)*, Routledge.

Beck, U. (1992) *Risk Society, Towards a New Modernity*, Sage Publications.

Brown, K. (2011) *An Introduction to Sociology*, 4th edition, Polity Press.

Fisher, A. *et al.* (2012) *Applied A2 Health & Social Care for OCR*, revised edition, Oxford.

Moonie, N. *et al.* (2007) *Core Themes – Health and Social Care*, Heinemann.

Putnam, R. (2001) *Bowling Alone: The Collapse and Revival of American Community*, 2nd edition, Simon & Schuster.

Taylor, S. and Field, D. (2007) *Sociology of Health and Health Care*, 4th edition, Blackwell.

Townsend, P. (1979) *Poverty in the United Kingdom*, Allen Lane and Penguin Books.

Walsh, M. and Tait, D. (2014) *Introduction to Sociology for Health Carers*, 2nd edition, CENGAGE Learning.

Wilkinson, R.G. (1997) Socioeconomic determinants of health. Health inequalities: relative or absolute material standards? *British Medical Journal* (Volume 314).

Glossary

Acute psychiatric settings – residential and hospital settings that provide care with intensive medical and nursing support for individuals in periods of acute psychiatric illness or mental health needs.

ADHD – attention deficit hyperactivity disorder, symptoms include a short attention span, constant fidgeting and impulsive behaviour.

Advance care plan – a plan to discuss and record in advance an individual's choices, decisions and wishes with respect to their care and treatment in case they are unable to express their preferences at a later stage.

Advocates – those who represent the views, needs and interests of individuals who are unable to represent themselves.

Aerobic exercise – sustained, rhythmic activity that involves large muscle groups.

Agreed ways of working – an organisation's policies and procedures.

Allied health professionals – a profession that includes non-medical and non-clinical professionals with expertise in specific fields, such as dieticians, therapists, and speech and language therapists. Allied health professionals work in partnership with health and social care professionals and practitioners.

Alzheimer's – the most common cause of dementia and causes damage to the brain. Signs and symptoms include memory loss in the early stages; individuals may then develop difficulties with their communication, thinking, reasoning and perception skills.

Amniotic sac – a 'bag' of liquid (mainly water) in the uterus, this is filled with amniotic fluid and provides a protective cushion for the foetus.

Angiogram – a type of X-ray that involves a dye visible in X-ray photographs that is injected into the blood system so that narrowing of coronary arteries can be seen.

Angioplasty – a microscopic deflated balloon is passed into a narrowed artery and inflated, pushing the artery open. Sometimes a microscopic mesh tube or stent is inserted at the same time, keeping the artery open for longer.

Anti-psychotic medication – a type of medication that is used to treat some mental health conditions.

Aspiration – a strong desire to achieve something.

Assumptions – ideas that are formed without any proof that they are true.

Asthma – a condition that can cause wheezing, coughing, chest tightness and breathlessness. It can develop in both young children and older people.

Authorised or nominated person – someone who acts on behalf of an individual to allocate their direct payment, with local authority agreement.

Autism – a condition that is also known as autism spectrum disorder (ASD). It affects children, young people and adults with respect to their communication, social interaction and behaviour.

Autonomy – self-rule, independence or freedom to do as an individual wishes.

Barred list – a list of individuals held by the DBS who are unsuitable for working with children and/or adults.

Beliefs – ideas that are accepted as true and real by the person that holds them.

'Big C' creativity – a process linked to new ideas, sudden understandings and creative excellence.

Biopsy – a sample of tissue that is taken from the body for examination under a microscope.

Body language – a form of non-verbal communication in which thoughts, feelings and intentions are expressed through the movement and position of the body.

Body mass index – a calculation of a person's weight in kilograms divided by the square of their height in metres to determine if they are overweight or underweight.

Break away techniques – techniques that do not involve aggression or force, and aim to promote safety and mutual respect.

Breech position – when the baby is 'bottom down' rather than head down in the uterus before birth.

Briefings – meetings that provide up-to-date information.

Capitalist – the Marxist term for industrialists, factory and business owners who provide employment for others.

Carbohydrate – sugar and starches that provide energy for humans and animals.

Cardiac output – the amount of blood being pumped by the heart.

Cardiovascular disease – a disease of the heart or blood vessels.

Care Quality Commission (CQC) – an independent regulator of health and social care in England. They monitor, inspect and regulate services to make sure they meet fundamental standards of quality and safety.

Carrier – a person without obvious signs or symptoms of disease who harbours the bacteria or virus, and acts as a vehicle transmitting the pathogen to others.

Centre for Independent Living – centres that promote the principles of independent living and provide services for individuals who use direct payments.

Child care environment – practitioners and organisations that work with children from birth–13 years in their own homes, in nursery or pre-school settings, schools, out-of-school clubs and activity clubs.

Child-initiated activities – enabling children to make decisions about their own activities and to lead the play or activity.

Chromosomes – thread-like structures located inside the nucleus of animal and plant cells. Each chromosome is made of protein and a single molecule of deoxyribonucleic acid (DNA). Passed from parents to offspring, DNA contains the specific instructions that make each type of living creature unique.

Chronic obstructive pulmonary disease (COPD) – a collection of lung diseases.

Clinical Commissioning Groups (CCGs) – most of the NHS commissioning budget is now managed by 209 CCGs. These are groups of general practices that come together in each area to commission the best services for their patients and population.

Closed question – a question with a limited number of answers to choose from.

Clostridium difficile – a bacterium infectious agent that causes infections in the digestive system. It is also referred to as *C. difficile* or *C. diff.*

Cochlear implant – a small electronic device that detects sounds and sends impulses to the brain.

Code of conduct – a document that contains guidance on the behaviours and attitudes that reflect best practice and are expected from workers.

Cognitive – relating to the mental processes of perception, memory, judgement and reasoning.

Communicable disease – an illness spread through fluid exchange, for example sneezing or coughing, or contact with a carrier.

Communication board – a board with symbols and pictures that enables individuals to communicate by pointing to or looking at them

Conception – occurs when the egg is fertilised by the sperm.

Consent – permission for something to happen or agreement to do something.

Contamination – to have made something dirty, polluted or poisonous by adding a chemical, waste or infection.

Continuing professional development – opportunities for professionals to maintain and develop their knowledge and skills, not just through training but also through experience, self study and sharing best practice.

Contraception – a method of deliberately preventing pregnancy

Coronary bypass – Using a piece of artery from the chest to bypass or bridge a blocked region of coronary artery, allowing blood to flow beyond the blockage.

CT scan – a 'computerised tomography' scan of the brain, internal organs, blood vessels or bones. Sometimes called a CAT scan.

Deafblind – individuals who have a level of hearing and sight loss that, combined, severely impacts their daily life.

Defendant – someone accused of an offence.

Degenerative condition – medical problems that worsen over time.

Dementia – a condition that is caused when the brain is damaged by diseases such as Alzheimer's or a stroke.

Depression – a mood disorder that affects how you feel, think and behave, and causes a persistent feeling of sadness, hopelessness and loss of interest.

Developmental stages – the natural progression in which children grow and develop. Not all children will develop at the same rate, but most children will follow the same pattern of milestones in development.

Dialect – a form of language that is associated with a specific region or group of people.

Dialysis – devices used to clean blood of impurities such as urea.

Dietician – a trained professional who provides advice and guidance on diet and nutrition.

Disclosures – when an individual or another person tells you either directly, or indirectly through their behaviour, that they have been, or are being, abused.

Discrimination – when people judge others based on their differences and use these differences to create disadvantage or oppression.

Disease – a disorder or incorrectly functioning organ, part or body system in a human especially one that produces specific symptoms or that affects a specific location and is not simply a direct result of physical injury.

Diuretics – drugs that flush out excess water from the body by increasing urination.

Diversity – accepting and respecting that each individual is unique and different.

DNA (deoxyribonucleic acid) – the carrier of genetic information and unique to each individual. A sample of any body fluid or tissue can be analysed and compared to identify an individual.

Duty of care – the legal obligation professionals have to safeguard individuals who they care for and support from danger, harm and abuse.

Dynavox – software that provides words and messages that can be accessed by touching a screen that contains text, pictures and symbols. It then converts those that are touched into speech.

Ectopic pregnancy – where the foetus develops outside the womb, usually in a fallopian tube.

Eligible – fit the criteria for, be suitable for or be entitled to something

Embryo – the fertilised egg divides to form a ball of cells called the embryo.

Empower – to give someone the authority or control to do something; the way a health, social care or early years worker encourages an individual to make decisions and to take control of their own life.

End of life care – the care provided for individuals who are likely to die within the next 12 months.

Endocrine system – a collection of glands that produce hormones and release them directly into the circulatory system to be transported around the body in the blood.

Endoscopy – inserting a microscopic light source and video camera at the end of a long flexible tube through either end of the gut. Images are relayed to a screen.

Environmental control – reducing the chance of infection in a location, e.g. via thorough cleaning. It is a fundamental principle of infection prevention in health care settings.

Epilepsy – a medical condition that affects the brain, causing seizures.

Epistemic play – acquiring knowledge through play. It is often associated with questions such as 'What does this object do?'

Fallopian tube – there are two, one each side of the uterus. They connect the ovaries to the uterus.

Fine motor skills – actions that require small movements, e.g. writing, threading and playing with dough.

Foetus – from eight weeks after fertilisation until birth the embryo is called a foetus.

Foodborne illness – (food poisoning) any illness resulting from contaminated food containing pathogenic bacteria, viruses or parasites, or from chemical or natural toxins such as poisonous mushrooms.

Genes – segments of DNA that contain information about the different characteristics of growth, development or appearance.

Glucose – a simple sugar that is an energy source in living organisms and a component of many carbohydrates.

Gross motor skills – actions that require large movements, e.g. running, jumping and skipping.

GUM clinic – a clinic specialising in genitourinary medicine.

Hazard – a potential source of harm or adverse health effect.

Hazardous substance – a substance that can be harmful to your health if inhaled, ingested or absorbed through your skin.

Health and Safety Executive (HSE) – the national independent regulator or official supervisory body for the health, safety and welfare of people in work settings in the UK.

Health environment – practitioners and organisations that provide diagnostic, preventative, remedial and therapeutic services in different settings.

Healthwatch England – the national consumer champion in health and care, with statutory powers to ensure the voice of the consumer is heard by those who commission, deliver and regulate health and care services.

Hearing aid – small digital or analogue amplification device worn in or behind the ear(s) to magnify sounds.

Hearing loss – refers to individuals who are unable to hear, as well as to individuals who are able to partially hear, for example just low tones.

HIV/AIDS – a virus which attacks the immune system, and weakens the ability to fight infections and disease.

Home adaptations – changes to the home to make it safer for the individual to live independently, e.g. a stair-lift to enable an individual to go upstairs in their home, making it accessible.

Hospice – a setting that provides support and end-of-life care to individuals and their families. Hospice care can be provided where individuals choose, for example at home, or in a hospice room in a hospital or nursing home.

HRT (hormone replacement therapy) – prescribing the hormones oestrogen and/or progesterone to post-menopausal women. There is some evidence that links this treatment to a potential increased risk of strokes, blood clots and certain cancers.

HSV – herpes simplex virus.

Hygiene – conditions or practices that help to maintain health and prevent disease, especially through cleanliness to reduce the spread of germs.

Hypertension – a term that is used to refer to high blood pressure.

Identifier – a tool that is used to match people to their records, e.g. to their health records.

Imaginative play – involves children pretending to be, or making up stories about, something or someone else, e.g. pretending to be a cat.

Immune system – the body's natural protection against pathogens that cause infections.

Immunisation – administering a vaccine to make an individual immune or resistant to an infectious disease.

Immuno-suppressants – medication that suppresses the types of white blood cell involved in rejection, slowing down or preventing the destruction of the donated organ. Also suppresses the response to viruses and cancers.

In utero – something that occurs in the womb, before birth.

Inclusive environment – somewhere where everyone feels valued, their differences respected, and able to reach their full potential.

Induction training – the training an employee receives when they first start working with an organisation.

Infection – the process of bacteria or viruses invading the body and making someone ill or diseased.

Informal or unstructured interview – an interview where the interviewer does not keep to a prepared list of questions.

Inhaler – a method of getting medication directly into the lungs. May be pressurised. Two types – relievers (blue) that dilate the bronchii during an attack and preventers (red, brown or orange) that reduce sensitivity and inflammation of the bronchii.

Interpreters – trained professionals who take a spoken or signed message and convert it from one language into another, ensuring they express its meaning and intent as accurately as possible.

Interpretivist – a sociological perspective that focuses on understanding the motivation and meaning of individual behaviour.

Interventionist role – being actively involved in children and young people's play, creativity and learning.

IQ (intelligence quotient) – an attempt to measure intelligence by representing a person's reasoning ability with a number.

Keyhole surgery – minimally invasive surgery. A laparoscope is inserted into a small incision and relays images of the inside of the abdomen or pelvis to a television monitor so that the surgeon can see the operation without exposing the area.

Kosher – food that is prepared according to Jewish law

Lacking mental capacity – when individuals are unable to make their own decisions about their care and treatment. This may be due to having a mental health condition or being unconscious due to a sudden illness or accident.

Legionella bacteria – a type of bacteria that causes diseases such as Legionnaire's disease that affect the lungs.

Legislation – provides individuals with rights to which they are entitled through laws passed by parliament. Law is upheld through the courts.

LGBT – an acronym used to describe the different groups that exist within the gay culture: lesbian, gay, bisexual and transgender.

Ligament – a short band of tough, flexible fibrous connective tissue which connects two bones or cartilages or holds together a joint.

Lightwriter – a text-to-speech device for individuals who cannot speak but who are able to type a message on the keyboard, which is then displayed. The message is then converted into speech.

Lithotripsy – using high-frequency sound waves to vibrate apart solid objects like gall stones.

'Little c' creativity – an everyday process whereby children and young people are able to be resourceful and problem solve.

Local authority – the governing body of a county or district officially responsible for all public services and facilities in that area.

Looked after children – children who are looked after by or under the care of the local authority.

Low-impact aerobics – slow and steady exercise, lessening the strain on joints.

Ludic play – a spontaneous type of play that draws on past experiences and often involves a range of symbolic or imaginary features. It can encourage a child to consider 'What can I do with this object?'

Mandatory training – the training an organisation requires an employee to undertake to be able to work safely.

Manual handling – the transporting or supporting of a person or object by hand or bodily force.

Means-tested payments – payments based on an individual's financial circumstances to determine whether an individual is eligible or has the right to claim assistance.

Mental capacity – being able to make a reasoned decision by understanding information, remembering it for long enough to make a decision and communicating this to others.

Mental health units – hospital-based settings that provide specialised care and treatment to individuals with mental health needs

Mentoring – a process where one person, such as a manager, transfers their knowledge and experience to another person to enable them to develop their skills and improve their performance.

Metabolism – the process the body uses to get or make energy from the food eaten. Food is made up of proteins, carbohydrates and fats. Chemicals in the digestive system break the food parts down into sugars and acids, the body's fuel.

Methicillin-resistant *Staphylococcus aureus* **(MRSA)** – a bacterium infectious agent that causes infections in different parts of the body where the risk of it occurring is higher in people with open wounds, invasive devices and weakened immune systems.

Milestones – key points in development, for example when a baby sits, crawls or walks for the first time.

Minerals – classed as micronutrients as they are needed in small quantities. They work with other nutrients so the body functions properly.

Monitor – the sector regulator for health services in England. Monitor's job is to make the health sector work better for patients.

Monitoring – to measure and check the progress or quality of something over time. Methods of monitoring can involve observations, inspections, analysis of surveys given to service users or staff, for example.

MRI scan – magnetic resonance imaging scan. A strong magnetic field and radio waves are used to produce detailed images of almost all parts of the body.

Nebuliser – a mouthpiece or facemask that introduces medication to the lungs as a fine spray.

Need to know basis – when information is given to people only if and when it is needed.

Needs assessment – the overall process for identifying and recording the health and social care risks and needs of an individual and evaluating their impact on daily living and quality of life so that appropriate action can be planned.

Nervous system – the communication network of the body. It is made up of the brain, spinal cord, nerves and sense organs. It co-ordinates the body's responses to external stimuli and controls everything an individual does: breathing, walking, thinking and feeling by sending messages around the body.

Neural tube defect – a condition that develops when the baby's spinal cord and spinal column do not form properly in the womb.

Neurofibrillary tangles – twisted protein fibres in brain cells; commonly recognised as a primary marker for Alzheimer's.

Non-interventionist role – not being actively involved in children and young people's play and creativity.

Non-judgemental – respecting a person's feelings, experiences and values, even though they may be different from yours. Not judging or criticising someone because of your own attitudes or beliefs.

Normative – relating to, or deriving from, a standard or norm, especially of behaviour.

Nurture – to care for and protect something as it grows.

Omega 3 oils – well known for their health benefits and important for normal metabolism.

Osteoporosis – a condition that weakens bones, causing them to break and fracture easily.

Ovaries – produce female hormones and produce 'ovum' also known as eggs.

Palliative care – an approach to providing care for individuals in the later stages of a terminal illness.

Pancreatitis – a medical condition where the pancreas becomes inflamed over a short period of time.

Parkinson's – a neurological condition in which symptoms usually develop gradually. Signs and symptoms can include tremors or shaking, body rigidity or stiffness, feeling tired and weak, pain and depression.

Pathogenic bacteria – bacteria that can cause infection.

Pathogens – infective agents, commonly known as 'germs' that can cause infections and diseases.

Peak flow – the rate of expired air, measured on a hand-held device.

Perceptual skills – the ability to become aware of things around us, mainly through our senses.

Performance management – an ongoing process between a care worker and their supervisor involving meetings and observations over time to provide feedback on performance and identify targets for improvement where appropriate.

Personal budget – the amount of money an individual is awarded by the local authority to spend on the help they need to achieve what is important to them.

Personal development plan – a way of staff recording their past achievements and future learning objectives.

Physical environment – surroundings or conditions, such as the space available, the positioning of furniture, amount of lighting and the level of noise.

Physiological – anything to do with the body and its systems, such as your heart beating faster and getting sweaty hands if you are scared.

Pitch – the quality of a vocal sound made by a person in a communication or situation, e.g. low or high.

Placenta – provides the foetus with oxygen and nourishment from the mother via the umbilical cord.

Policies – clear statements of intent of how an organisation intends to conduct its services.

Positive relationships – meaningful interactions that result in positive emotions such as happiness, enjoyment, peace and a sense of wellbeing. They are constructive and beneficial for all those involved.

Postnatal – refers to the period after a woman has given birth, the first few weeks. 'Post' means after and 'natal' means birth.

Postnatal depression – a mental condition that some mothers develop after giving birth. It is a serious mental disorder that requires help and support.

Preconception health – consideration of health, fitness and lifestyle before trying to conceive a baby, to improve chances of becoming pregnant and to give the baby a good start.

Precursor behaviours – changes in mood or behaviours that indicate that an individual is becoming anxious; these can be identified by those who know an individual well.

Premature labour – when labour starts before the 37th week of pregnancy.

Preventative measures – using methods to stop or prevent something, e.g. providing a jar-opening device for an individual to allow them to open jars safely and prevent injury.

Pride – the name given to the events celebrating lesbian, gay, bisexual and transgender (LGBT) culture.

Proactive – when a person creates or controls a situation by causing something to happen rather than responding to it after it has happened.

Procedures – the way in which the service or organisation expects its employees to put its policies into action.

Professional development – the process of improving and increasing the skills and capabilities of staff.

Proletariat – the Marxist term for workers who sell their labour to earn an income.

Protected time – a period of time where staff spend one-to-one time with individuals.

Psychiatrists – medical practitioners that specialise in diagnosing, treating and preventing mental health conditions.

Psychologists – practitioners that specialise in studying how people behave – how they think, act and react.

Race – a group of people classified together on the basis of common history, nationality or geography, for example Asian, Black, White, Traveller.

Reflective practitioner – a professional who looks back over the work they do on a regular basis, and spends time thinking about and making improvements to their working practices.

Reflexes – inborn and involuntary movements, not voluntary movements.

Regulator – the official supervisory body that monitors a specific industry or activity.

Religion – a system of beliefs, faith and worship, such as Buddhism, Christianity, Hinduism and Judaism. Religion can also include a lack of belief.

Restrictive interventions – actions that deliberately limit an individual's movement and/or freedom to immediately reduce danger or harm to the individual or others.

Review – a formal meeting where an individual's care or support plan is reviewed.

Risk assessments – the framework for identifying, avoiding, minimising and controlling risks so that day-to-day duties can be carried out safely.

Safeguarding – proactive measures to reduce the risks of danger, harm and abuse.

Safeguarding alert – concern that a vulnerable adult may have been, is or might be, a victim of abuse.

Screening – process of identifying healthy people who may be at risk of disease; for example, the breast screening programme.

Secure units – low, medium and high security facilities that provide specialised care and treatment to individuals with mental health needs and pose a risk to others.

Sedentary – inactive, not moving around a lot, tending to spend time sitting.

Segregated – to be set apart from others.

Self-esteem – the value an individual gives themselves.

Septicaemia – a potentially life-threatening illness caused by an infection.

Service led – a service-led provision is where an individual has to fit into existing traditional services such as day centres.

Shabbat – the Jewish day of rest

Sight loss – individuals who are unable to see, i.e. 'blind', as well as individuals who are able to partially see, for example, shadows.

Signers – trained professionals who take a message and convert it from one language into another using signs, ensuring they express its meaning and intent as accurately as possible.

Social care environment – professionals and organisations that provide care, support and protection to adults, young people and children at risk, or with needs arising from illness, disability, old age or other circumstances that place people at a disadvantage in society.

Social care outcomes – the results of receiving social care that is desired by the individual, e.g. living independently, finding employment.

Social class – the classification of people according to their occupation and income to be working class, middle class or upper class.

Social environment – the social conditions that influence building relationships, such as individuals and professionals' backgrounds, education, interactions with others.

Social groupings – the classification of people by, for example, their gender, social class, ethnicity, age, locality.

Social institutions or structures – the elements that make up society, e.g. family, school, workplace, judicial system, health and social care services.

Socialisation – the process where people learn the values, attitudes and norms of their society.

Specialist assessment and treatment units – residential units that provide assessment and treatment in a therapeutic environment and are run by NHS Trusts and independent organisations.

Speech and language teams – trained teams of professionals who provide support with enabling individuals to develop effective communication skills, and can also provide training and support to those working with individuals.

Speech therapists – trained professionals who assess an individual's communication difficulties and provide advice on how to address them.

Spirometer – equipment that measures the volume of the lungs and how much air can be exchanged per breath.

SRE – sex and relationship education.

Standard precautions – the minimum infection prevention practices that apply to all patient care, regardless of suspected or confirmed infection status of the patient, in any setting where health care is delivered.

Statutory service – a service provided by local authority as laid down by legislation/law.

Stereotypes – generalisations that are made, which are often offensive and exaggerated, about a particular group of people.

Sterilising – a process that involves removing all pathogens that cause infections.

Steroids – drugs used to reduce inflammation brought about by overactive immune systems.

Stillbirth – a baby that is not born alive after 24 weeks. It can be linked to placenta complications.

Stressor – any event or situation that causes an individual to feel pressured or threatened, e.g. an exam, moving house, receiving a diagnosis or being ill.

Stroke – a serious and life-threatening medical condition that occurs when blood supply to part of the brain is cut off.

Structuralist – a sociological perspective that is concerned with the overall organisation or 'structure' of society.

Structured interview – an interview where the interviewer asks pre-prepared questions and records the answers.

Subjective – based on or influenced by personal feelings, tasks or opinions

Supervision – a process in which more experienced workers monitor and support their colleagues to improve their working practices.

Support plan – the document where day-to-day requirements and preferences for care and support are detailed to enable an individual to live with dignity and respect in the community. It may be known by other names e.g. care plan, or an individual plan.

Suspicions of abuse – when you suspect an individual is likely to be at risk of being harmed or abused, or when you suspect harm or abuse has occurred.

Symbolic play – involves children using one thing to represent something else, e.g. using a banana as a phone.

Tendon – a flexible but inelastic cord of strong fibrous collagen tissue attaching a muscle to a bone.

Tone – the strength of a vocal sound made by a person in a communication or situation, e.g. quiet or loud.

Translators – trained professionals who take a written message and convert it from one language into another, ensuring they express its meaning and intent as accurately as possible.

Ultrasound – using high-frequency sound to generate internal images of structures within the body. Echoes from the objects are interpreted by a computer.

Umbilical cord – this connects the baby to the placenta.

Universal services – services that are available to everyone, such as transport and housing.

Values – ideas that form the system by which a person lives their life. Often people's beliefs can develop into their values.

Values of care – core principles that underpin care work. They aim to eliminate discrimination, reduce inequalities and help to ensure individuals' care needs are met.

Vitamins – a group of organic compounds that are essential for normal growth and nutrition, and are required in small quantities in the diet because they cannot be synthesised in the body.

Virus – tiny organisms that may cause illnesses in humans ranging from flu or a cold to life-threatening conditions like HIV/AIDS. They cannot grow or multiply on their own and need to take over a human or animal cell to help them multiply.

Working in partnership – a way of working that involves developing positive relationships between individuals, carers and professionals where individuals remain at the centre. Good quality care and support is developed through mutual respect and open and honest communication.

Index